T0319662

The Environmental Impact of COVID-19

The Environmental Impact of COVID-19

Edited by

Deepak Rawtani
National Forensic Sciences Univ.
Gujarat
India

Chaudhery Mustansar Hussain
New Jersey Inst. of Technology
U.S.A

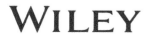

Registered Offices
John Wiley & Sons, Inc., 111 River Street, Hoboken, NJ 07030, USA
John Wiley & Sons Ltd, The Atrium, Southern Gate, Chichester, West Sussex, PO19 8SQ, UK

For details of our global editorial offices, customer services, and more information about Wiley products visit us at www.wiley.com.

Library of Congress Cataloging-in-Publication Data
Names: Rawtani, Deepak, editor. | Hussain, Chaudhery Mustansar, editor.
Title: The environmental impact of COVID-19 / Deepak Rawtani, Chaudhery Mustansar Hussain.
Description: Hoboken, NJ : Wiley, 2024. | Includes index.
Identifiers: LCCN 2022055656 (print) | LCCN 2022055657 (ebook) | ISBN
    9781119777373 (cloth) | ISBN 9781119777380 (adobe pdf) | ISBN
    9781119777397 (epub)
Subjects: LCSH: COVID-19 (Disease)–Environmental aspects.
Classification: LCC RA644.C67 E595 2023(print) | LCC RA644.C67(ebook) |
    DDC 614.5/924144–dc23/eng/20221202
LC record available at https://lccn.loc.gov/2022055656
LC ebook record available at https://lccn.loc.gov/2022055657

Cover image: © Andrii Vodolazhskyi/Shutterstock
Cover design by Wiley

Set in 9.5/12.5pt STIXTwoText by Straive, Pondicherry, India

Contents

Foreword

"All outstanding work, in art as well as in science, results from immense zeal applied to a great idea" this quote by "Santiago Ramón y Cajal" aptly defines the cadence of the editors with their artwork titled **"The Environmental Impact of COVID-19"**. This book is a complete guide to the influence of the pandemic COVID-19 that changed the world and its impact on the environment.

The book is smartly divided into 18 chapters ranging from topics like environmental factors, Viability, and strategies for curbing COVID-19, to traditional, modern, and digital techniques for analysis of COVID. Apart from the topics mentioned earlier, this book also sheds light on case studies of COVID-19 and its impact on the environment, waste management strategies and implications on pandemic on climate change.

The challenges in the environmental management of COVID are both problematic and fascinating. People are working on them with enthusiasm, tenacity, and dedication to develop new methods to manage and mitigate pandemic level threats and provide novel solutions to keep up with dynamic threats. In this new age of interdependence and globalization, it is necessary for practitioners, students and professionals to have state of the art know how about factors influencing the environment concerning COVID-19.

This book provides very useful information and guidance in handling various environment-related issues with regard to COVID-19.

Dr. J.M. Vyas
(Vice Chancellor)
National Forensic Sciences University

1

COVID-19: A Pandemic - Introduction

Pratik Kulkarni[1], Tejas Barot[1], Piyush Rao[1], Aayush Dey[1],
and Deepak Rawtani[2]

[1] *School of Doctoral Studies & Research (SDSR), National Forensic Sciences University (Ministry of Home affairs, GOI),*
Gandhinagar, Gujarat, India
[2] *School of Pharmacy, National Forensic Sciences University (Ministry of Home affairs, GOI), Gandhinagar, Gujarat, India*

1.1 Introduction: Sources and Chemical Activities of COVID-19

Coronavirus or COVID-19 is an infectious disease caused by a novel virus known as extreme coronavirus-2 respiratory syndrome (SARS-CoV-2). It began to spread as a disease from Wuhan, the capital of the province of Hubei in China, in December 2019. It has since spread worldwide, contributing to an ongoing pandemic, as announced by the WHO on 11 March 2020 (Hui et al. 2020; Hui and Zumla 2019; Tang et al. 2020b). With more than 9 months under the pandemic, more than 70 million people have been tested positive for infection and more than a million deaths and counting worldwide. Its primary source was identified in the respiratory tract of patients in Wuhan undergoing treatment for pneumonia, which was then identified as the new SARS-CoV-2 virus.

The original source of the virus is still unknown, but the first cases were related to the Huanan Seafood Market in Wuhan. There are also some wild animals known to be sold on the market, including birds, marmots, bats, and snakes. It was shown that market samples were positive for the novel virus, but the animal was not specified (Astuti 2020; Guo et al. 2020; Tian et al. 2020). However, recent reports have suggested that bats could be the potential host of the virus as they shared96 % homology of the entire genome-wide sequence with the bat CoV. From the genetic analysis, a region of RNA-dependent RNA polymerase (RdRP) gene in SARS-CoV-2 was confirmed to be similar to a region of RdRP found in bat coronavirus RaTG13 with an astounding 96% homology of the genome sequence. Of more than 100 strains sequenced till the end of March, a 99.9% sequence match was observed but since then several changes in the genome have been discovered, which show a high probability of sequence diversity in the virus. Pangolin CoV genomes have also been found to have an 85.5–92.4 % homology with SARS-CoV-2, indicating that SARS-CoV-2 could be a potential intermediate host. How the virus transmits from either bats or pangolins needs to be studied more for a better confirmation (Harapan et al. 2020; Shereen et al. 2020; Udugama et al. 2020; ul Qamar et al. 2020).

1.1.1 Sources and Transmission

Currently, the source of transmission is known to be from human to human through respiratory droplets. Yet, not the only probable source of transmission is the respiratory tract. As a source of transmission, close contact has also been confirmed (Figure 1.1). For example, the virus can be transmitted by direct or indirect contact with the mucous membranes of the eye, mouth, or nose (Hui and Zumla 2019; Hui et al. 2020; Tang et al. 2020b). In a closed environment with relatively high aerosol concentrations, the possibility of aerosol transmission also exists (Astuti 2020). Some gastrointestinal symptoms have also been reported including diarrhea, nausea, and vomiting. All populations are vulnerable to the virus. Mostly elderlies and people with a weak immune function or underlying diseases are likely to become severely affected by the virus. Additionally, pregnant women and new-born babies infected with the virus can develop severe pneumonia. This group of patients should therefore be considered to be of primary importance in preventing and managing SARS-CoV-2 attacks (Astuti 2020; ul Qamar et al. 2020).

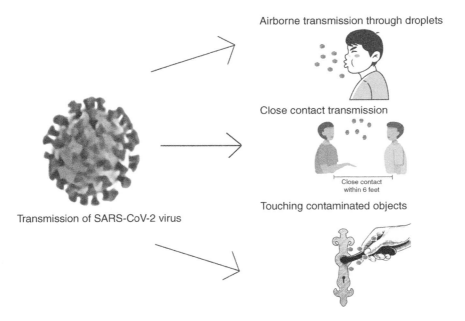

Figure 1.1 A schematic diagram showing SARS-CoV-2 transmission through different routes.

1.1.2 Structure of SARS-CoV-2

The virus is recognized as a non-segmented, enveloped, positive-sense RNA virus that is part of the subfamily of sarbecovirus, orthocoronavirinae, widely distributed in humans and other mammals. SARS-CoV-2 is about 60–140 nm in diameter and contains single-stranded RNA with 30,000 nucleotides in length (Wu et al. 2020). It is characterized by a distinct crown-like spikes on its outer surface, and its genome has 27 encoded proteins which also includes RdRP and 4 structural proteins with different functions namely Spike surface glycoprotein (S), which is involved in the coding for proteins that form receptor-binding spikes that help the virus to infect cells by binding to the receptors via embrane fusion (Sexton et al. 2016; Tang et al. 2020a; Wrapp et al. 2020). This binding also determines its host tropism and transmission capabilities. The other three proteins – Nucleocapsid protein (N), Small envelope protein (E), and Matrix protein (M) – are more conserved than the S protein and are essential for proper virus functioning. These proteins are involved in the encapsulation of RNA and/or proteins into protein assemblies, envelope formation, budding, and pathogenesis (Bauch and Orabyet al. 2013; Lim et al. 2016; Neuman et al. 2011; Schoeman and Fielding 2019).

SARS-CoV-2 is considered to have a long transmission period as its mean incubation time is estimated within three to seven days. It has also been reported that asymptomatic patients of the virus could be effective carriers during their incubation period (Udugama et al. 2020). This property is different from other SARS-CoV as most of those cases are transmitted via agents known as "superspreaders" and those who cannot infect others during their incubation period. These data thus support the current WHO guidelines of a 14-day quarantine period for active monitoring (Udugama et al. 2020; Yi et al. 2020).

1.1.3 Common Symptoms, Immune Reaction to the Virus, and Mechanism of Entry

Fatigue, fever, dry cough, dyspnea, and myalgia are key manifestations of the disease. Nasal congestion, sore throat, runny nose, headache, vomiting, and diarrhea are some less common symptoms (Figure 1.2). Patients termed under severe category often have dyspnea and/or hypoxia after a week of onset which is followed by septic shock, acute respiratory distress syndrome (ARDS), metabolic acidosis which is difficult to correct, and coagulation

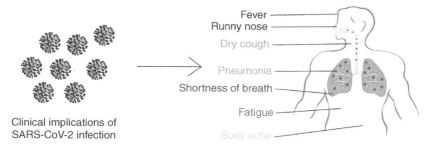

Figure 1.2 Clinical manifestations of infection with SARS-CoV-2 in humans.

dysfunction that develops rapidly. Patients with mild fatigue, low fever, and absence of pneumonia can be considered asymptomatic but can still spread the virus between humans (Udugama et al. 2020; Zhou et al. 2020).

Invasion of the virus into the host cell triggers an immune response which the innate immune system encounters through antigen presenting cells (APC), e.g. macrophages, dendritic cells (Chen et al. 2020; Guo et al. 2020; Huang et al. 2020). This APCs have specific receptors known as Pattern Recognition Receptors (PRR) located in several regions in the host cells like plasma and endosomal membranes, lysosomes, cytosol, and endocytolysosomes. Now, recognition of pathogen-associated molecular patterns (PAMP) comprising viral structural components including nucleic acid, carbohydrate moieties, glycoproteins induces cascade signaling to produce immune cell effectors which trigger a different biological response following protein activation. For instance, Toll-like receptor 4 (TLR-4) might induce the protein spikes of CoV to produce proinflammatory cytokines like IFN-α, IFN-γ, IL-1β, IL-6, TNF-α, TGFβ and chemokines like CCL2,3,5, CXCL8,9,10. Their excessive release from the cells of the immune effector leads to hyperinflammation, resulting in ARDS eventually (Chen et al. 2010, 2020; Cheung et al. 2005; Huang et al. 2020; Li et al. 2020a, 2020c; Rabi et al. 2020).

Various studies have shown that SARS-CoV-2 host cell entry is regulated by its interaction with the angiotensin-converting enzyme 2 (ACE-2) (Zhou et al. 2020). A critical finding stated that in comparison to SARS-CoV, SARS-CoV-2 spikes bind to the ACE-2 enzyme with 10–20 times higher affinity, thereby making it easier to spread among the humans. Therefore, upon entry into the respiratory epithelial cells, the virus replicates quickly, along with triggering a strong immune response characterized by cytokine storm syndromes known as hypercytokinaemia. This group of disorders is characterized by an uncontrollable increase in cytokine production, which leads to ARDS and ultimately leading to multiple organ failure. Studies have revealed that many patients succumbed to multiple organ failure indicating a substantial decrease in T-cell population, whereas surviving T-cell population being functionally exhausted, indicated decreased immunity in the patients with secondary infections, worsening the respiratory failure even further (Li et al. 2020b).

1.1.3.1 Immuno-evasion of Coronaviruses

Viruses including the novel SARS-CoV-2 have several ways to avoid the immune defense mechanisms to survive and infect the host cells (Janeway et al. 2008; Li et al. 2020a). The state of the cell before and after the entry of the virus is very crucial in determining the immune evasion potential of the virus.

The virus can form double vesicles outside the cells to evade recognition processes which acts as shields of cytosolic PRRs to dsRNA as intermediate products (Li et al. 2020). Apart from double vesicle formation, blocking INF is also a part of virus immune evasion. A non-structural protein group termed as nsp1 from SARS-CoV acts as INF-I suppressors via inactivating host translational machinery, RNA and inhibiting STAT1 phosphorylation. At an early stage, failure of INF-I leads to initiation of viral replication and subsequent dissemination, thus increasing the severity of disease (Prompetchara et al. 2020; Totura and Baric 2012). SARS-CoV lack a 5' cap in its structure making it easier for the immune system to recognize it. However, SARS-CoV-2 has developed a host mimicking property by using two nonstructural proteins, namely nsp 14, which is a protein-forming cap followed by a nsp 16 modification. This mechanism makes viral RNA similar to host cell RNA and prevents recognition of any PRR (Chen et al. 2009; Daffis et al. 2010; Totura and Baric 2012).

1.1.3.2 World at Loss due to COVID-19

COVID-19 has become a pandemic of a major scale which has impacted the lifestyle of all the nations globally. The pandemic has contributed to significant socioeconomic instability, resulting in the largest global recession in history. All social meeting events, including sports, religious, political, and cultural meetings, have been postponed or cancelled with one-third of the global population being under lockdown (Evans 2020; Nicas 2020; Nicola et al. 2020). Also, schools, universities, and colleges have been closed until further notice in more than 197 countries (Nicola et al. 2020). Moreover, misinformation related to the virus and its spread has caused incidents of discrimination and xenophobia against Chinese people. On the contrary, there has been a significant decrease in environmental pollution and carbon emissions due to travel bans in most nations and the closure of heavy industries (Brief 2020; Sui 2020; UNESCO 2020).

Impact on political systems has been prominent as it caused suspensions of legislative meetings, rescheduling of elections due to fear of virus spread, and isolation or deaths of multiple political leaders (Evans 2020). The pandemic has affected the educational systems of all schools, colleges, and universities worldwide, leading to near closure. According to UNESCO monitoring, more than 192 countries have implemented national closures. Some countries have applied for local closures and collectively this has impacted more than 90% of world's student population (Chen et al. 2020). Apart from impacting students, teachers, and their families, the pandemic has also caused far-reaching socioeconomic consequences. The pandemic has shed light on various social and economic issues, including student debt, food insecurity, disability and digital learning services, and access to housing and the internet. This has affected the disadvantaged children and their families the most due to problems like interrupted learning, childcare problems, nutritional problems, and economic burden on the families of the children who cannot work. In response to curb this, UNESCO has suggested distance learning program via open educational applications and facilities to provide remote learning to the students (Boseley 2020; Chen et al. 2020; Strumpf 2020).

Owing to the pandemic, worries have moved from supply-side manufacturing problems to a downturn in enterprises in the services sector from a socioeconomic perspective. Owing to panic purchasing and shortages of food and other supermarket products, supply shortages have been affected a lot. Shortage of face masks and common drugs was also seen due to panic buying and insufficient supply of the stocks (Bachman 2020; Strumpf 2020). The technology industry has also warned about the delays in delivery of electronic goods. Global stock markets saw the largest fall in the history since the 2008 financial crisis and lead to crash of the stock markets. Global conferences and events across sports, fashion, and technology industries have been postponed or cancelled due to the pandemic (Wilson and Campus 2020). There is also an approximate monetary effect on the travel and trade market, which is expected to be in the billions and is still growing. The International Labor Organization reported an approximate loss of 30 million jobs, compared to 25 million during the 2008 financial crisis. On 18 March, the WHO published a study on mental health and psychosocial problems and discussed advice on various social considerations during the outbreak.

The sectors of performing arts and cultural heritage have had a profound effect on their organizational activities as well as on people who are working, autonomous, or both. Organizations have continued to preserve their publicly supported missions in order to provide communities with the requisite access to cultural heritage and to maintain public safety and promote artists worldwide. There has been a striking impact on the environment and the climate due to the pandemic as well. A significant drop in air pollution due to imposing of travel ban has been observed globally. Approximately 25% reduction has been witnessed in carbon emissions in China. However, this has also affected the environmental diplomacy efforts worldwide, thereby postponing of the United Nations Climate Change Conference. Its impact is also presumed to be seen in an economic fallout leading to a lesser investment in green energy and renewable technologies (Jin et al. 2020; National UNESCO 2020).

1.1.3.3 Incubation Period

The incubation period of the infection is 2–14 days, with an average incubation period of 3–7 days, indicating a long duration of transmission. The latency period of the virus is estimated to be consistent with other known human viruses, for instance, non-SARS human CoVs, SARS CoV, and Middle East respiratory syndrome (MERS)-CoV, which has a range of 2–5 transmission for non-human CoV and 2- to 14-day transmission rate for SARS and MERS-CoV, along with a mean rate of 3, 5, and 5.7 days, respectively (Assiri et al. 2013; Lessler et al. 2009). Asymptomatic patients with COVID-19 are reported to transmit the virus at a similar effectiveness during their incubation period which increases its transmission at a much faster rate (Quilty et al. 2020; Rothe et al. 2020). This behavior of SARS-CoV-2 is different from SARS-CoV, as the latter is caused mostly due to "superspreaders" and they do not infect the susceptible persons during their incubation period (Lipsitch et al. 2003). Therefore, with this data available, the current period as recommended by WHO is of 14 days, for active monitoring of the patients (Udugama et al. 2020; Yi et al. 2020).

1.1.3.4 SARS-CoV-2 and Basic Reproduction Number (R0)

To evaluate the transmissibility of SARS-CoV-2, a basic reproduction number is available, expressed as R nought (R0) and is defined as the average number of infections (secondary) spread by an active SARS-CoV-2 patient. As per reports, an R0 value >1 indicates an exponential spread of the virus and can cause an epidemic or pandemic. The R0 of this virus has been reported to be in the range of 1.4–6.49 (mean: 3.28), which is significantly higher than the SARS-CoV range of R0 2–5 (Liu et al. 2020).

1.1.3.5 Pathological Characteristics

Biopsy reports from the very first patient infected and died from the infection have revealed pathological characteristics of the virus similar to ARDS. Pneumocyte desquamation and hyaline membrane formation were evident from histological analysis of lung tissue, indicating ARDS. Also, the lung tissues were found to be infiltrated by interstitial mononuclear activity. Moreover, the intra-alveolar spaces were found to have giant multinucleated cells with enlarged atypical pneumocytes having large nuclei and a prominent nucleolus with amphophilic granular cytoplasm which suggested changes of viral cytopathic nature (Xu et al. 2020). These pathological features are similar to that of SARS-CoV and MERS-CoV infected patients (Ding et al. 2003; Ng et al. 2014). Hence, understanding the pathology of the virus and its comparison with its familial counterparts could help physicians develop a timely strategy for their treatment and reduce their mortality rate.

1.1.3.6 Case Definitions

The case definitions are currently based on the provisional guidance documents provided by the WHO (Chatterjee et al. 2020; WHO 2020a). An acute respiratory infection called SARI is an example of a history of fever with a measured temperature of >38°C and cough, an initiation of infection within a 10-day period, and hospitalization is required.

For SARS-CoV-2 infection, surveillance case descriptions include a person with SARI and no other etiology with one of the following:

  i) travel history in the last 14 days to Wuhan, Hubei Province, China; and
 ii) a healthcare worker (HCW) looking after an SARI patient and patients of uncertain etiology.

In addition, patients with acute respiratory disease and one of the following conditions:

  i) direct contact with an infected individual or a possible case within 14 days of the onset of SARS-CoV-2; and
 ii) visited or operated within 14 days before the onset of symptoms in a healthcare facility where positive cases of infection have been identified.

There remains the elusiveness of a delicate and precise concept of community-based oversight. The referral metrics and their impact-based results have yet to be determined. Concerns regarding the current outbreak, such as the need to quarantine children, the minimum quarantine time, and its impact on mental and socioeconomic costs, also need to be addressed.

1.1.3.7 Prevention of Transmission

Respiratory droplets and physical contact are the chief sources of SARS-CoV-2 transmission. Hence, precautionary measures are of prime importance and standard methods include hand hygiene, using personal protective equipment (PPE) kits, and respiratory etiquettes. Use of alcohol-based hand rubs, having 60–80% alcohol, is recommended currently as a part of hand hygiene. A proper hand wash with soap and water following the correct steps have proved to suffice. For hand drying, the use of cloth towels must be avoided and disposable tissue paper has been recommended. A PPE kit comprises medical grade face masks or particulate respirators, face shields, goggles, gloves, gowns, and shoe covers (Chang et al. 2020, Chatterjee et al. 2020). Face or procedure masks along with a head strap should be sufficient for droplet and contact-based transmission. When entering the patient's room, utmost care must be taken and the kits must be worn before entering and removed only after leaving it. For those in group settings and who are symptomatic, it is mandatory. Due to an increased risk of exposure, it is mandatory for patients in home care environments, suspected cases of moderate respiratory symptoms with COVID-19, and even HCWs to always wear medical masks, along with observing hand hygiene and proper disposal (Chang et al. 2020). National Institute for Occupational Safety and Health (NIOSH)-certified N-95 masks and EU standard FFP2 or equivalent are examples of particulate respirators which must be compulsorily used by the HCWs in aerosol-generating procedures (AGPs). In addition to wearing long-sleeved, waterproof, sterile gowns made of non-absorbent materials, face shields or goggles must also be worn when performing AGPs. Waterproof aprons, where gowns are not appropriate, should be sufficient. Latex, powder-free gloves must be used when handling infectious materials from the patient. In order to follow the respiratory and cough labels, the nose and mouth must be covered while sneezing and coughing through disposable tissue paper, not a cotton cloth. Flexing the elbow to cover the nose and mouth must be done if nothing is available, followed by appropriate hand hygiene. Most importantly, symptomatic patients should not be allowed to congregate in public places and crowded areas while in the community settings. Self-deferral and containment must be encouraged using the Information, education, and communication (IEC) messages, especially for the symptomatic patients. For patients advised for home care, a well-ventilated room must be arranged and for those in the healthcare settings, a negative pressure room must be arranged (Chang et al. 2020, Chatterjee et al. 2020).

1.1.3.8 Quarantine

WHO has stated that, "The International Health Regulations (IHR) being an international legal instrument binds 194 countries worldwide, including all the WHO member States. They aim to assist the international community in preventing and responding to acute public health risks with the potential to cross borders and threaten people globally, according to the official statement" (WHO 2020b). In order to establish procedures that must be followed by the WHO to maintain global public health security, the IHR is also defined as "the rights and obligations of nations to report public health events" (WHO 2020b). The Department of Health and Family Welfare around the world has issued travel restrictions and additional advice from time to time, taking into account the rise in cases, in line with the outlined IHR principles. Travelling by all means (air, ship, etc.) was regulated and open only for rescue missions such as "Vande Bharat Mission" of India and for supply of necessary goods like medical equipment and food around the world. Currently, many countries like India, the United States, the United Kingdom have gradually started to and fro travel of foreign nationals and travelers. However, tourists are still exempted from travelling to other countries (MOHFW 2019). Upon returning to any country, a mandatory 14-day quarantine period has been established for everyone, except under medical emergencies (MOHFW 2019). The impact of such travel ban is yet to be seen on the economy and other sectors; however, it is estimated to be a loss in millions of dollars (Chinazzi et al. 2020). Until the pandemic outbreak is staunched, such bans may only provide a symbolic shield. Moreover, imposition of such travel bans has also raised many ethical concerns (Habibi et al. 2020). In an example, a cruise named Diamond Princess, docked off from Yokohama in Japan, was subjected to quarantine for a period two weeks, after a tourist tested positive after disembarking at Hong Kong (Dooley and Rich 2020; The Japan Times 2020). Out of 3700 passengers and aboard, 705 were tested positive for the virus. At one point, this incident became the second largest site of outbreak outside China. The worldwide imposition of lockdown has been viewed as a drastic measure of public health (Habibi et al. 2020; Sands et al. 2016). The benefits of such a decision continue to be addressed, but it is not appropriate to underplay the long-term adverse effects induced by it (Stone 2020). This has inevitably led to economic, social, and psychological stress on the whole population and has a certain detrimental effect on long-term health (Poletto et al. 2014). Such government-led interventions remain debatable and coercive in terms of top-down quarantine approaches; population-controlled and civil society-controlled self-quarantine and monitoring could establish more sustainable and implementable approaches in a pandemic of this scale (Li et al. 2020).

1.1.3.9   Global Response by WHO

WHO and the Global Research Collaboration for Infectious Disease Preparedness held a meeting at its headquarters in Geneva on 11 and 12 February 2020 to bring together research funders and leading scientists around the world to evaluate current information on the novel coronavirus disease, identify weaknesses, and develop a collaborative effort to fund the priority-based research needed (WHO 2020c).

Following this, a Global Surveillance for COVID-19 infection in humans was established by WHO, and 16 laboratories globally were selected for referral testing on confirmatory basis. For laboratory diagnosis, interim guidance documents have been prepared by the WHO (WHO 2020d, 2020e). Home care for suspected patients with the infection and practice of hand and face hygiene at healthcare settings, clinical management, risk communication and engagement with the community, preventing further infection, and global surveillance are also included in the documents (WHO 2020f, 2020g). Moreover, an online course has also been developed by the WHO to educate people and HCWs regarding the emerging respiratory viruses including the novel coronavirus. Also, a commodity package has been established for a quick set-up of emergency isolation and quarantine facilities, which includes a list of essential biomedical equipment (WHO 2020h, 2020i). As per reports, the SARS outbreak back in 2003 was originated from mutation in coronavirus spread from small carnivorous animals sold at the live market in Guangdong, China. Mask palm civets, Chinese ferret badgers, and racoon dogs were the likely sources (Bell et al. 2004; Cyranoski and Abbott 2003; Guan et al. 2003). Likewise, for the 2012 MERS-CoV outbreak, dramedy camels were found to be the virus sources (Azhar et al. 2014).

Assuming that the increase in COVID-19 cases could be due to exposure to the live animal market, WHO has since prohibited its business with immediate effect from 21 January 2020. Thus, the importance of adopting the One Health Framework in prevention against deadly pathogens is indicated by such spill over events (Chatterjee et al. 2016; McKenzie et al. 2016). As evident during previous outbreaks, Nipah and Ebola virus diseases, HCWs are always at a risk of contacting the infection and may contribute to the disease morbidity and mortality (Arunkumar et al. 2019; Evans et al. 2015; Hewlett and Hewlett 2005; Kumar et al. 2019; Pallivalappil et al. 2020). Transmission from an asymptomatic patient has always been a major concern. For example, before the onset of fever, more than 10 HCWs were infected by a patient undergoing surgery (WHO 2020j). In several early case examples of hospital-associated transmission, 40 HCWs and 17 hospitalized patients were infected with the novel virus and represented a total of 29% and 12% of all the cases, respectively (Wang et al. 2020).

Mental health issues have also been a substantial threat during such infections which includes generalized anxiety disorders, depression, and poor sleep (Huang et al. 2020; Zhu et al. 2020). There have also been increasing reports of stigma surrounding people of Asian origin globally (CDC et al. 2020). In order to prevent such stigmas, a guide has been developed by WHO by collaborating with the International Federation of Red Cross and Red Crescent Societies and United Nations Children's Fund. In addition, during the second meeting of the IHR Emergency Committee, a statement was issued highlighting the caution of the member states against creating any policies that promote stigma and discrimination in accordance with the principles of the IHR set out in Article 3.

1.1.4 Treatments

Currently there is no treatment available for the disease, and there are many potential anti-viral drug therapies along with some other combinations which have proven effectiveness against the viral infection. Individuals suspected and confirmed as positive for the infection are recommended to be treated in hospitals or at home under specific isolation and protective settings. Suspected patients can be isolated and treated in a private room, and similarly, the confirmed ones can be treated in the same ward. However, critical cases need to be transferred to the intensive care unit as quickly as possible.

1.1.4.1 General Treatment Strategies for COVID-19

These include bed rest and supportive consultation, maintaining a stable constant inner environment such as providing water electrolytes, ensuring sufficient energy intake, and monitoring vital health signs for instance heart rate, pulse, blood pressure, respiratory rate, and oxygen saturation (Figure 1.3).

1.1.4.2 Antiviral Therapy

Being a member of the type 1 IFN family, Interferon-alpha (IFN α) plays an important role in host resistance to viral infection. As demonstrated by some in vitro experiments, IFN α promotes both innate and adaptive immune responses by suppressing viral infection by inhibiting its replication (Ströher et al. 2004; Zorzitto et al. 2006). Protection from the SARS-CoV-2 virus has also been shown in cynomolgus monkeys after treatment with IFN α (Haagmans et al. 2004). Furthermore, synthetic recombinant IFN α showed its therapeutic benefits for patients in a pilot clinical trial (Loutfy et al. 2003). IFN α should therefore be considered as a potential drug candidate for therapy with COVID-19.

1.1.4.3 COVID-19 Convalescent Plasma for Prophylaxis

Convalescent plasma (CP) is well known as a treatment option for infectious diseases, including severe viral infections of the lower respiratory tract (Mair-Jenkins et al. 2015). Generation of neutralizing antibodies may be possible from recovered SARS-CoV-2 patients (Nie et al. 2020; Ou et al. 2020) that could have applications in preventing SARS-CoV-2 infection in patients with underlying conditions and high-risk individuals. Monoclonal antibodies have been shown to be protective during hospitalization for other respiratory viruses in specific high-risk patients (Feltes et al. 2003; The IMpact-RSV Study Group 1998). Also, animal models have suggested a prophylactic utility against

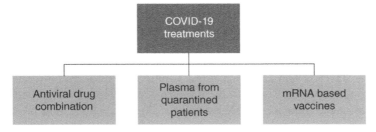

Figure 1.3 A schematic chart showing the treatment options for COVID-19.

SARS-CoV-1 (ter Meulen et al. 2004). However, there are some risks with the use of CP such as acute lung injury during transfusion or a hypothetical risk of antibody-dependent enhancement of the viral infection (ADE). ADE from viral infection can occur in several other diseases and, due to the presence of certain antibodies, is characterized by disease enhancement (Casadevall and Pirofski 2020). Clinical trials from SARS-CoV-2 recovered patients have been ongoing as of now (Shoham 2020).

1.1.4.4 FDA-Approved Drug/Agents for Emergency Use Authorization (EUA)

As of now, there is no specific drug/vaccine treatment available for combatting the viral spread. Recently, the use of widely studied potential candidate hydroxychloroquine has been stopped with immediate effect as it lacks efficacy against the virus. The following combinations have been recently given approval by the United States Food and Drug Administration (FDA) for emergency use with proven clinical benefits:

Currently, a combination of drugs Casirivimab and Imdevimab have been approved for EUA. These two agents are recombinant human IgG1 monoclonal antibodies that act by targeting the receptor-binding domain of the spike protein of SARS-CoV-2. This combination has been approved for the treatment of mild-to-moderate COVID-19 in adults and pediatric patients (aged 12 years and older with a weight of at least 40 kg) with positive results for direct testing. The combination has also been recommended for those at high risk for progressing to severe infection by the virus and/or hospitalization.

Another recently approved combination therapy consists of Baricitinib (Olumiant) along with Remdesivir (Veklury). This combination has been recommended for the treatment of suspected or laboratory-confirmed COVID-19 patients in hospitalized adults and pediatric patients of 2 years of age or older for emergency use by healthcare providers; and requires O_2 supplementation, invasive mechanical ventilation, or oxygenation of the extracorporeal membrane (ECMO).

REGIOCIT has also been approved by the FDA on the basis of scientific evidence to be used as a substitute for suspected or known COVID-19 adult patients in critical care settings receiving continuous renal replacement therapy (CRRT) and for whom Regional Citrate Anticoagulation (RCA) is appropriate. This replacement solution is composed of citrate for RCA of the extracorporeal circuit and is intended for a continuous use with venovenous hemofiltration (CVVH) and continuous venovenous hemodiafiltration (CVVHDF) modalities (FDA et al. 2020).

1.1.4.5 Vaccines

Several groups are working on potential COVID-19 vaccines, with some backed by the non-profit Coalition for Epidemic Preparedness Innovations (CEPI). Currently, >50 projects around the globe are centered on developing a vaccine for COVID-19 treatment. Till now, more than five candidate vaccines have been undergoing human clinical trials. Reports suggest the availability of the vaccine by January 2021, while some also suggest it to be available by Summer or Fall 2021 (Radcliffe 2020).

Some notable projects are from BioNTech/Fosun Pharma/Pfizer, Moderna, and the University of Oxford in England (in partnership with AstraZeneca, USA) where the FDA has given the approval for Phase 3 clinical trials after initial success in preventing the infection and has also indicated the safety of the vaccines. Moderna has developed an mRNA-based vaccine and the University of Oxford has developed a vaccine based on the modified virus that can trigger immune responses (Radcliffe 2020). Very recently, the vaccine developed by BioNTech/Fosun Pharma/Pfizer was approved by the UK government to roll out first doses to the volunteers and have started shipping it to other countries around the globe. With an effectivity of >95% by Pfizer and Moderna and some other companies, it remains to be seen how the demands for the vaccine are met and how fast they are distributed efficiently given their specific conditions for storage under deep freeze and so on.

Another potential vaccine candidate is from Inovio, which has been working on a DNA-based vaccine for MERS, allowing the company to develop a COVID-19 vaccine quickly. A Phase 3 trial has already started. Advances in genetic sequencing and other technological developments have increased the speed for vaccine development. However, experts suggest that widespread use of the vaccine will not be possible for at least another year for completing a Phase 3 trial successfully that takes around 12–18 months (Radcliffe 2020).

1.1.5   Conclusion

In conclusion, the COVID-19 pandemic has impacted the world as we know in every possible way and its overall implications in all the sectors need to be carefully addressed in order to prevent another pandemic of this scale. With almost 10 months in pandemic, there is no perfect treatment available yet, for its prevention and control. As of now, practicing the safety and prevention guidelines as laid down by the governmental authorities remains mainstay for its control. Also, as the vaccine development is under an emerging stage, it remains to be seen how it changes the dynamics of the spread of this novel virus. This chapter discussed all the introductory parameters regarding the outbreak of SARS-CoV-2 virus and laid a brief emphasis on its control and prevention. The upcoming chapters will deal more with the diagnosis and the imminent socioeconomic and environmental impact of the pandemic and the collective efforts needed to prevent it in the distant future.

References

Arunkumar, G., Chandni, R., Mourya, D.T. et al. (2019). Outbreak investigation of Nipah virus disease in Kerala, India, 2018. *The Journal of infectious diseases* 219 (12): 1867–1878.

Assiri, A., Al-Tawfiq, J.A., Al-Rabeeah, A.A. et al. (2013). Epidemiological, demographic, and clinical characteristics of 47 cases of Middle East respiratory syndrome coronavirus disease from Saudi Arabia: a descriptive study. *The Lancet infectious diseases* 13 (9): 752–761.

Astuti, I. (2020). Severe acute respiratory syndrome coronavirus 2 (SARS-CoV-2): an overview of viral structure and host response. *Diabetes & Metabolic Syndrome: Clinical Research & Reviews* 14 (2): 407–412.

Azhar, E.I., El-Kafrawy, S.A., Farraj, S.A. et al. (2014). Evidence for camel-to-human transmission of MERS coronavirus. *New England Journal of Medicine* 370 (26): 2499–2505.

Bachman, D. (2020). The economic impact of COVID-19 (novel coronavirus). Deloitte Insights (accessed 28).

Bauch, C.T. and Oraby, T. (2013). Assessing the pandemic potential of MERS-CoV. *The Lancet* 382 (9893): 662–664.

Bell, D., Roberton, S., and Hunter, P.R. (2004). Animal origins of SARS coronavirus: possible links with the international trade in small carnivores. *Philosophical Transactions of the Royal Society of London. Series B: Biological Sciences* 359 (1447): 1107–1114.

Boseley, S., 2020. WHO warns of global shortage of face masks and protective suits. *The Guardian*, 7. https://www.theguardian.com/world/2020/feb/07/who-warns-global-shortage-face-masks-protective-suits-coronavirus.

Brief, C. (2020). Analysis: Coronavirus temporarily reduced China's CO_2 emissions by a quarter. Retrieved April, 27, p. 2020.

Casadevall, A. and Pirofski, L.A. (2020). The convalescent sera option for containing COVID-19. *The Journal of clinical investigation* 130 (4): 1545–1548.

Centers for Disease Control and Prevention (2020). Reducing stigma. www.cdc.gov/coronavirus/2019-ncov/about/related-stigma.html (accessed 13 December 2020).

Chang, D., Xu, H., Rebaza, A. et al. (2020). Protecting health-care workers from subclinical coronavirus infection. *The Lancet Respiratory Medicine* 8 (3): e13.

Chatterjee, P., Kakkar, M., and Chaturvedi, S. (2016). Integrating one health in national health policies of developing countries: India's lost opportunities. *Infectious diseases of poverty* 5 (1): 1–5.

Chatterjee, P., Nagi, N., Agarwal, A. et al. (2020). The 2019 novel coronavirus disease (COVID-19) pandemic: a review of the current evidence. *Indian Journal of Medical Research* 151 (2): 147.

Chen, Y., Cai, H., Xiang, N. et al. (2009). Functional screen reveals SARS coronavirus nonstructural protein nsp14 as a novel cap N7 methyltransferase. *Proceedings of the National Academy of Sciences* 106 (9): 3484–3489.

Chen, J., Lau, Y.F., Lamirande, E.W. et al. (2010). Cellular immune responses to severe acute respiratory syndrome coronavirus (SARS-CoV) infection in senescent BALB/c mice: CD4+ T cells are important in control of SARS-CoV infection. *Journal of virology* 84 (3): 1289–1301.

Chen, N., Zhou, M., Dong, X. et al. (2020). Epidemiological and clinical characteristics of 99 cases of 2019 novel coronavirus pneumonia in Wuhan, China: a descriptive study. *The Lancet* 395 (10223): 507–513.

Cheung, C.Y., Poon, L.L., Ng, I.H. et al. (2005). Cytokine responses in severe acute respiratory syndrome coronavirus-infected macrophages in vitro: possible relevance to pathogenesis. *Journal of virology* 79 (12): 7819–7826.

Chinazzi, M., Davis, J.T., Ajelli, M. et al. (2020). The effect of travel restrictions on the spread of the 2019 novel coronavirus (COVID-19) outbreak. *Science* 368 (6489): 395–400.

Cyranoski, D. and Abbott, A., 2003. Virus detectives seek source of SARS in China's wild animals 423, 463.

Daffis, S., Szretter, K.J., Schriewer, J. et al. (2010). 2′-O methylation of the viral mRNA cap evades host restriction by IFIT family members. *Nature* 468 (7322): 452–456.

Ding, Y., Wang, H., Shen, H. et al. (2003). The clinical pathology of severe acute respiratory syndrome (SARS): a report from China. *The Journal of Pathology: A Journal of the Pathological Society of Great Britain and Ireland* 200 (3): 282–289.

Dooley, B. and Rich, M. (2020). Cruise ship's coronavirus outbreak leaves crew nowhere to hide. The New York Times. www.nytimes.com/2020/02/10/business/coronavirus-japan-cruise-ship.html (accessed 13 December 2020).

Evans, O. (2020). Socio-economic impacts of novel coronavirus: The policy solutions. *BizEcons Quarterly* 7: 3–12.

Evans, D.K., Goldstein, M., and Popova, A. (2015). Health-care worker mortality and the legacy of the Ebola epidemic. *The Lancet Global Health* 3 (8): e439–e440.

Feltes, T.F., Cabalka, A.K., Meissner, H.C. et al. (2003). Palivizumab prophylaxis reduces hospitalization due to respiratory syncytial virus in young children with hemodynamically significant congenital heart disease. *The Journal of pediatrics* 143 (4): 532–540.

Guan, Y., Zheng, B.J., He, Y.Q. et al. (2003). Isolation and characterization of viruses related to the SARS coronavirus from animals in southern China. *Science* 302 (5643): 276–278.

Guo, Y.R., Cao, Q.D., Hong, Z.S. et al. (2020). The origin, transmission and clinical therapies on coronavirus disease 2019 (COVID-19) outbreak–an update on the status. *Military Medical Research* 7 (1): 1–10.

Haagmans, B.L., Kuiken, T., Martina, B.E. et al. (2004). Pegylated interferon-α protects type 1 pneumocytes against SARS coronavirus infection in macaques. *Nature medicine* 10 (3): 290–293.

Habibi, R., Burci, G.L., de Campos, T.C. et al. (2020). Do not violate the International Health Regulations during the COVID-19 outbreak. *The Lancet* 395 (10225): 664–666.

Harapan, H., Itoh, N., Yufika, A. et al. (2020). Coronavirus disease 2019 (COVID-19): a literature review. *Journal of Infection and Public Health* 13 (5): 667–673.

Hewlett, B.L. and Hewlett, B.S. (2005). Providing care and facing death: nursing during Ebola outbreaks in central Africa. *Journal of Transcultural Nursing* 16 (4): 289–297.

https://gisanddata.maps.arcgis.com/apps/opsdashboard/index.html#/bda7594740 fd40299423467b48e9ecf6 (accessed 13 December 2020).

https://www.gov.uk/government/publications/coronavirus-covid-19-maintaining-educational-provision/guidance-for-schools-colleges-and-local-authorities-on-maintaining-educational-provision (accessed 13 December 2020).

https://www.mayoclinic.org/diseases-conditions/coronavirus/symptoms-causes/syc-20479963 (accessed 13 December 2020).

https://www.worldometers.info/coronavirus/ (accessed 13 December 2020).

Huang, C., Wang, Y., Li, X. et al. (2020). Clinical features of patients infected with 2019 novel coronavirus in Wuhan, China. *The Lancet* 395 (10223): 497–506.

Hui, D.S. and Zumla, A. (2019). Severe acute respiratory syndrome: historical, epidemiologic, and clinical features. *Infectious Disease Clinics* 33 (4): 869–889.

Hui, D.S., Azhar, E.I., Madani, T.A. et al. (2020). The continuing 2019-nCoV epidemic threat of novel coronaviruses to global health—the latest 2019 novel coronavirus outbreak in Wuhan, China. *International Journal of Infectious Diseases* 91: 264.

IMpact-RSV Study Group* (1998). Palivizumab, a humanized respiratory syncytial virus monoclonal antibody, reduces hospitalization from respiratory syncytial virus infection in high-risk infants. *Pediatrics* 102 (3): 531–537.

Janeway, C., Murphy, K.P., Travers, P., and Walport, M. (2008). *Janeway's Immuno biology*. Routledge Taylor and Francis Group.

Jin, Y.H., Cai, L., Cheng, Z.S. et al. (2020). A rapid advice guideline for the diagnosis and treatment of 2019 novel coronavirus (2019-nCoV) infected pneumonia (standard version). *Military Medical Research* 7 (1): 4.

Kumar, C.G., Sugunan, A.P., Yadav, P. et al. (2019). Infections among contacts of patients with Nipah virus, India. *Emerging infectious diseases* 25 (5): 1007.

Lessler, J., Reich, N.G., Brookmeyer, R. et al. (2009). Incubation periods of acute respiratory viral infections: a systematic review. *The Lancet infectious diseases* 9 (5): 291–300.

Li, G., Fan, Y., Lai, Y. et al. (2020a). Coronavirus infections and immune responses. *Journal of medical virology* 92 (4): 424–432.

Li, H., Liu, S.M., Yu, X.H. et al. (2020b). Coronavirus disease 2019 (COVID-19): current status and future perspective. *International Journal of Antimicrobial Agents* 55: 105951.

Li, X., Geng, M., Peng, Y. et al. (2020c). Molecular immune pathogenesis and diagnosis of COVID-19. *Journal of Pharmaceutical Analysis*. 10.

Lipsitch, M., Cohen, T., Cooper, B. et al. (2003). Transmission dynamics and control of severe acute respiratory syndrome. *Science* 300 (5627): 1966–1970.

Liu, Y., Gayle, A.A., Wilder-Smith, A., and Rocklöv, J. (2020). The reproductive number of COVID-19 is higher compared to SARS coronavirus. *Journal of Travel Medicine* 27 (2): https://doi.org/10.1093/jtm/taaa021.

Loutfy, M.R., Blatt, L.M., Siminovitch, K.A. et al. (2003). Interferon alfacon-1 plus corticosteroids in severe acute respiratory syndrome: a preliminary study. *Jama* 290 (24): 3222–3228.

Mair-Jenkins, J., Saavedra-Campos, M., Baillie, J.K. et al. (2015). The effectiveness of convalescent plasma and hyperimmune immunoglobulin for the treatment of severe acute respiratory infections of viral etiology: a systematic review and exploratory meta-analysis. *The Journal of infectious diseases* 211 (1): 80–90.

McKenzie, J.S., Dahal, R., Kakkar, M. et al. (2016). One Health research and training and government support for One Health in South Asia. *Infection ecology & epidemiology* 6 (1): 33842.

Ministry of Health and Family Welfare, Government of India (2019). Revised travel advisory. www.mohfw.gov.in (accessed 13 December 2020).

Neuman, B.W., Kiss, G., Kunding, A.H. et al. (2011). A structural analysis of M protein in coronavirus assembly and morphology. *Journal of structural biology* 174 (1): 11–22.

Ng, D.L., Al Hosani, F., Keating, M.K. et al. (2014). Ultrastructural findings of a fatal case of Middle East respiratory syndrome coronavirus infection in the United Arab Emirates. *The American journal of pathology* 186 (3): 652–658.

Ng, D.L., Al Hosani, F., Keating, M.K. et al. (2016). Clinicopathologic, immunohistochemical, and ultrastructural. Findings of a fatal case of Middle East respiratory syndrome coronavirus infection in the United Arab Emirates. *The American Journal of Pathology* 186 (3): 652–658. doi: 10.1016/j.ajpath.2015.10.024. PMID: 26857507; PMCID: PMC7093852.

Nicas, J. (2020). He has 17,700 bottles of hand sanitizer and nowhere to sell them. *The New York Times*. March, 14.

Nicola, M., Alsafi, Z., Sohrabi, C. et al. (2020). The socio-economic implications of the coronavirus and COVID-19 pandemic: a review. *International Journal of Surgery*. 78: 185–193.

Nie, J., Li, Q., Wu, J. et al. (2020). Establishment and validation of a pseudovirus neutralization assay for SARS-CoV-2. *Emerging microbes & infections* 9 (1): 680–686.

Ou, X., Liu, Y., Lei, X. et al. (2020). Characterization of spike glycoprotein of SARS-CoV-2 on virus entry and its immune cross-reactivity with SARS-CoV. *Nature communications* 11 (1): 1–12.

Pallivalappil, B., Ali, A., Thulaseedharan, N.K. et al. (2020). Dissecting an outbreak: a clinico-epidemiological study of Nipah virus infection in Kerala, India, 2018. *Journal of Global Infectious Diseases* 12 (1): 21.

Poletto, C., Gomes, M.F., Piontti, A.P. et al. (2014). Assessing the impact of travel restrictions on international spread of the 2014 West African Ebola epidemic. *Eurosurveillance* 19 (42): 20936.

Prompetchara, E., Ketloy, C., and Palaga, T. (2020). Immune responses in COVID-19 and potential vaccines: Lessons learned from SARS and MERS epidemic. *Asian Pac J Allergy Immunol* 38 (1): 1–9.

Quilty, B.J., Clifford, S., Flasche, S., and Eggo, R.M. (2020). Effectiveness of airport screening at detecting travellers infected with novel coronavirus (2019-nCoV). *Eurosurveillance* 25 (5): 2000080.

Rabi, F.A., Al Zoubi, M.S., Kasasbeh, G.A. et al. (2020). SARS-CoV-2 and coronavirus disease 2019: what we know so far. *Pathogens* 9 (3): 231.

Radcliffe, S. (2020). Here's exactly where we are with vaccines and treatments for COVID-19. *Health News*. www.healthline.com/health-news/heres-exactly-where-were-at-with-vaccines-and-treatments-for-covid-19 (accessed 13 December 2020).

Rothe, C., Schunk, M., Sothmann, P. et al. (2020). Transmission of 2019-nCoV infection from an asymptomatic contact in Germany. *New England Journal of Medicine* 382 (10): 970–971.

Sands, P., Mundaca-Shah, C., and Dzau, V.J. (2016). The neglected dimension of global security—a framework for countering infectious-disease crises. *New England Journal of Medicine* 374 (13): 1281–1287.

Schoeman, D. and Fielding, B.C. (2019). Coronavirus envelope protein: current knowledge. *Virology journal* 16 (1): 69.

Sexton, N.R., Smith, E.C., Blanc, H. et al. (2016). Homology-based identification of a mutation in the coronavirus RNA-dependent RNA polymerase that confers resistance to multiple mutagens. *Journal of virology* 90 (16): 7415–7428.

Shereen, M.A., Khan, S., Kazmi, A. et al. (2020). COVID-19 infection: origin, transmission, and characteristics of human coronaviruses. *Journal of Advanced Research* 24: 91–98.

Shoham, S. (2020). Efficacy and Safety Human Coronavirus Immune Plasma (HCIP) vs. Control (SARS-CoV-2 Non-immune Plasma) Among Adults Exposed to COVID-19 (CSSC-001). www.clinicaltrials.gov/ct2/show/NCT04323800 (accessed 13 December 2020).

Stone, J. (2020). Why travel bans don't work during an outbreak like coronavirus. www.forbes.com/sites/judystone/2020/02/01/why-travel-bans-dont-work-duringan-outbreak-like-coronavirus/#2f56450d53ea (accessed 13 December 2020).

Ströher, U., DiCaro, A., Li, Y. et al. (2004). Severe acute respiratory syndrome-related coronavirus is inhibited by interferon-α. *Journal of Infectious Diseases* 189 (7): 1164–1167.

Strumpf, D. (2020). Tech sector fears supply delays as effects of virus ripple through China. www.wsj.com/articles/tech-sector-fears-supply-delays-as-effects-of-virus-ripple-through-china-11580484181 (accessed 13 December 2020).

Sui, C. (2020). China's Racism is wrecking its success in Africa. www.foreignpolicy.com/2020/04/15/chinas-racism-is-wrecking-its-success-in-africa/ (accessed 13 December 2020).

Tang, X., Wu, C., Li, X. et al. (2020a). On the origin and continuing evolution of SARS-CoV-2. *National Science Review* (6): 1012–1023.

Tang, Y.W., Schmitz, J.E., Persing, D.H., and Stratton, C.W. (2020b). The laboratory diagnosis of COVID-19 infection: Current issues and challenges. *Journal of Clinical Microbiology* 58 (6): e00512–20.

Ter Meulen, J., Bakker, A.B., Van Den Brink, E.N. et al. (2004). Human monoclonal antibody as prophylaxis for SARS coronavirus infection in ferrets. *The Lancet* 363 (9427): 2139–2141.

The Japan Times (2020). 44 more on Diamond Princess Cruise Ship test positive for COVID-19. The Japan Times online. www.japantimes.co.jp/news/2020/02/13/national/coronavirus-diamond-princess/ (accessed 13 December 2020).

Tian, X., Li, C., Huang, A. et al. (2020). Potent binding of 2019 novel coronavirus spike protein by a SARS coronavirus-specific human monoclonal antibody. *Emerging microbes & infections* 9 (1): 382–385.

Totura, A.L. and Baric, R.S. (2012). SARS coronavirus pathogenesis: host innate immune responses and viral antagonism of interferon. *Current opinion in virology* 2 (3): 264–275.

Udugama, B., Kadhiresan, P., Kozlowski, H.N. et al. (2020). Diagnosing COVID-19: the disease and tools for detection. *ACS nano* 14 (4): 3822–3835.

ul Qamar, M.T., Alqahtani, S.M., Alamri, M.A., and Chen, L.L. (2020). Structural basis of SARS-CoV-2 3CLpro and anti-COVID-19 drug discovery from medicinal plants. *Journal of Pharmaceutical Analysis* 10 (4): 313–319.

UNESCO (2020). Education: From disruption to recovery.

Wang, D., Hu, B., Hu, C. et al. (2020). Clinical characteristics of 138 hospitalized patients with 2019 novel coronavirus–infected pneumonia in Wuhan, China. *Jama* 323 (11): 1061–1069.

Wilson, J. and Campus, S. (2020). The economic impact of coronavirus: analysis from Imperial experts. Imperial News | Imperial College London. Imperial News. www.imperial.ac.uk/news/196514/the-economic-impact-coronavirus-analysis-from/ (accessed 13 December 2020).

World Health Organization (2020a). Infection prevention and control during health care when novel coronavirus (nCoV) infection is suspected: interim guidance, 25 January 2020.

World Health Organization (2020b). Laboratory biosafety guidance related to coronavirus disease 2019 (COVID-19): interim guidance, 12 February 2020 (No. WHO/WPE/GIH/2020.1). World Health Organization.

World Health Organization (2020c). Laboratory testing for 2019 novel coronavirus (2019-nCoV) in suspected human cases, Interim guidance, 2 March 2020.

World Health Organization (2020d). Novel Coronavirus (2019-nCoV): situation report, 3.

World Health Organization (2020e). Risk communication and community engagement (RCCE) readiness and response to the 2019 novel coronaviruses (2019- nCoV): interim guidance, 26 January 2020.

World Health Organization (2020f). *World Health Organization, IFRC, UNICEF. COVID19 stigma guide*. Geneva: WHO.

World Health Organization (2020g). *Acute respiratory syndrome in China*. Geneva: WHO.

World Health Organization. Clinical management of severe acute respiratory infection when novel coronavirus (2019-nCoV) infection is suspected. Geneva: WHO; 2020h. www.who.int/docs/default-source/coronaviruse/clinical-management-of-novel-cov.pdf (accessed 13 December 2020).

World Health Organization (2020i). *Disease commodity package -Novel coronavirus (nCoV)*. Geneva: WHO.

World Health Organization (2020j). International health regulations. www.who.int/cholera/health_regulations/en/ (accessed 13 December 2020).

Wrapp, D., Wang, N., Corbett, K.S. et al. (2020). Cryo-EM structure of the 2019-nCoV spike in the prefusion conformation. *Science* 367 (6483): 1260–1263.

Wu, A., Peng, Y., Huang, B. et al. (2020). Genome composition and divergence of the novel coronavirus (2019-nCoV) originating in China. *Cell host & microbe.*

https://www.fda.gov/emergency-preparedness-and-response/mcm-legal-regulatory-and-policy-framework/emergency-use-authorization (accessed 13 December 2020).

www.ft.com/content/d78b8183-ade7-49c2-a8b5-c40fb031b801 (accessed 13 December 2020).

www.ifla.org/covid-19-and-libraries (accessed 13 December 2020).

www.theguardian.com/culture/2020/mar/13/coronavirus-culture-arts-films-gigs-festivals-cancellations (accessed 13 December 2020).

Xu, Z., Shi, L., Wang, Y. et al. (2020). Pathological findings of COVID-19 associated with acute respiratory distress syndrome. *The Lancet respiratory medicine* 8 (4): 420–422.

Yi, Y., Lagniton, P.N., Ye, S. et al. (2020). COVID-19: what has been learned and to be learned about the novel coronavirus disease. *International Journal of Biological Sciences.* 16 (10): 1753.

Zhou, P., Yang, X.L., Wang, X.G. et al. (2020). A pneumonia outbreak associated with a new coronavirus of probable bat origin. *Nature.* 579 (7798): 270–273.

Zhu, Z., Xu, S., Wang, H. et al. (2020). COVID-19 in Wuhan: immediate psychological impact on 5062 health workers. *MedRxiv* 24: 10443.

Zorzitto, J., Galligan, C.L., Ueng, J.J., and Fish, E.N. (2006). Characterization of the antiviral effects of interferon-α against a SARS-like coronavirus infection in vitro. *Cell research* 16 (2): 220–229.

2

Viability of COVID-19 in Different Environmental Surfaces

Saeida Saadat[1], Piyush K. Rao[1], Nitasha Khatri[2], and Deepak Rawtani[3]

[1] *School of Doctoral Studies & Research (SDSR), National Forensic Sciences University (Ministry of Home affairs, GOI), Gandhinagar, Gujarat, India*
[2] *Gujarat Environment Management Institute (GEMI), Gandhinagar, Gujarat, India*
[3] *School of Pharmacy, National Forensic Sciences University (Ministry of Home affairs, GOI), Gandhinagar, Gujarat, India*

2.1 Introduction

A novel coronavirus disease initially occurred in China in the year 2019 and therefore named COVID-19 (Lu and Shi 2020; Li et al. 2020). This virus caused a serious disease which quickly became a worldwide pandemic (Bae 2020; Onyema 2020). COVID-19 is in fact a coronavirus which causes an infectious respiratory illness called severe acute respiratory syndrome coronavirus 2 (SARS-CoV-2) (Boldog et al. 2020; Singhal 2020). A COVID-19 patient might experience symptoms within 2–14 days of incubation period. In rare cases, there has been a very long incubation time of up to 29 days, while this time the patients can be contagious (Jiang et al. 2020; Men et al. 2020). To avoid the spread of the virus, precautionary practices should be practiced by everyone around the world, including personal hygiene, frequently washing/sanitizing hands, and wearing face masks (Kucharski et al. 2020; Wang et al. 2020). This virus could attack the respiratory system, and a number of symptoms such as fever, dry cough, shortage of breath, tiredness, and muscle pain could be experienced by the patients (Huang et al. 2020; Lu and Shi 2020; Zhou et al. 2020). In severe cases, diarrhea, sepsis, and septic shock may also happen, which might even cause death (Yue et al. 2020; Zu et al. 2020). During the pandemic, the healthcare employees in China have been advised to wear surgical masks to prevent the spread of infection. More than any other groups of people, healthcare workers are exposed to possible infectious contacts. If they take care of all the necessary precautionary actions, it would be a great help to protect their co-workers and the public (Ather et al. 2020; Zhang et al. 2020a) Similarly, anyone who is not using personal precautionary tools will get a direct contact with infectious items and spread the virus quickly. In addition, it is crucial for the restaurants to take care of the hygiene in pandemic time and have separate sections for food and dishes (Fiorillo et al. 2020; Ng and Peggy 2020). Similarly, other public places such as airports, malls, and public transportation should take extra care of the hygiene and disinfect the surfaces to

The Environmental Impact of COVID-19, First Edition. Edited by Deepak Rawtani and Chaudhery Mustansar Hussain.
© 2024 John Wiley & Sons Ltd. Published 2024 by John Wiley & Sons Ltd.

prevent the spread of the virus. Ever since the pandemic started, there has been discussions about spreading of this virus through the surfaces and their decontamination techniques (Cavanagh and Wambier 2020). However, the survival of coronavirus on different surfaces including solid, liquid, and gas have not been well known so far. But there are many reports which indicate that this virus could survive on environmental surfaces for different time intervals starting from a few hours to several days (Bhardwaj and Agrawal 2020; Hemida and Abduallah 2020). Transmission of COVID-19 between people majorly occurs through the respiratory droplets of an infected individual via sneezing, coughing, or even talking. Therefore, it has been highly recommended to stay at home, wear face mask, and maintain physical distance during pandemic (Feng et al. 2020; Xu et al. 2020). Therefore, online trans-actions have been highly practiced in affected regions during pandemic. There is a high possibility to get infected by touching infected surfaces or objects. In case if someone touches the infected surfaces by this virus, and without washing hands touches their mouth, nose, or eyes, the virus could find its way to the respiratory organs through the mucus membranes and cause infection (Sanche et al. 2020). In normal conditions, COVID-19 can survive on different surfaces for few hours to several days. The surfaces which could be highly contami-nated with this virus are door handles, mobile phones, elevator buttons, and handholds of the public transport vehicles (Liu et al. 2020; Fiorillo et al. 2020).Therefore, it is very impor-tant to have knowledge about the survival time and infectivity of COVID-19 on different surfaces in order to disinfect the environmental surfaces properly and prevent spreading of this virus through different surfaces (Dennis et al. 2021; Garrido-molina et al. 2021). The aim of this article is to discuss about the transmission way of COVID-19 through the envi-ronmental surfaces, survival of this virus on solid, liquid, and gaseous surfaces, and proper disinfection of the surface to prevent spreading of this virus.

2.2 Transmission of COVID-19

COVID-19 transmits through droplets from person to person or through touching the infected surfaces (Hamblin and Rezaei 2020). Transmission through droplets could happen via cough-ing, sneezing, or even during talking while people stay close to each other without keeping distance at about 2 m. As droplets can travel up to 2 m and stay infectious for some time, insufficient disinfection of the air and surfaces might spread the virus (Han et al. 2020; Rothan and Byrareddy 2020). Therefore, appropriate disinfection of the surfaces and taking care of hygiene will prevent spreading the virus. This virus is quite complicated such that even if COVID-19 test of an infected person returned negative results, RT-PCR test of the same person returned positive after around 13 days from discharging from hospitals (Aboubakr 2021; Velavan and Meyer 2020). Although pregnant women are at high risk of getting infected by COVID-19, they cannot transmit it to their children (Rao and Rawtani 2022; Read and Wild 2020). There is a doubt that either COVID-19 can transmit from animals to people, but there is a probability that this virus has been transmitted from animals like snake, cat, or any other similar animals to humans (Csiszar et al. 2020; Lipsitch et al. 2020; Nghiem et al. 2020). Based on evidences, this virus and its spreading rate are more complicated rather than the past pandemics. The incubation period is long, and there have been patients with no symptoms while they could be carriers of the virus. These complications make this virus different from other pandemics, and therefore, a total lockdown implemented all around the world to prevent the spread of this virus (Anderson et al. 2020; Lotfi et al. 2020).

2.2.1   Influence of Environmental Factors on Transmission of COVID-19

Survival of micro-organisms such as bacteria, fungus, and viruses such as COVID-19 on environmental surfaces depends on a few factors such as temperature, relative humidity (RH), and the materials of the surfaces. Lower temperature and appropriate RH would help the virus to survive for long on different surfaces. However, the impact of the environmental factors on the stability and infectivity rate of viruses is very complicated and more exploration is needed (Kucharski et al. 2020). RH also affects the viability of the viruses, and the relationship between RH and temperature in combination on inactivation of the viruses has not been still clearly studied. However, it has been reported that the temperature could affect more on the survival of the viruses compared to RH (Rothan and Byrareddy 2020; Zhou et al. 2020). As tested in different types of water such as lake water and sewage, suitable temperature for COVID-19 survival has been shown to be between 4 and 25 °C. The effect of temperature (28–33 °C) and humidity (95%) on the spreading of COVID-19 have been studied which revealed that the aforesaid factors do not have significant impact on the spread of this virus (Kroumpouzos et al. 2020; Xie and Zhu 2020). However, raising the temperature of about 40 °C could decrease the survival duration of some pathogenic micro-organisms including Meddle East respiratory syndrome coronavirus (MERS-CoV) (Mccloskey and Heymann 2020). But the survival of COVID-19 has been reported to be higher with higher amount of inoculant. Other pathogen (HCoV-229E) could survive in RH 30–50% in room temperature. The viability of other pathogen (HuCoV-229E) has been studied in dissimilar environmental conditions. This virus could remain survival at 20 °C and a high RH of 50% for about 67 hours, and a 20% infectious virus could be detected after six days. At 30% RH, the survival rate of the virus was 26.76 hours, but at RH 80% the survival rate was only three hours and no infectious virus was detectable after 24 hours (Kucharski et al. 2020; Ren et al. 2020; Kroumpouzos et al. 2020). In a study, the relationship between temperature and COVID-19 has been studied. In this study, the average temperature and the average raise of new COVID-19 patients have been investigated. This study has been done in different countries including United States, Iran, Spain, Germany, and Italy. To reduce the effect of co-factors such as cultural variations between these countries or implementing of government procedures, different parts of each and every country have been compared individually. The results revealed that there is a significant variation in the average temperature and increasing of COVID-19 patients in all those areas (Bogoch et al. 2020). Additionally, the cities with a temperature between 5 and 11 °C and humidity ranging between 47 and 79% have been highly infected by COVID-19. However, the highest temperature for the viability of COVID-19 in vitro is reported to be 4 °C and the optimum humidity rate is 20–80%. Furthermore, in countries like South Korea, Japan, Iran, and Italy, the spread of COVID-19 in different temperatures ranging between 30 and 50 °C has happened. But in Southern China at the similar condition, this virus did not spread quickly (Hamblin and Rezaei 2020; Wu et al. 2020). However, the above-mentioned studies indicate a real relationship between the temperature and the transmission of the COVID-19 virus compared to global temperature. Therefore, there is no very close relationship between environmental factors (humidity/temperature) and the transmission of COVID-19 (Zheng 2020).

It has been reported that COVID-19 virus could be stable on different type of surfaces and can be transmitted via respiratory droplets (Sun and Ostrikov 2020). The stability of the dried virus on smooth surface remains viable for over five days at 22–25 °C and about 41–50% humidity. However, in some other research, it has also been reported that coronavirus loses its viability at higher temperature and humidity. It was hypothesized that the prolonged stability of the virus was probably linked to cold weather and high humidity of the environment (Xu et al. 2020). A study by Chan et al. have described that the cold temperature and dry environment increased the transmission of this virus in semitropical regions such as Hong Kong (Chan et al. 2011). It was also established that the countries in which there was intensive use of air conditioning, such as Hong Kong and Singapore had greater transmission rate and high transmission occurred in well air-conditioned environment such as hotels and hospitals. In a separate study, it was established that risk of transmission was 18 times more in cold days compared to warm days in Hong Kong (Cai et al. 2007; Lin et al. 2006; Tan et al. 2005; Yuan et al. 2006). The environmental factors such as sunlight, wind velocity, air pressure can also contribute to transmission of coronavirus (Cai et al. 2007; Yuan et al. 2006). Wang et al. has also established that high temperature and humidity reduce the transmission of the novel coronavirus. The findings were similar with the study that reported that the heat and humidity decrease the transmission of influenza (Lipsitch and Viboud 2009; Lowen et al. 2008; Shaman and Kohn 2009; Steel et al. 2011; Park et al. 2020). There could be two possibilities on the high or low transmission of this virus; first, survival rate of this virus is high in cold environment and the respiratory droplets that have virus remain suspended in air for longer duration (Lowen and Steel 2014; Tellier 2009). Second reason can be cold and dry weather weakens the immunity of the host, and therefore, host is more prone to infection (Eccles 2002; Kudo et al. 2019). Wang et al. established that these findings are consistent with the hypothesis that high temperature and high humidity reduce viability of coronavirus in the environment (Chan et al. 2011; Yuan et al. 2006). The researchers selected a temperature range from −21 to 21 °C and relative humidity from 47 to 100%. The environmental conditions such as temperature does not have any impact on the transmission of the coronavirus. The transmission of the virus has happened on the extreme hot/cold or dry geographical locations and vice versa (Chan et al. 2011; Yuan et al. 2006). The previous relationship between the respiratory disease and temperature indicated that the SARS and influenza need specific temperature for their survival and by increasing the temperature the viability of the virus can be reduced (Chan et al. 2011; Jaakkola et al. 2014). Aranow hypothesized that warmer season tends to reduce the spread of virus and which might be somehow co-related to higher vitamin D levels which results in stimulating the immune system (Aranow 2011). In another report, it was found that high level of UV application can also decrease transmission of coronaviruses (Yao et al. 2020). The literature has shown that the cumulative incidence rate of COVID-19 had no close association with temperature. Therefore, it has been suggested that the temperature could not have major impact on transmission of this virus (Jamil et al. 2020). Similar kind of results with MERS-CoV suggested that the virus can survive at the temperature above 45 °C. The limitations of the study was that the whole meteorological data was not included and further studies would be required for concrete

Table 2.1 Survival of coronavirus on difference environmental surfaces.

Virus	Surfaces	Time	Temperature (°C)	RH (%)
SARS-CoV-2	Aerosol	24 h	21–23	65
	Paper	4–5 d	22	65
	Banknote paper	2 d	22	65
	Tissue paper	30 min	22	65
	Plastic	4–5 d	22	65
	Stainless steel	4 d	22	65
	Copper	8 h	—	—
	Cardboard	24 h	—	—
	Phosphate buffer saline	14 d	20 °C	—
SARS-CoV-1	Aerosol	3 h	21–23	65
	Paper	1 d	20	—
	Plastic	1 d	38	80–89
	Stainless steel	2 d	—	—
	Copper	8 h	—	—
	Cardboard	8 h	—	—

Source: Based on Aboubakr et al. (2020).

proof (Ather et al. 2020; Hemida and Abduallah 2020; Yao et al. 2020). Survival of COVID-19 on different environmental surfaces is shown in Table 2.1.

2.3 Survival of COVID-19 on Different Environmental Surfaces

During the pandemic, fomites are considered one of the key transformants of the viruses (Schwartz et al. 2020). Existing literature reports that COVID-19 survives in environmental surfaces for quite a long time starting from a few hours to many days (Jamal et al. 2021). COVID-19 could survive on plastic and other solid surfaces for many days, that means that domestic waste and the waste from quarantined places could be the source of infection. In the beginning of this pandemic, the generated waste from different sources has not been processed in a proper manner (Kooraki et al. 2020; Luis et al. 2020). The infected domestic waste as well as the waste from the quarantined places could be called medical waste. Therefore, the surfaces of the waste materials which are majorly plastic materials could be the key vehicle of the spread of this virus (Nghiem et al. 2020). As mentioned before, COVID-19 can survive in the environment on different surfaces for several days. There are several factors that could affect the duration of the survival of this virus on different surfaces (Zuniga and Cortes 2020). These factors are humidity, surface type, temperature, and the density of the viral particles in the air (Casanova et al. 2010). In a study, the survival of the SARS-CoV-1 has been compared to that of the SARS-CoV-2 on different surfaces such as cardboard, copper, plastic, and stainless steel. It has been confirmed that the stability of the SARS-CoV-2 is similar to SARS-CoV-1 (Doremalen et al. 2020). In another study, the survival of SARS-CoV-2 has been studied in different environmental conditions. The results revealed that this virus can survive in aerosol form for about 24 hours in low temperature and humidity. Therefore, the infected surface could contain virus for around four days (Lipsitch et al. 2020). In paper and plastic surfaces, the stability of this virus is around four to five days; hence, in infected gloves and gowns, this virus could survive for several days. The study of the stability of COVID-19 in different temperature has revealed that this virus is highly stable in cold temperatures at around 4°C but not likely stable in hot temperatures (Araújo and Naimi 2020). The disinfectant effects tested on COVID-19 have shown that this virus can remain viable up to five minutes incubation with hand soap and after five minutes the virus could not be detected. Therefore, it is obvious that environmental conditions have a direct effect on the stability of COVID-19 (Wang et al. 2020). Fomites are the best spreaders of human viruses such as noroviruses during pandemics. These viruses can survive on different surfaces for different time intervals starting from few hours to several days (Guzman 2021). Coronaviruses can survive on hard surfaces and plastic-based materials for several days, which means that wastes from quarantine facilities could be the infection source (Ashour et al. 2020; Nghiem et al. 2020). In a study by Yao et al. (2020), the stability of SARS-CoV-2 and SARS-CoV-1 have been evaluated in aerosols and other environmental surfaces. In this study, two strains SARS-CoV-2 (MN985325.1) and SARS-CoV-1 (AY274119.3) have been selected for evaluation. Several surfaces such as aerosols, plastic, stainless steel, copper, and cardboard have been selected for survival of this virus. SARS-CoV-2 could survive in aerosols for three hours but the infectivity of this virus reduced. COVID-19 have been more survival on plastic and stainless-steel surfaces compared to copper and cardboard. This virus could survive on plastic surfaces for 72 hours, and the infectivity reduction was observed. On stainless steel, the survival rate has been 48 hours with high infectivity reduction (Yao et al. 2020). On copper surface, this virus was not detectable after four hours (Lai et al. 2020) and SARS-CoV-1 was not detectable after eight hours. Also, on cardboard surface, SARS-CoV-2 could not survive after 24 hours and SARS-CoV-1 could not survive after eight hours (Doremalen and Bushmaker 2020). In the following section, the survival of COVID-19 on households, hospitals, and liquid surfaces are discussed. In the Figure 2.1. the survival of COVID-19 on different environmental media is shown.

2.3.1 Survival of COVID-19 on Households and Hospitals Surfaces

COVID-19 cannot survive for long on dry or less humid (Kooraki et al. 2020; Xu et al. 2020) During the SARS-CoV-2 pandemic, dealing with paper documents, paper currency, and envelopes have been a huge concern for employees handling these documents, due to infection risks. While returning home after visiting healthcare centers, people would panic that their clothes carry fomites and infect home with the virus. Human coronavirus can survive on different surfaces up from 2 to 14 days (Araújo and Naimi 2020; Guzman 2021; Lai et al. 2020). On other surfaces such as polyvinyl chloride, glass, and stainless steel, this virus can remain viable up to five days, and on silicon surface the viability of this virus is up to three days (Fiorillo et al. 2020). HuCoV-229E could not be

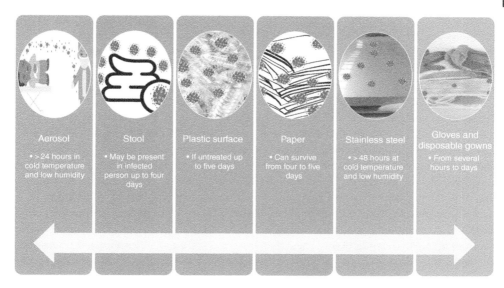

Figure 2.1 Survival of COVID-19 on different environmental media.

detectable post drying the aluminum, surgical gloves at room temperature for up to three hours. Cotton materials can absorb contaminated droplets quicker rather than other fluids. Therefore, droplets on nonabsorbent gown or gloves may be more dangerous to the environment due to the contamination issue (Mccloskey and Heymann 2020). The infectivity of a strain of SARS-CoV on paper/cotton gown could not be detected within five minutes at room temperature which reveals that the infectivity of the virus disappears on cotton gowns faster than other surfaces. On an experiment, a sterilized piece of paper has been contaminated with high concentration of 105TCD50/ml, and left to be absorbed for about three hours at room temperature. Then, this sample has been placed into a culture tube but no viral infection has been detectable. In a similar experiment with 106TCID50/mL, the viral infection disappeared within 24 hours (Aboubakr 2021; Purohit et al. 2022). The concentrated form of 104 viral infection on paper after drying it at room temperature showed no viral infection for up to five minutes. Normally the infection risk of viral contamination on paper materials is less and hence washing hands after handling contaminated materials would be highly effective against viral transmission (Dey et al. 2022; Ren et al. 2020).

2.3.2 Stability of COVID-19 in Liquid Media

The stability duration of coronavirus depends on the virus strain, the solution type in which the virus stayed, and the temperature of the environment (Chan et al. 2011). In dechlorinated normal water or sewage, this virus can remain stable for up to 14 days at 4 °C and at 20 °C for only two days. In PBS (phosphate buffer saline), this virus can survive up to 14 days at 20 °C. P9 strain of SARS-CoV is reported to be able to survive in serum for at least 96 hours and the same strain can survive in urine for around 72 hours, but in the urine, this strain has shown low level of infectivity. The level of infectivity of SARS-CoV P9 remains active at room temperature for up to 60 hours and falls at about 72 hours and at 120 hours could not be detectable (Li et al. 2020). This strain could well survive in different temperatures such as 4, 20, and 37 °C with high infectivity level in cells for about two hours. The highest temperature and particular time period for inactivation of SARS-CoV are reported to be 56 °C for 1.5 hour, 67 °C for one hour, and 75 °C for half of an hour. A study reports that coronaviruses could remain infectious for many months at 4 °C. GVU6109 which is a strain of coronaviruses can stay infective in respiratory samples for about one week at room temperature, and about 20 days at 4 °C (Lai et al. 2005). Another strain of coronaviruses (CoV HKU 39849) possesses better survival rate compared to that of HuCoV 229E and other respiratory viruses like RSV or OC43. This strain is stable in liquid media for around 5–14 days at about 25 °C and a relative humidity of 50%. This condition is similar to that of air conditioner in closed environment. This strain cannot survive at 56 °C for more than 15 minutes. CoVHKU 39849 could be highly affected by high level of humidity such as 95% or above at temperatures of about 33 °C, and in this condition, increasing the temperature up to 38 °C would highly affect the virus. At 38 °C and 95% humidity, this virus has not been able to survive. In pasteurized sewage, this virus could be reduced up to 99% within nine days. Therefore, it has been suggested that the contaminated water could be a highly possible vehicle of this virus to human exposure (Parikh and Rawtani 2022; Ren et al. 2020).

2.4 Disinfection of the Surfaces as an Efficient Weapon Against Coronaviruses

During a pandemic such as COVID-19, efforts to stop the spread of the virus is highly advisable due to the high transmission and mortality rate of this virus. In fact, there are very few actions which could help the basic public help to control the spreading of the virus. These actions include fast detection of the cases, quarantine regulations, and significant precautionary measurements such as frequent washing of hands and using face masks (Luan and Ching 2020; Rothan and Byrareddy 2020). In addition, the WHO has highly recommended certain traveling regulations from infected regions including screening of the cases and stopping suspected cases from traveling. Also, disinfecting of the aircraft has advised to be taken care of during pandemic time. Therefore, along with these precautionary measurements, we should improve our knowledge about the impact of disinfectants on the pathogenic micro-organism which causes pandemic, in order to apply this preventive tool against these viruses in a proper manner (Doremalen et al. 2020; WHO 2020; Zhang et al. 2020b). We have been using disinfectants during the pandemic, but we should know what disinfectant is and how to evaluate its effectiveness. As mentioned earlier, due to the lack of treatment during the pandemic, there is a serious necessity to prevent the spread of virus and one of the most important materials which can contribute in prevention of the viruses is disinfectants (Quan et al. 2017). During the pandemic time, the availability of disinfectants for public is very important. It may be advisable to develop new ones in order to make them available for everyone. Not only the availability of disinfectants is important but also the quality and effectiveness of these materials on the viruses should properly get checked in order to disinfect the environmental surfaces and prevent the spread of the virus (Meo et al. 2020). In case of developing novel disinfectant/sanitizer, their activity on viral cells as well as on humans' cells should be evaluated to ensure that they are not toxic to humans' cells. In addition, neutralization of these tools is crucial; as well as the contact time evaluation, means when they are applied on the viruses and after sometimes the viruses could get back their viability. Therefore, it is important to find out a particular contact time of the disinfectants on the surfaces to grant the complete degradation of the viral cells on the surfaces (Anderson et al. 2020; Hassan and Harekrishna 2020; Ilyas et al. 2020). These measurements need proper control in order to ensure the complete removal of the infectivity of the viruses, significant of neutralization, and non-toxicity of the disinfectants under different environmental conditions such as temperature and contact time. Thus, a disinfectant/sanitizer could be defined as an antiseptic which has antiviral properties in a specific period of time and decreases the viral titer to a high extent (WHO 2020).

2.5 Conclusion

This article highlighted the viability and infectivity of COVID-19 on different environmental surfaces including solid, liquid, and gas. COVID-19 could spread through respiratory droplets of the patient while coming in close contact with a healthy person or via touching the infected surfaces. Through respiratory droplets by coughing/sneezing and talking, the viruses spread on the air and inhaled by the healthy person which can cause infection. This type of transmission can occur during incubation period, showing the symptoms or even after recovery of the patients. It is also highly possible to get infected by touching the infected surfaces. COVID-19 could remain viable on different surfaces for quite a long time. In case if someone touches the infected surfaces by this virus, and without washing hands touches their mouth, nose, or eyes, the virus could find its way to the respiratory organs through the mucus membranes and cause infection. Therefore, it is very important to have knowledge about the survival and infectivity rate of COVID-19 on different environmental surface in order to disinfect these surfaces in a proper manner and avoid spreading viruses. Depending on the environmental conditions (temperature and RH) as well as the material type, COVID-19 can remain viable on surfaces for quite a long time (few hours to several days). For example, COVID-19 is able to survive on glasses and copper for four hours, cardboards and gloves for 24 hours, hard plastic such as water bottles for three days, stainless steel for two to three days, and silicon materials up to five days. This time period could change depending on the environmental conditions such as temperature and humidity. Therefore, it is very necessary to disinfect the surfaces to ensure the prevention of the virus through touching the infected surfaces. Disinfection of the surfaces should be done properly by using means of proper disinfectant materials and correct amount of this materials must be used to ensure that the viruses have been completely killed on the surfaces. While using disinfectant on solid surfaces as well spraying in air, it is very important to apply the non-toxic materials as they can directly or indirectly come in contact with human body.

References

Aboubakr, H. A. (2021) Stability of SARS-CoV-2 and other coronaviruses in the environment and on common touch surfaces and the influence of climatic conditions: a review, *Transboundary and Emerging Diseases* 68.2 pp. 296–312. doi: https://doi.org/10.1111/tbed.13707.

Anderson, R.M., Heesterbeek, H., Klinkenberg, D., and Hollingsworth, T.D. (2020). How will country-based mitigation measures influence the course of the COVID-19 epidemic? *The Lancet* 395 (10228): 931–934.

Aranow, C. (2011) Vitamin D and the immune system, *Journal of Investigative Medicine. BMJ*, 59(6), pp. 881–886. doi: https://doi.org/10.2310/jim.0b013e31821b8755.

Araújo, M.B. and Naimi, B. (2020). Spread of SARS-CoV-2 coronavirus likely constrained by climate. *MedRxiv* 1–26.

Ashour, H., M., Elkhatib, W., F., Rahman, Md M., et al. (2020). Insights into the recent 2019 novel coronavirus (SARS-CoV-2) in light of past human coronavirus outbreaks. *Pathogens* 9 (3): 2–15.

Ather, A., Patel, B., Ruparel, N., B. *et al.* (2020) Coronavirus Disease 19 (COVID-19): implications for clinical dental care, *Journal of Endodontics*. Elsevier Inc, 19, pp. 1–12. doi: https://doi.org/10.1016/j.joen.2020.03.008.

Bae, J. (2020). A Chinese case of Coronavirus Disease 2019 (COVID-19) did not show infectivity during the incubation period: based on an epidemiological survey. *Journal of Preventive Medicine and Public Health* 53 (2): 67.

Bhardwaj, R. and Agrawal, A. (2020) Likelihood of survival of coronavirus in a respiratory droplet deposited on a solid surface Likelihood of survival of coronavirus in a respiratory droplet deposited on a solid surface *Physics of Fluids* 32.6 (2020): 061704, 061704. doi: https://doi.org/10.1063/5.0012009.

Bogoch, I. I., Watts, A., Thomas-Bachli, A., Huber, C., Kraemer, M. U., & Khan, K (2020) Pneumonia of unknown aetiology in Wuhan, China: potential for international spread via commercial air travel, *Journal of Travel Medicine*, 27(2), taaa008. doi: https://doi.org/10.1093/jtm/taaa008.

Boldog, P., Tekeli, T., Vizi, Z. et al. (2020) Risk assessment of novel coronavirus COVID-19 outbreaks outside China. *Journal of Clinical Medicine* 9.2: 571. doi: https://doi.org/10.3390/jcm9020571.

Cai, Q.-C., Lu, J., Xu, Q.-F. *et al.* (2007) Influence of meteorological factors and air pollution on the outbreak of severe acute respiratory syndrome, *Public Health*. 2007/02/20. The Royal Institute of Public Health. Published by Elsevier Ltd., 121(4), pp. 258–265. doi: https://doi.org/10.1016/j.puhe.2006.09.023.

Casanova, L. M., Jeon, S., Rutala, W., A. *et al.* (2010) Effects of air temperature and relative humidity on coronavirus survival on surfaces, *Applied and Environmental Microbiology* 76(9), pp. 2712–2717. doi: https://doi.org/10.1128/AEM.02291-09.

Cavanagh, G. and Wambier, C.G. (2020). Rational hand hygiene during the coronavirus 2019 (COVID-19) pandemic. *Journal of the American Academy of Dermatology* 82 (6): e211.

Chan, K. H., Peiris, J., S. M, Lam, S., Y. *et al.* (2011) The effects of temperature and relative humidity on the viability of the SARS coronavirus, *Advances in Virology*, 2011. doi: https://doi.org/10.1155/2011/734690.

Csiszar, A., Jakab, F., Valencak, T., G. et al. (2020). Companion animals likely do not spread COVID-19 but may get infected themselves. *GeroScience* 42 (5): 1229–1236.

Dennis, J. M., McGovern, A., P., Vollmer, S., J., & Mateen, B., A. (2021) Improving survival of critical care patients with coronavirus disease 2019 in England: a National Cohort Study, March to June 2020, *Critical Care Medicine* 49.2 209. doi: https://doi.org/10.1097/CCM.0000000000004747.

Dey, A., Rao, P.K., and Rawtani, D. (2022). Risk management of COVID-19. In: *COVID-19 in the Environment*, 217–230. https://doi.org/10.1016/B978-0-323-90272-4.00018-X.

van Doremalen, P. D.N and Bushmaker, B. S.T (2020) Aerosol and surface stability of SARS-CoV-2 as compared with SARS-CoV-1, *Advances in Colloid and Interface Science*, 275. doi: https://doi.org/10.1016/j.cis.2019.102063.

van Doremalen, Neeltje, Dylan H. Morris, Myndi G. Holbrook, A. Gamble. et al. (2020) Aerosol and surface stability of SARS-CoV-2 as compared with SARS-CoV-1, *The New England Journal of Medicine*, 728. doi: https://doi.org/10.1016/j.scitotenv.2020.138870.

Eccles, R. (2002) 'An explanation for the seasonality of acute upper respiratory tract viral infections, *Acta Oto-Laryngologica*. Informa UK Limited, 122(2), pp. 183–191. doi: https://doi.org/10.1080/00016480252814207.

Fiorillo, L., Cervino, G., Matarese, M. et al. (2020). COVID-19 surface persistence: a recent data summary and its importance for medical and dental settings. *International Journal of Environmental Research and Public Health* 17 (9): 3132.

Garrido-molina, J. M., Márquez-Hernández, V., V., Alcayde-García, A. *et al.* (2021) Disinfection of gloved hands during the COVID-19 pandemic. *Journal of Hospital Infection*. 107 5–11. doi: https://doi.org/10.1016/j.jhin.2020.09.015.

Guzman, M.I. (2021). Bioaerosol size effect in COVID-19 transmission.

Qingmei Han, Qingqing Lin, Zuowei Ni, L. Y. (2020) Uncertainties about the transmission routes of 2019 novel coronavirus *Influenza and Other Respiratory Viruses* 14.4 470. doi: https://doi.org/10.1111/irv.12735.

Hassan, M. and Harekrishna, K. (2020) Sanitization during and after COVID - 19 pandemic: a short review, *Transactions of the Indian National Academy of Engineering*. Springer Singapore, 5(4), pp. 617–627. doi: https://doi.org/10.1007/s41403-020-00177-9.

He, F., Deng, Y., and Li, W. (2020). Coronavirus disease 2019: What we know? *Journal of medical virology* 92 (7): 719–725.

Hemida, M. G. and Abduallah, M. M. B. (2020) The SARS-CoV-2 outbreak from a one health perspective *One Health* 10, p. 100127. doi: https://doi.org/10.1016/j.onehlt.2020.100127.

Huang, C. *et al.* (2020) Clinical features of patients infected with 2019 novel coronavirus in Wuhan, China, *The Lancet* 395.10223, pp. 497–506. doi: https://doi.org/10.1016/S0140-6736(20)30183-5.

Ilyas, S., Srivastava, R. R. and Kim, H. (2020) Disinfection technology and strategies for COVID-19 hospital and bio-medical waste management, *Science of the Total Environment*. Elsevier B.V, p. 141652. doi: https://doi.org/10.1016/j.scitotenv.2020.141652.

Jaakkola, K., Saukkoriipi, A., Jokelainen, J. *et al.* (2014) 'Decline in temperature and humidity increases the occurrence of influenza in cold climate, *Environmental Health*: a global access science source. BioMed Central, 13(1), p. 22. doi: https://doi.org/10.1186/1476-069X-13-22.

Jamal, M., Shah, M., Almarzooqi, S., M. *et al.* (2021) Overview of transnational recommendations for COVID-19 transmission control in dental care settings, *Oral Diseases* 27 (2021) pp. 655–664. doi: https://doi.org/10.1111/odi.13431.

Jamil, T., Alam, I., Gojobori, T., and Duarte, C.M. (2020). No evidence for temperature-dependence of the COVID-19 epidemic. *Frontiers in Public Health* 436.

Jiang, X., Niu, Y., Li, X. et al. (2020). Is a 14-day quarantine period optimal for effectively controlling coronavirus disease 2019 (COVID-19)? *MedRxiv.*

Kooraki, S., Hosseiny, M., Myers, L. et al. (2020). Coronavirus outbreak: what the department of radiology should know acknowledgments. *Journal of the American College of Radiology.* American College of Radiology. doi: https://doi.org/10.1016/j.jacr.2020.02.008.

Kroumpouzos, Z., Gupta, M., Jafferany, M. *et al.* (2020) COVID-19: a relationship to climate and environmental conditions?, *Dermatologic Therapy* 33.4 pp. e13399–e13399. doi: https://doi.org/10.1111/dth.13399.

Kucharski, A. J., Russell, T., W., Diamond, C. *et al.* (2020) Articles early dynamics of transmission and control of COVID-19 : a mathematical modelling study, *The Lancet Infectious Diseases* 20.5 (2020): 553–558 20(5), pp. 553–558. doi: https://doi.org/10.1016/S1473-3099(20)30144-4.

Kudo, E., Song, E., Yockey, L., J., and Iwasaki, A. (2019) Low ambient humidity impairs barrier function and innate resistance against influenza infection, *Proceedings of the National Academy of Sciences of the United States of America.* 2019/05/13. National Academy of Sciences, 116(22), pp. 10905–10910. doi: https://doi.org/10.1073/pnas.1902840116.

Lai, M.Y.Y., Cheng, P.K.C., and Lim, W.W.L. (2005). Survival of severe acute respiratory syndrome coronavirus. *Clinical Infectious Diseases* 41 (7): e67–e71.

Lai, C., Shih, T.-P, Wen-Chien Ko, W.-C. *et al.* (2020) Severe acute respiratory syndrome coronavirus 2 (SARS-CoV-2) and corona virus disease-2019 (COVID-19): the epidemic and the challenges, *International Journal of Antimicrobial Agents.* Elsevier B.V., 2, p. 105924. doi: https://doi.org/10.1016/j.ijantimicag.2020.105924.

Li, M., Lei, P., Zeng, B. *et al.* (2020) Spectrum of CT findings and temporal progression of the disease, *Academic Radiology.* Elsevier Inc., (10), pp. 1–6. doi: https://doi.org/10.1016/j.acra.2020.03.003.

Li, Q., Guan, X., Wu, P., Wang, X., Zhou, L., Tong, Y., . . . & Feng, Z. (2020) Early transmission dynamics in Wuhan, China, of novel coronavirus–infected pneumonia, *New England Journal of Medicine* pp. 1199–1207. doi: https://doi.org/10.1056/NEJMoa2001316.

Lin, K., Fong, D., Y.-T., Zhu, B. and Karlberg, J. (2006) Environmental factors on the SARS epidemic: air temperature, passage of time and multiplicative effect of hospital infection, *Epidemiology and Infection*, 134(2), pp. 223–230. doi: https://doi.org/10.1017/S0950268805005054.

Lipsitch, M. and Viboud, C. (2009) Influenza seasonality: lifting the fog, *Proceedings of the National Academy of Sciences of the United States of America.* National Academy of Sciences, 106(10), pp. 3645–3646. doi: https://doi.org/10.1073/pnas.0900933106.

Lipsitch, M., Swerdlow, D.L., and Finelli, L. (2020). Defining the epidemiology of Covid-19 — studies needed. *New England Journal of Medicine* 382 (13): 1194–1196.

Liu, Z., Magal, P., Seydi, O. and Webb, G. (2020) Understanding unreported cases in the COVID-19 epidemic outbreak in Wuhan, China, and the importance of major public health interventions. *Biology* 9.3 50. doi: https://doi.org/10.3390/biology9030050.

Lotfi, M., Hamblin, M. R. and Rezaei, N. (2020) COVID-19: Transmission, prevention, and potential therapeutic opportunities, *Clinica Chimica Acta* 508, pp. 254–266. doi: https://doi.org/10.1016/j.cca.2020.05.044.

Lowen, A. C. and Steel, J. (2014) Roles of humidity and temperature in shaping influenza seasonality, *Journal of Virology*. American Society for Microbiology, 88(14), pp. 7692–7695. doi: https://doi.org/10.1128/JVI.03544-13.

Lowen, A. C., Steel, J., Mubareka, S. and Palese, P. (2008) High temperature (30 degrees C) blocks aerosol but not contact transmission of influenza virus, *Journal of Virology*. 2008/03/26. American Society for Microbiology (ASM), 82(11), pp. 5650–5652. doi: https://doi.org/10.1128/JVI.00325-08.

Lu, Q. and Yuan Shi (2020) Coronavirus disease (COVID - 19) and neonate: what neonatologist need to know, *Journal of Medical Virology* 92.6 pp. 564–567. doi: https://doi.org/10.1002/jmv.25740.

Luan, P. T. and Ching, C. T. (2020) A reusable mask for Coronavirus Disease 2019 (COVID-19), *Archives of Medical Research*. Instituto Mexicano del Seguro Social (IMSS), 2019. doi: https://doi.org/10.1016/j.arcmed.2020.04.001.

Luis, J., Cole, D. C., Ravasi, G. *et al.* (2020) Exaggerated risk of transmission of COVID-19 by fomites, *The Lancet Infectious Diseases*. Elsevier Ltd, 20(8), pp. 892–893. doi: https://doi.org/10.1016/S1473-3099(20)30561-2.

Mccloskey, B. and Heymann, D.L. (2020). SARS to novel coronavirus – old lessons and new lessons. *Epidemiology & Infection* 148.

Men, K., Li, Y., Wang, X. et al. (2020). Estimate the incubation period of coronavirus 2019 (COVID-19). *MedRxiv*.

Meo, S.A., Al-Khlaiwi, T., Usmani, A., M. et al. (2020). Biological and epidemiological trends in the prevalence and mortality due to outbreaks of novel coronavirus COVID-19. *Journal of King Saud University - Science*. King Saud University. doi: https://doi.org/10.1016/j.jksus.2020.04.004.

Ng, Y. and Peggy, P. L. (2020) Coronavirus disease (COVID-19) prevention: virtual classroom education for hand hygiene, *Nurse Education in Practice*. Elsevier Ltd, p. 102782. doi: https://doi.org/10.1016/j.nepr.2020.102782.

Nghiem, L. D., Morgan, B., Donner, E. and Short, M., D. *et al.* (2020) The COVID-19 pandemic: considerations for the waste and wastewater services sector, *Case Studies in Chemical and Environmental Engineering*. Elsevier Ltd, p. 100006. doi: https://doi.org/10.1016/j.cscee.2020.100006.

Onyema, E. M. (2020) Impact of coronavirus pandemic on education, *Journal of Education and Practice* 11(13), pp. 108–121. doi: https://doi.org/10.7176/JEP/11-13-12.

Parikh, G. and Rawtani, D. (2022). Environmental impact of COVID-19. In: *COVID-19 in the Environment*, 203–216. https://doi.org/10.1016/B978-0-323-90272-4.00001-4.

Park, J.-E., Son, W.-S., Ryu, Y. *et al.* (2020) Effects of temperature, humidity, and diurnal temperature range on influenza incidence in a temperate region, *Influenza and Other Respiratory Viruses*. 2019/10/21. John Wiley and Sons Inc., 14(1), pp. 11–18. doi: https://doi.org/10.1111/irv.12682.

Purohit, S., Rao, P.K., and Rawtani, D. (2022). Sampling and analytical techniques for COVID-19. In: *COVID-19 in the Environment*, 75–94. https://doi.org/10.1016/B978-0-323-90272-4.00008-7.

Quan, F.S, Rubino, I., Lee, S.-H. *et al.* (2017) Universal and reusable virus deactivation system for respiratory protection *Scientific Reports* 7.1, pp. 1–10. doi: https://doi.org/10.1038/srep39956.

Rao, P.K. and Rawtani, D. (2022). Modern digital techniques for monitoring and analysis. In: *COVID-19 in the Environment*, 115–130. https://doi.org/10.1016/B978-0-323-90272-4.00015-4.

Read, S. H. and Wild, S. H. (2020) What are the risks of COVID-19 infection in pregnant women ?, *The Lancet*. Elsevier Ltd, 395(10226), pp. 760–762. doi: https://doi.org/10.1016/S0140-6736(20)30365-2.

Ren, S.Y., Wang, W.B., Hao, Y.G. et al. (2020). Stability and infectivity of coronaviruses in inanimate environments. *World Journal of Clinical Cases* 8 (8): 1391.

Rothan, H. A. and Byrareddy, S. N. (2020) The epidemiology and pathogenesis of coronavirus disease (COVID-19) outbreak, *Journal of Autoimmunity*. Elsevier, (February), p. 102433. doi: https://doi.org/10.1016/j.jaut.2020.102433.

Sanche, S., Lin, Y., T., Xu, C. et al. (2020). High contagiousness and rapid spread of severe acute respiratory syndrome coronavirus 2. *Emerging Infectious Diseases* 26 (7): 1470.

Schwartz, J., King, C. and Yen, M. (2020) Protecting healthcare workers during the Coronavirus Disease 2019 (COVID-19) outbreak: lessons from Taiwan's severe acute respiratory syndrome response, *Clinical Infectious Diseases* 71.15 pp. 858–860. doi: https://doi.org/10.1093/cid/ciaa255.

Shaman, J. and Kohn, M. (2009) Absolute humidity modulates influenza survival, transmission, and seasonality, *Proceedings of the National Academy of Sciences of the United States of America*. 2009/02/09. National Academy of Sciences, 106(9), pp. 3243–3248. doi: https://doi.org/10.1073/pnas.0806852106.

Singhal, T. (2020). A review of Coronavirus Disease-2019 (COVID-19). *The Indian Journal of Pediatrics* 87: 281–286.

Steel, J., Palese, P. and Lowen, A. C. (2011) Transmission of a 2009 pandemic influenza virus shows a sensitivity to temperature and humidity similar to that of an H3N2 seasonal strain, *Journal of Virology*. 2010/11/17. American Society for Microbiology (ASM), 85(3), pp. 1400–1402. doi: https://doi.org/10.1128/JVI.02186-10.

Sun, Z. and Ostrikov, K. (2020) 'of', *Sustainable Materials and Technologies*. Elsevier B.V, p. e00203. doi: https://doi.org/10.1016/j.susmat.2020.e00203.

Tan, J., Mu, L., Huang, J. et al. (2005) An initial investigation of the association between the SARS outbreak and weather: with the view of the environmental temperature and its variation, *Journal of Epidemiology and Community Health*. BMJ Group, 59(3), pp. 186–192. doi: https://doi.org/10.1136/jech.2004.020180.

Tellier, R. (2009) Aerosol transmission of influenza A virus: a review of new studies, *Journal of the Royal Society, Interface*. 2009/09/22. The Royal Society, 6(Suppl 6), pp. S783–S790. doi: https://doi.org/10.1098/rsif.2009.0302.focus.

Velavan, T. P. and Meyer, C. G. (2020) The COVID-19 epidemic, *Tropical Medicine & International Health* 25(3), pp. 278. doi: https://doi.org/10.1111/tmi.13383.

Wang, D., Hu, B., Hu, C. et al. (2020) Clinical characteristics of 138 hospitalized patients with 2019 novel coronavirus-infected pneumonia in Wuhan, China, *JAMA*. American Medical Association, p. e201585. doi: https://doi.org/10.1001/jama.2020.1585.

WHO (2020). Coronavirus disease 2019 (COVID-19) Situation Report – 30, 2019 (February).

Wu, Y., Jing, W., Liu, J. et al. (2020) Effects of temperature and humidity on the daily new cases and new deaths of COVID-19 in 166 countries. *Science of the Total Environment* 729 139051 doi: https://doi.org/10.1016/j.scitotenv.2020.139051.

Xie, J. and Zhu, Y. (2020) Association between ambient temperature and COVID-19 infection in 122 cities from China, *Science of the Total Environment*. Elsevier B.V., 724, p. 138201. doi: https://doi.org/10.1016/j.scitotenv.2020.138201.

Xu, Z., Shi, L., Wang, Y. *et al*. (2020) Case report pathological findings of COVID-19 associated with acute respiratory distress syndrome, *The Lancet Respiratory*. Elsevier Ltd, 8(4), pp. 420–422. doi: https://doi.org/10.1016/S2213-2600(20)30076-X.

Yao, Y., Pan, J., Liu, Z. et al. (2020). No association of COVID-19 transmission with temperature or UV radiation in Chinese cities. *The European Respiratory Journal*. NLM (Medline). doi: https://doi.org/10.1183/13993003.00517-2020.

Yuan, J., Yun, H., Lan, W. *et al*. (2006) A climatologic investigation of the SARS-CoV outbreak in Beijing, China, *American Journal of Infection Control*. Association for Professionals in Infection Control and Epidemiology, Inc. Published by Mosby, Inc., 34(4), pp. 234–236. doi: https://doi.org/10.1016/j.ajic.2005.12.006.

Yue, P., Korkmaz, A.G., and Zhou, H. (2020). Household financial decision making amidst the COVID-19 pandemic. *Emerging Markets Finance and Trade* 56 (10): 2363–2377.

Zhang, H., Yu, J., Xu, H.-J. *et al*. (2020a) Corona virus international public health emergencies: implications for radiology management, *Academic Radiology*. Elsevier Inc., 27(4), pp. 463–467. doi: https://doi.org/10.1016/j.acra.2020.02.003.

Zhang, W., Du, R.-H., Li, B. *et al*. (2020b) Molecular and serological investigation of 2019-nCoV infected patients: implication of multiple shedding routes. *Emerging Microbes & Infections* 9.1 386–s doi: https://doi.org/10.1080/22221751.2020.1729071.

Zheng, Y.-Y. (2020) COVID-19 and the cardiovascular system *Nature Reviews Cardiology* 17.5 (2020): 259–260 doi: https://doi.org/10.1038/s41569-020-0360-5.

Zhou, P., Yang, X.-L., Wang, X.-G. *et al*. (2020) A pneumonia outbreak associated with a new coronavirus of probable bat origin, *Nature*. Springer US, 2019. doi: https://doi.org/10.1038/s41586-020-2012-7.

Zu, Z.Y., Di Jiang, M., Peng Peng, X. et al. (2020). Coronavirus Disease 2019 (COVID-19): a perspective from China. *Radiology* 296 (22): E15–E25.

Zuniga, J. M. and Cortes, A. (2020) The role of additive manufacturing and antimicrobial polymers in the COVID-19 pandemic, *Expert Review of Medical Devices*. Taylor & Francis, 17(6), pp. 477–481. doi: https://doi.org/10.1080/17434440.2020.1756771.

3

Influence of Environmental Factors in Transmission of COVID-19

Aayush Dey[1], Piyush K. Rao[1], and Deepak Rawtani[2]

[1] School of Doctoral Studies and Research, National Forensic Sciences University (Ministry of Home affairs, GOI), Gandhinagar, Gujarat, India
[2] School of Pharmacy, National Forensic Sciences University (Ministry of Home affairs, GOI), Gandhinagar, Gujarat, India

3.1 Introduction

The global pandemic of COVID-19 poses a grave risk to the well-being of the human population. The SARS-CoV-2 causes the COVID-19. The genetic constituency of a positive-sense single-stranded RNA makes up the coronavirus disease causing SARS-CoV-2 virus, which tends to be extremely contagious and causes the respiratory system to cease (Swerdlow and Finelli 2020). Different time series models claim that chronic exposure to the SARS-CoV-2 virus has caused a sharp spike in the death rate of the global human population in huge numbers (Maleki et al. 2020). The Global Emergency Committee preceding the announcements made by WHO regarding the novel coronavirus disease, recognized the requirement for prompt detection, quarantine, and treatment (Sohrabi et al. 2020). Such steps were implemented by the committee because during the initial phases of COVID-19 infection, patients are asymptomatic, i.e. symptoms such as fever, cough are not visible. Due to the aforementioned reason, optimum insight on how to maintain cleanliness and hygiene in the surrounding environment and different types of surfaces have been repeatedly relayed to the general public. Also a proper information regarding transference of the virus among humans via mediums such as air, food, and water is not available. There are various aspects that are responsible for the spread of the novel coronavirus (Figure 3.1). Human population distribution, communal interaction, climate change due to deforestation and habitat invasion, agriculture, and interaction with animals (domestic and wild) are some of the dynamics that have not been extensively studied regarding the transmission of COVID-19 (Barratt et al. 2019; Dehghani and Kassiri 2020). The proper mechanism regarding how the novel coronavirus gains access to the body, or whether the viral strain gains access via orifices of ears and nose or via oral passage and the eyes, is still not established, though findings related to earlier epidemic due to a virus very analogous to the SARS-CoV-2 can be referred to (Sun et al. 2020).

The Environmental Impact of COVID-19, First Edition. Edited by Deepak Rawtani and Chaudhery Mustansar Hussain.
© 2024 John Wiley & Sons Ltd. Published 2024 by John Wiley & Sons Ltd.

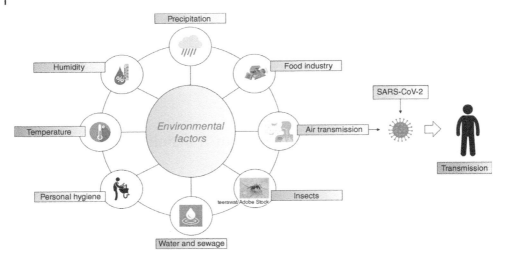

Figure 3.1 Transmission of COVID-19 accounting to different environmental factors.

Since the means of the viral spread is unknown, protection with glasses, face shields, and masks are recommended by the Centre of Disease Control and Prevention (CDC) (CDC 2020a). According to some studies, contracting the coronavirus infection is still possible even with the use of personal protective equipments (PPEs), and according to Yang (2020), there is no substantial proof regarding inhibiting disease contraction by the use of PPE. Conferring to the estimates made by the World Health Organization (WHO), no conclusion has been made regarding the survival or perseverance of the SARS-CoV-2 in different mediums such as metal surfaces. All of the viral strains in the beta-coronavirus family can persist on any plane or medium for quite a few hours (Parry 2004), and the same is speculated for the novel coronavirus. It is because of this reason, several spots in public places, such as eateries and vendor markets, infirmaries, and other residential and commercial areas have to play an equal part in keeping their surroundings clean (WHO 2020a). Stopping and preventing the swift transmittal of the coronavirus disease has now become a global challenge; hence healthcare facilities and manpower and their respective management must be coordinated on a global scale. The coronavirus has a potent variability; and considering the type of climate and environmental factors (Saadat et al. 2020), it is rather important that more focus must be given to its prevention and control and the process must be rapid and thorough (Askari et al. 2018). Nonetheless a hierarchy has been postulated regarding how to deal with SARS-CoV-2 virus. The hierarchy involves three steps namely, self-care, regulation of environmental factors, and the absolute utilization of PPEs (Lai et al. 2020). This chapter further discusses in detail the several environmental factors and their impact on COVID-19 transmission that include weather dynamics i.e., temperature and humidity, the effects of precipitation on the spread of COVID-19, transmission through water sources, air as a medium for COVID-19 transmission, and the effects of food industry in transmission of COVID-19, etc. Also various aspects regarding personal hygiene and disinfection of surfaces against the prevalence of COVID-19 have been discussed in detail.

3.2 Temperature, Humidity, and Transmission of COVID-19

A very crucial aspect for the well-being of the human population is temperature. Various researches have been carried out which have evidently related the development and spread of the COVID-19 epidemic and its regulation to environmental temperature and humidity. A study conducted in Barcelona, Spain (Tobías and Molina 2020) exhibits that higher temperatures during the summer season has an inverse relationship with the survivability of the novel coronavirus spread and contamination. A basic incidence rate was calculated relating the environmental temperature levels and the prevalence degree of positive COVID-19 infection cases. It was inferred that per 1 °C rise in temperature, the incidence rate decreased by 7.5%. A research by Wang et al. (2020a) evidently enumerates the association amidst the spread of the novel coronavirus and the dynamics of the weather, i.e. temperature and humidity. This study by Wang et al. (2020a) portrays a consistent association to the rapport between ambient temperature and spread of the novel coronavirus. According to this study, 1 °C rise in temperature exhibited reduction in the effective reproductive number value (R values) which denotes the spread of COVID-19. Furthermore, the association amidst humidity and the transmission of COVID-19 is not so substantial. Another study was conducted that established an association between the per day increase in the cases of COVID-19 infection and maximum surrounding temperature. The occurrence of COVID-19 was observed to be negligible to moderate in places with maximum surrounding temperature. It was also observed that with the increase in temperature, the prevalence of the disease decreased (Bhattacharjee 2020). At colder temperatures, i.e. around 4 °C, SARS-CoV-2 showed exhibited the most prevalence, and at temperatures around 70 °C, resistance of the virus is reduced to precisely 5 minutes (Chin et al. 2020). For 1 °C increase of the minimum surrounding temperature, 0.86% reduction in COVID cases was observed (Wang et al. 2020b). According to a report published by WHO (2020b), heat, extremely acidic and basic pH, and daylight assist in the neutralization of the SARS-CoV-2 virus. Nonetheless a study conducted by Chin et al. (2020) stated that at room temperature coronavirus is stable at pH range 3–10. Analogous with other researches and studies, another work by Chiyomaru and Takemoto (2020) positively indicates that greater temperatures of the summer season is responsible for substantial decrement in the COVID-19 case statistics.

A study conducted in New South Wales, Australia (Ward et al. 2020) stated that an increase in the relative ambient humidity was directly linked to the decline in COVID-19 cases, and that the relationship between the relative ambient humidity and the number of confirmed cases were constantly negative. This study also stated that an increase of about 7–8% in the number of confirmed cases were observed with 1% decrease in relative humidity. COVID-19 prevalence with respect to maximum air humidity is not negligible and is statistically significant. Another study showed that with increase in air humidity levels, the COVID-19 prevalence decreases (Eslami and Jalili 2020).

3.3 Precipitation and Its Effects on COVID-19 Transmission

Apart from core ambient dynamics, i.e. temperature and humidity, the study by Chiyomaru and Takemoto (2020) also states an association between COVID-19 transmission and the amount of periodic precipitation. It states that higher precipitation rates have a somewhat linear relationship to the spread in COVID-19 cases, i.e. very low transmission rates of COVID-19 were observed in areas with high precipitation. Another study backing this proposition is the study by Chien and Chen (2020) which clearly states that higher precipitation rates substantially diminish the chances of COVID-19 infection. It states that areas with more than 1.77 inches of rainfall observed a steep decline in the relative transmission risk percentage.

3.4 Food Industry and COVID-19 Transmission

The novel coronavirus disease is a respiratory ailment and its transmission occurs mainly when a healthy individual is in direct contact with another infected person. A healthy individual can also contract the COVID-19 infection if respiratory droplets from an infected individual is inhaled while coughing and sneezing. It has been rendered highly unlikely that a healthy human being can contract the novel coronavirus disease from food and food packaging materials (WHO 2020c). According to CDC, no significant evidence regarding the transmission of COVID-19 through food, food packaging materials, and food workers, hence rendering them risk free. Washing and disinfection of food packaging surfaces have been suggested by the CDC, because SARS-CoV-2 can persist on surfaces ranging from a few hours to few days, approximately accounting to 72 hours (van Doremalen et al. 2020). Hygiene care is a crucial recommendation while preparing food and separation of raw meat from other foods (Rizou et al. 2020). Other steps for personal hygiene have also been recommended, for example, winding the elbow around the nose and mouth while sneezing or coughing, hence shielding other individuals in vicinity from the respiratory droplets. Symptomatic patients must be isolated along with people who have been in direct contact with them. Maintaining a distance of 6 ft or 1.8 m (social distancing) at confined places with significant number of people is another step that ensures the non-prevalence of COVID-19 (Seymour et al. 2020a). Being considerate about the current viral pandemic, it becomes imperative for the food industry to implement guidelines of personal hygiene upon its working personnel and ensure that they follow the implemented guidelines. Proper implementation can also be ensured by an obligatory drill on hygiene principles. This must be done in order to reduce or completely eliminate any chances of food or packaging materials getting contaminated with the novel coronavirus. Enforcing utilization of PPE, i.e. masks, gloves, face shields, etc., in addition with strict rules regarding the maintenance of physical distancing, hand-washing, and sanitation at different phases of food processing, manufacturing, and advertising will ensure the elimination of viral spread. Maintaining a healthy workforce, detection, and exclusion of infected workers or handlers and their immediate contact from the workplace will also help in reducing the viral spread (WHO 2020c).

In order to reduce the viral spread, food industries must follow the five-step good staff hygienic practices which include the following steps:

- Appropriate hand sanitization – hands must be washed meticulously for roughly 20 seconds and soap must be applied, after that wash out the lather with water.
- Recurrent use of hand sanitizers (alcohol based).

- Appropriate respiratory hygiene – covering of mouth and nose with bent elbows while coughing and sneezing.
- Frequent disinfecting of surfaces where an individual works and other places of touch, for example, door knobs.
- Keeping a safe distance from symptomatic people.

3.5 Water and Sewage as a Medium for COVID-19 Transmission

There are a few factors that play a significant part in assisting human health and well-being, which includes safe water supply, proper sewage collection and disposal, and maintaining ambient and personal hygiene (Khatri et al. 2020; WHO 2020d). The probability of novel coronavirus transmission tends to be relatively absent via stools of an infected individual. Although diarrhea is one the extensive occurring symptom of COVID-19 infection, according to a statistical approach demonstrated by D'Amico et al. (2020), the incidence rate of diarrhea ranges between 2 and 50% of established COVID-19 cases. Whereas another statistical reproach reveals that the general recurrence rate of diarrhea in Chinese cities is about 5.8% (Li et al. 2020). Evidences of occurrence of the viral RNA residues of the novel coronavirus disease in stools of patients with coronavirus disease have been confirmed (Chen et al. 2020). Medema et al. (2020) confirms the perseverance of the novel coronavirus in sewage even though it does not pose as a risk factor confirms the survivability of the virus in sewage, and this is a very important piece of information as this can be used as a tool to monitor and track the frequency of the novel coronavirus recurrence in different sets of populations (Lodder and de Roda Husman 2020; Rao and Rawtani 2022). A study by Qu et al. (2020) stated that the novel coronavirus can prevail in water mediums as well as sewage for a varying time period that may extend from days to a few weeks. Since many studies have proved the prevalence of the novel coronavirus in an aqueous and sewage environment, a number of factors have been outlined that is important for its survivability, which includes temperature of the ambience, sunlight availability, presence of organic compounds, and occurrence of hostile micro-organisms. All the aforementioned factors have a variable effect on the transmission of COVID-19 via water and wastewater sources. A study by WHO stated that there are no prevailing evidence regarding the transmission of SARS-CoV-2 virus via contaminated water sources (Naddeo and Liu 2020). Since viruses with protein coats are hostile to the environment, they become readily susceptible to oxidants such as chlorine and other hostile micro-organisms. The human intestinal viruses significantly neutralizes the SARS-CoV-2 virus at a rapid rate (WHO 2020b; Purohit et al. 2022).

3.6 COVID-19 Transmission via Air

Clinical symptoms of the novel coronavirus disease are not visible in an individual in the preliminary stages of the coronavirus infection. Such individuals are also known as asymptomatic patients and are the most responsible for the transmittal of the novel coronavirus disease. This transmission routes may vary, i.e. via respiratory droplets, being in a close contact with infected individuals, and also through foul airflow (Zhi 2020). The principle reasons behind the transmittal of SARS-CoV-2 via aerosol and airflow include cardiopulmonary resuscitation, introduction of phlegm, sack and mask airflow, bronchoscopy, and non-invasive ventilation along with intubation/extubation (CDC 2020a). During the MERS-CoV pandemic in 2015 which broke out in Korea, studies and researches evaluated the prevalence of MERS-CoV in air and surface of the aforementioned complex instruments (Bin et al. 2016). This depicts the likelihood of novel coronavirus occurrence in air. Therefore, the viral filters must be utilized with closed suctioning in confined and closed environments that ensures least likelihood of contamination for treating a patient with respiratory ailment is suggested (Phua et al. 2020). It should be evident that the individuals residing in polluted ambience must utilize masks, and if masks are unavailable the use of face mask is strongly recommended (Bowdle and Munoz-Price 2020). Utilizing non-standard masks might aggravate the prevalence of the novel coronavirus (Greenhalgh et al. 2020). Apart from the protective perks that a mask provides, some people have faced issues or indications of claustrophobia, discomfort, distress in the respiratory pathway, and excessive itchiness of the skin, etc.,(Barratt et al. 2019). The most frequently used mask is the N95 mask, and these masks can be decontaminated and used again. Ethylene oxide, H_2O_2, γ-rays of cobalt isotope, i.e. ^{60}CO and heat application are some of the approaches to neuter the N95 masks (Card et al. 2020; Cramer et al. 2020; Kenney et al. 2020). γ-rays of the aforementioned cobalt isotope can easily sterilize and efficiently neutralize the novel coronavirus (Feldmann et al. 2019), but utmost care must be taken regarding the radiation levels, as high levels of γ-radiation can cause impairments in the fibers of the mask rendering it useless, which will ultimately result in the passage of air without filtration. This method is perfectly safe to use and there are no side effects of the radiation (Cramer et al. 2020). H_2O_2 is another antiviral that tends to prevent viral replications and exhibits no antagonistic effects upon the respiratory tract when used in adequate volumes (Kelly et al. 2020). The application of enhanced traffic control bundling (eTCB) was very efficient during MERS outbreak and due to its similarity with the current SARS-CoV-2 outbreak, it can prove to be a great strategy in preventing the spread of the novel coronavirus disease via air (Yen et al. 2020). The strategy of eTCB included the isolation and quarantine of people indicating the clinical symptoms of COVID-19, and other asymptomatic people get to wear PPEs and apply disinfectants during their hospital visits. This strategy has been approved and is currently being used to control the novel coronavirus disease epidemic (Yen et al. 2015; Ong et al. 2020; Schwartz et al. 2020). Droplets released from an infected individual that can travel to a distance of 6 feet via air as a medium has been accounted for in the internal environment of ophthalmologists (CDC 2020b), for ventilation or airflow purposes high efficiency particulate air (HEPA) filters have been introduced.

3.7 Transmission of COVID-19 Through Insects

Since the spread of the novel coronavirus disease is taking place on a global scale, many factors have contributed to its transmittal. To name a few, ecology, demographic conditions, and human behavior are some inclusions in the list of such aspects. So far, almost seven strains of coronaviruses have been discovered (Gorbalenya et al. 2020). A study by Dehghani and Kassiri (2020) reported a particular chronology regarding the spread and advancement of COVID-19 virus from bats to ant-eaters also known as pangolins and then to humans. The spread of the novel coronavirus disease occurs via aerosols in human. Apart from the transmission via aerosols, no studies have illustrated insects or arthropods as a medium of COVID-19 transmittal (Shankar et al. 2020; Wu and McGoogan 2020). There have been researches that particularly state that domestic bugs and pests or beetles are the chief vectors of infectious pathogens, and these insects do transmit diseases by coming in contact with polluted surfaces or patient's respiratory and excretory discharges that are primarily associated with the spread of diseases (Kobayashi et al. 1999; Graczyk et al. 2005). Since genetic residues of viral SARS-CoV-2 have been found in stools of infected patients, the feeding off stools of infected patients by the domestic mosquitoes and beetles seems to pose a significant reason behind the transmission of the novel coronavirus disease and this risk factor must not be neglected (Eslami and Jalili 2020; Dey et al. 2022). These insects can transmit hundreds of pathogens via the appendages, body hair, mouth, vomit, and feces. Due to the aforementioned reasons, the elimination of such mechanical vectors is essential in domestic households and also in open communities. In addition to improving environmental hygiene several strategies have been devised to control the growth of such organisms. These strategies include placing domestic wastes and trash in proper garbage cans, monitoring salubrious landfills, cleaning of household and public restrooms, following appropriate steps for sewage disposals, and prevention of aggregation of manure and pesticides in ambient residential areas. Secretions from individuals who are suspected to have contracted the novel coronavirus disease infection, such as blood and feces are clinical and laboratory wastes and they can act as a point source of viral infections (Peng et al. 2020). However, no research has evidently confirmed the occurrence of the SARS-CoV-2 virus in urine samples of infected individuals (Frithiof et al. 2020). To conclude, waste management is necessary, and if not properly managed and completely overlooked, it is a possibility that the COVID-19 infection can be spread via insects (CDC 2020a).

3.8 Personal Hygiene Amidst COVID-19 Transmission

The first and foremost advice amidst a spreading pandemic is to practice hand and eye hygiene and utilize PPEs. Most of the drawbacks for not following the guidelines for the pandemic happen in a discrete individual or a group or at the communal stages. These drawbacks are well known to the personnel working at a healthcare unit. Use of decontaminating agents is necessary amidst the COVID-19 pandemic and not just any disinfectant. Some disinfectants are not that effective for neutralizing pathogens, and if put in simpler terms an individual must use disinfectants that actually neutralizes the infection causing organism and in this case, SARS-CoV-2. Alcohol-based sanitizers have proven to be very useful amidst the COVID-19 pandemic, and its effectiveness has helped in prevention of the viral spread to a great extent. Also the fact must be taken into consideration that amidst the lockdown, public access of such materials have been limited, and this has emerged as a noteworthy issue. Mixture of alcohol, glycerine, and hydrogen peroxide make up home-made disinfectants and its effectiveness have been examined by WHO (Seymour et al. 2020b). Lack of application of hand sanitizers and interaction with respiratory droplets from nose and mouth from an infected individual can infect a healthy individual with the novel coronavirus. It is very evident that hand sanitization and hygiene are effective in reduction and prevention of respiratory illness. In individuals infected with SARS-CoV-2, speculations regarding ailments of the eye such as conjunctivitis have been made (Qing et al. 2020). Although not many viral strains have been reported in the conjunctical discharge of an individual, and non-consistent with the above stated fact, a study by Loffredo et al. (2020) suggests that eye probably can be a medium for COVID-19 infection. Nonetheless, ailments of the respiratory and the nasopharyngeal tract may result into eye infections. When coming in contact with an infected individual, nasopharyngeal and respiratory infections may be very efficient and hence causing eye infections, and this phenomenon is more prominent in the clinical staff of a hospital or a health clinic. The use of masks, goggles, PPE kits, and hand disinfectants have exhibited a noteworthy decrease in individual-to-individual viral spread (Pradhan et al. 2020). Infected people do contaminate any surface they might touch, and it may include all kinds of household items and other appliances; hence explaining the importance of hand sanitizers and disinfectants (Eslami and Jalili 2020).

3.9 Prevalence of SARS-CoV-2

When the novel coronavirus infects a healthy individual and reaches the communal phase of the disease, the chances of individual-to-individual spread of the SARS-CoV-2 is very high. The transmission rate is also high when the infected individual exhibits mild symptoms. The primary modes of the viral transmission include respiratory droplet transmission via air, unclean hands, inanimate surface, and close contact to an infected individual (Kampf et al. 2020). The novel coronavirus, like other members of the coronavirus family, can have a viable period of nine days on any surface at normal environmental conditions. Despite the environmental conditions, if the temperature lies in the range of 30–40 °C, the viability of other members of the coronavirus family, for example, SARS-CoV, Human coronavirus (HCoV), Middle east respiratory syndrome coronavirus (MERS-CoV), and Canine coronavirus (CCV) reduces significantly (Kampf et al. 2020). Persistence of HCoV is lesser at about 30% relative humidity on any inanimate surface when compared to 50% relative humidity at normal room temperature (Ijaz et al. 1985). According to a study by van Doremalen et al. (2020), the survivability rate of the novel coronavirus, i.e. SARS-CoV-2 in aerosols with temperature ranging between 21 and 23 °C and relative humidity pertaining at 65% is about 15.8% with a time duration of 3 hours. The persistence of different members of the coronavirus family in different kinds of surfaces has been studied extensively and has been compiled in Table 3.1.

Table 3.1 Prevalence of coronaviruses on different surfaces.

Medium	Coronavirus type	Initial viral concentration	Environmental condition		Persistence time period	Time period for complete neutralization (hours)	Reduction in viral concentration	References
			Temperature range (°C)	Relative humidity (%)				
Aerosols	SARS-CoV-2	3.5 $\log_{10}$/ml	21–23	65	3 h	—	84.2%	van Doremalen et al. (2020)
		2.0 $\log_{10}$/ml	Room temperature	—	16 h	—	45%	Fears et al. (2020)
	SARS-CoV-1	4.3 $\log_{10}$/ml	21–23	65	3 h	—	84.2%	van Doremalen et al. (2020)
	MERS-CoV	6.0 $\log_{10}$/ml	20	40	10 min	—	7%	van Doremalen et al. (2013)
		6.0 $\log_{10}$/ml	20	70	10 min	—	89%	van Doremalen et al. (2013)
		5.5 $\log_{10}$/ml	25	79	60 min	—	37%	Pyankov et al. (2018)
		5.5 $\log_{10}$/ml	38	24	60 min	—	95.3%	Pyankov et al. (2018)
	HCoV	7.5 $\log_{10}$/ml	6	30	24 h	—	30%	Ijaz et al. (1985)
		7.5 $\log_{10}$/ml	6	50	24 h	—	10%	Ijaz et al. (1985)
		7.5 $\log_{10}$/ml	6	80	24 h	—	10%	Ijaz et al. (1985)
		7.5 $\log_{10}$/ml	20	30	72 h	—	50%	Ijaz et al. (1985)
		7.5 $\log_{10}$/ml	20	50	72 h	—	40%	Ijaz et al. (1985)
		7.5 $\log_{10}$/ml	20	80	72 h	48 h	90%	Ijaz et al. (1985)

(Continued)

Table 3.1 (Continued)

Medium	Coronavirus type	Initial viral concentration	Environmental condition		Persistence time period	Time period for complete neutralization (hours)	Reduction in viral concentration	References
			Temperature range (°C)	Relative humidity (%)				
Plastics	SARS-CoV-2	$10^{3.6}$ TCID$_{50}$/ml	21–23	40	72 h	96 h	$10^{0.6}$ log$_{10}$	van Doremalen et al. (2020)
		$10^{6.8}$ TCID$_{50}$/ml	22	65	96 h	1 wk	Complete reduction	Chin et al. (2020)
	SARS-CoV-1	10^{7} TCID$_{50}$/ml	22–25	40–50	28 d	—	~5 log$_{10}$	Chan et al. (2011)
		10^{7} TCID$_{50}$/ml	33	80–89	24 h	—	0.75 log$_{10}$	Chan et al. (2011)
		10^{7} TCID$_{50}$/ml	38	>95	24 h	—	2 log$_{10}$	Chan et al. (2011)
	MERS-CoV	10^{6} TCID$_{50}$/ml	20	40	48 h	72 h	7%	van Doremalen et al. (2013)
		10^{6} TCID$_{50}$/ml	30	80	8 h	24 h	89%	van Doremalen et al. (2013)
	HCoV-229E	10^{3} PFU	21	30–40	5 d	—	~ 2–5 log$_{10}$	Warnes et al. (2015)
Stainless steel	SARS-CoV-2	$10^{6.8}$ TCID$_{50}$/ml	22	65	96 h	1 wk	Complete reduction	Chin et al. (2020)
		$10^{3.6}$ TCID$_{50}$/ml	21–23	40	72 h	96 h	5.8 log$_{10}$	van Doremalen et al. (2020)
	SARS-CoV-1	$10^{6.75-7}$ TCID$_{50}$/ml	21–23	40	48 h	72 h	3.2 log$_{10}$	van Doremalen et al. (2020)

Material	Virus	Concentration						Reference
	MERS-CoV	$6.0\ \log_{10}$/ml	30	30	24 h	48 h	~5.5 $\log_{10}$	van Doremalen et al. (2013)
		$6.0\ \log_{10}$/ml	20	40	48 h	72 h	~5.5 $\log_{10}$	van Doremalen et al. (2013)
		$6.0\ \log_{10}$/ml	30	80	8 h	24 h	~5.5 $\log_{10}$	van Doremalen et al. (2013)
	HCoV-229E	10^3 PFU	21	30–40	5 d	—	2 $\log_{10}$	Warnes et al. (2015)
Glass	SARS-CoV-2	$10^{6.8}$ TCID$_{50}$/ml	22	65	48 h	96 h	5.8 $\log_{10}$	Chin et al. (2020)
	HCoV-229E	10^3 PFU	21	30–40	5 d	—	2.5 $\log_{10}$	Warnes et al. (2015)
Cloth	SARS-CoV-2	$10^{6.8}$ TCID$_{50}$/ml	22	65	24 h	48 h	4.8 $\log_{10}$	Chin et al. (2020)
Paper	SARS-CoV-2	$10^{6.8}$ TCID$_{50}$/ml	22	65	30 min	3 h	4.8 $\log_{10}$	Chin et al. (2020)
Wood	SARS-CoV-2	$10^{6.8}$ TCID$_{50}$/ml	22	65	24 h	48 h	5.6 $\log_{10}$	Chin et al. (2020)
Cardboard	SARS-CoV-2	$10^{3.6}$ TCID$_{50}$/ml	21–23	40	24 h	48 h	2 $\log_{10}$	van Doremalen et al. (2020)
	SARS-CoV-1	$10^{3.6}$ TCID$_{50}$/ml	21–23	40	8 h	24 h	2 $\log_{10}$	van Doremalen et al. (2020)

SARS-CoV-2, Severe Acute Respiratory Syndrome Coronavirus-2; SARS-CoV-1, Severe Acute Respiratory Syndrome Coronavirus-1; MERS, Middle East Respiratory Syndrome; HCoV, Human Coronavirus; TCID, Tissue Culture Infectious Dose; PFU, Plaque Forming Units.

3.10   Disinfection of Surfaces – SARS-CoV-2

To ensure environmental cleanliness a few guidelines have been issued by the WHO (WHO 2020e). The guidelines stated the use of sodium hypochlorite solution (0.1% dilution ratio – 1 : 50) (Henwood 2020). Sodium hypochlorite solution is one of the most exploited disinfectant for sterilization of different surfaces. Other alternatives to sodium hypochlorite are ethanol with concentrations ranging from 62 to 70% or 0.5% concentrated H_2O_2 (Eslami and Jalili 2020). Benzalkonium chloride and chlorhexidine digluconate are biocidal agents that can be used for surface disinfection, but are not optimally effective. According to a study by Chin et al. (2020), efficacy of hand soap regarding surface disinfection was examined, and it was affirmed that for a contact time of five minutes the SARS-CoV-2 virus is rendered inactive. According to CDC, water temperatures above 65 °C can be used as a surface disinfectant (Seymour et al. 2020a).

Apart from suspension and carrier tests, for a quite long time now neutralization of different virulent microbes in surfaces, air and water sources via UV radiation has been in practice (Kowalski 2009a; Raeiszadeh and Adeli 2020). The spectrum of wavelength ranging between 200 and 280 nm is the particular UV radiation region that has been exploited for germicidal activities. This particular wavelength range is also termed as the ultraviolet (UV-C) spectrum. The intercellular components of micro-organisms, i.e. the RNA, DNA, and the proteins absorb photons from the UV-C spectrum. These photons in turn cause immediate damages to the genomic system of the microbes hence stopping their replication mechanism and hence ensuring their non-survivability. This outlines the basic disinfection of micro-organisms via UV radiation. Although greater decline in the spread of the novel coronavirus has been observed with the usage of the UV-C spectrum, there are some safety considerations that have to be taken into account, as this spectrum has proved itself to be carcinogenic for humans if there is any direct contact (Raeiszadeh and Adeli 2020). Acute effects of UV radiation include the introduction of a rapid sunburn in the skin, and since it is a mutagen, it consists of characteristics of a tumor originator and promoter, hence the carcinogenic activity of UV rays. Chronic exposure of the human eye to the UV rays can cause serious illnesses such as photokeratitis, cataracts, solar retinopathy, and retinal damage (van Kuijk 1991).

3.10.1   Suspension Tests for Surface Disinfection

In order to evaluate the efficacy of surface disinfectants, suspension tests have been carried out (Kampf et al. 2020). Suspension tests are generally performed in order to measure the efficiency of surface disinfectants in neutralization of corona viruses within a given contact time in a suspension. 4 $\log_{10}$ reduction in the concentration of coronavirus was observed when it was treated with 78–95% ethanol and 70–100% 2-propanol. A blend of 45% concentrated 2-propanol and 30% concentrated 1-propanol with glutardialdehyde, formaldehyde, and povidone iodine with respective concentrations of 2.5, 1, and 7.5% also neutralized coronavirus, and similar neutralization results were obtained when compared to the blend of ethanol and 2-propanol disinfectant. Among all disinfectants, only a minimal concentration of 0.21% of sodium hypochlorite is required to neutralize coronaviruses. In case of H_2O_2, i.e. hydrogen peroxide, only 0.5% of concentration is required in addition to an incubatory period (time period of exposure to the viral strain) of one minute in suspension tests. Chlorhexidine digluconate has been effectively used for the neutralization of mouse hepatitis virus and canine coronavirus but remained absolutely ineffective against the novel coronavirus. In contrary, lower concentrations of benzalkonium chloride with an exposure period of 10 minutes exhibited greater efficacy against the novel coronavirus. A concentration of 0.05% benzalkonium chloride exhibited a greater efficiency when compared to 0.2% concentrated benzalkonium chloride which was practically ineffective. A compilation of data acquired in suspension tests regarding different disinfectants on the novel coronavirus as well as different strains of coronaviruses and other viral strains is depicted in Table 3.2.

3.10.2 Carrier Tests for Surface Disinfection

In a carrier test, a carrier for example a penicylinder is contaminated by submersion in a liquid culture. The liquid culture here belongs to SARS-CoV-2. Further steps include the drying of the carrier and bringing the carrier in contact to a suitable disinfectant for a given exposure time. The carrier is further cultured in a nutrient broth and the growth of test micro-organism (SARS-CoV-2) is examined. Nil growth of test micro-organism depict the efficacy of the disinfectant, whereas growth indicates a failed test. Efficacy of ethanol was observed under one minute exposure to the SARS-CoV-2 virus. A concentration of around 62–71% of ethanol in carrier test neutralized 2.0–4.0 $\log_{10}$ of the SARS-CoV-2 virus. Both sodium hypochlorite and glutardialdehyde exhibited great reduction of the SARS-CoV-2 strain with concentrations of sodium hypochlorite ranging from 0.1 to 0.5% and 0.2% concentrated glutardialdehyde. In carrier test, benzalkonium chloride and ortho-phthalaldehyde were the least effective.

3.10.3 Ultraviolet (UV-C) Radiation-Mediated Disinfection of SARS-CoV-2

The coronavirus family and their reaction to UV-C spectrum is pre-determined. Several studies have established a well-defined kinetics regarding the neutralization of SARS-CoV-2 via UV-C irradiation (Table 3.3). These kinetics were procured by the previously available data regarding the response of SARS-CoV-1 to UV-C inactivation. The novel coronavirus and SARS-CoV-1 are very much alike when genomic characteristics are considered. Both the strains of viruses consist of positive-sense ssRNA as the genetic material and are protein coated. The genetic materials are of animal origin and belong to the β-CoV group. In addition to the similarity in the genetic materials, SARS-CoV-2 has 76.47% similarity in the amino acid sequence in the spike protein. The structural conformation and the electrostatic characteristics of both the viral strains are similar too (Scheller et al. 2020; Xie and Chen 2020).

The coronavirus family unlike commonly studied bacteria such as *Escherichia coli* (Kowalski 2009b) exhibits marginally more resistance when exposed to the specific UV-C spectrum. The responses of the coronavirus family against the UV-C radiation is analogous to that of a bacteriophage (Kowalski 2009b) which exhibit more sensitivity of SARS-CoV-2 toward UV radiation. Experimental studies exhibit that neutralization rate constant for SARS-CoV-2 virus was 1.49 and 0.13 cm^2 mJ^{-1} (Table 3.4).

Table 3.2 Suspension test – inactivation of coronaviruses by different disinfecting solutions.

Coronavirus family	Class of disinfectant	Disinfectant used	Concentration of disinfectant used (%)	Viral strain	Time of exposure (seconds)	Viral reduction (log10)	References
SARS-CoV	Alcohol	Ethanol	78	Isolate FFM-1	30	≥5.0	Rabenau et al. (2005a, b)
			80	Isolate FFM-1	30	≥4.3	Rabenau et al. (2005a, b)
			85	Isolate FFM-1	30	≥5.5	Rabenau et al. (2005a, b)
			95	Isolate FFM-1	30	≥5.5	Rabenau et al. (2005a, b)
		2-Propanol	70	Isolate FFM-1	30	≥3.3	Rabenau et al. (2005a, b)
			75	Isolate FFM-1	30	≥4.0	Siddharta et al. (2017)
			100	Isolate FFM-1	30	≥3.3	Rabenau et al. (2005a, b)
		2-Propanol + 1-Propanol	30	Isolate FFM-1	30	≥2.8	Rabenau et al. (2005a, b)
			45	Isolate FFM-1	30	≥4.3	Rabenau et al. (2005a, b)
	Aldehydes	Glutaraldehyde	0.5	Isolate FFM-1	120	>4.0	Rabenau et al. (2005a, b)
			2.5	Hanoi	300	>4.0	Kariwa et al. (2006)
		Formaldehyde	0.7	Isolate FFM-1	120	>3.0	Rabenau et al. (2005a, b)
			1	Isolate FFM-1	120	>3.0	Rabenau et al. (2005a, b)
	Others	Povidone iodine	0.23	Hanoi	15	≥4.4	Kariwa et al. (2006)
			0.23	Isolate FFM-1	60	>4.0	Eggers et al. (2018)
			0.25	Hanoi	60	>4.0	Kariwa et al. (2006)
			0.47	Hanoi	60	3.8	Kariwa et al. (2006)
HCoV	Others	Hydrogen peroxide	0.5	229E	60	>4.0	Omidbakhsh and Sattar (2006)
		Benzalkonium chloride	0.2	ATCC VR-759 (strain OC43)	10 min	>3.7	Wood and Payne (1998)
MERS-CoV	Alcohol	Ethanol	80	EMC Strain	30	>4.0	Siddharta et al. (2017)

		2-Propanol	75	EMC Strain	30	≥4.0	Siddharta et al. (2017)
	Others	Povidone iodine	0.23	Isolate HCoV-EMC/2012	15	≥4.4	Eggers et al. (2018)
			1	Isolate HCoV-EMC/2012	15	4.3	Eggers et al. (2015)
			4	Isolate HCoV-EMC/2012	15	5.0	Eggers et al. (2015)
			7.5	Isolate HCoV-EMC/2012	15	4.6	Eggers et al. (2015)
CCV	Alcohol	Ethanol	70	Strain I-71	10min	>3.3	Saknimit et al. (1988)
		2-Propanol	50	Strain I-71	10min	>3.7	Saknimit et al. (1988)
	Aldehyde	Formaldehyde	0.7	Strain I-71	10min	>3.7	Saknimit et al. (1988)
			0.009	Strain I-71	24h	>4.0	Pratelli (2008)
	Others	Benzalkonium chloride	0.00175	Strain S378	3d	3.0	Pratelli (2008)
			0.05	Strain I-71	10min	>3.7	Saknimit et al. (1988)
		Didecyldimethyl ammonium chloride	0.0025	Strain S378	3d	>4.0	Pratelli (2008)
		Chlorhexidine digluconate	0.02	Strain I-71	10min	0.3	Saknimit et al. (1988)
		Sodium hypochlorite	0.001	Strain I-71	10min	0.9	Saknimit et al. (1988)
			0.01	Strain I-71	10min	1.1	Saknimit et al. (1988)

SARS-CoV-2, Severe Acute Respiratory Syndrome Coronavirus-2; HCoV, Human Coronavirus; MERS-CoV, Middle East Respiratory Syndrome Coronavirus; CCV, Canine Coronavirus.

Table 3.3 Carrier test – inactivation of coronaviruses by different disinfecting solutions.

Coronavirus family	Class of disinfectant	Disinfectant used	Concentration of used disinfectant (%)	Viral strain	Time of exposure (seconds)	Viral reduction (log10)
SARS-CoV	Alcohol	Ethanol	70	Isolate FFM-1	60	>3.0
	Aldehydes	Glutaraldehyde	2	Isolate FFM-1	60	>3.0
	Others	Sodium hypochlorite	0.01	Isolate FFM-1	60	<3.0
			0.1	Isolate FFM-1	60	>3.0
			0.5	Isolate FFM-1	60	>3.0
		Benzalkonium chloride	0.04	Isolate FFM-1	60	<3.0

SARS-CoV, Severe Acute Respiratory Syndrome Coronavirus.
Source: Based on Kampf et al. (2020).

3.11 Conclusion

Culmination of various studies have shown that the perseverance of coronavirus on any kind of surface and the rate of transmission can be reduced. This reduction can be achieved by plummeting the regularity of coming in contact with surfaces by hands and utilizing disinfectants efficaciously. Even if an individual comes in contact to different kinds of surfaces or mediums, it should be made sure that hand gloves should be worn at all times. The most important and the easiest way to sterilize different surfaces is to clean them with detergents and disinfecting agents. Thorough disinfection with alcohols such as ethanol with a concentration of about 62–70% or H_2O_2 and sodium hypochlorite with a concentration of 0.5 and 0.1%, respectively, must be done. Contact time must vary between 30 and 60 seconds. Temperature and humidity has an important impact in the transmittal of the novel coronavirus disease. Various studies suggest an inversely proportional relationship between the factors and the transmission rate of COVID-19. However food and food packaging material do not pose as much of a risk factor for COVID-19 transmission. As long as good manufacturing practices are followed by the professionals and other personnel in the food industry, COVID-19 transmission rates will remain at a minimal level. Effect of transmission by factors such as water sources and wastewater is minimal; however, the same cannot be stated for the air transmission routes. Although blood-borne arthropods, i.e. mosquitoes and beetles are evident in transmitting pathogens, SARS-CoV-2 can be excluded, but there is a need in keeping checks regarding insects being a probable dynamic in the spread of the novel coronavirus. Personal hygiene has the most crucial effect on the transmission of COVID-19. Regular washing and disinfection of body parts especially hands after coming in contact with a surface or symptomatic people is necessary. Environmental factors may or may not have an effect in the transmission of COVID-19, but it is up to an individual to tackle the spread of COVID-19 by practicing appropriate regulatory measures.

Table 3.4 Kinetics of SARS-CoV-2 and SARS-CoV-1 neutralization by the means of UV-C irradiation.

Virus	UV radiation wavelength (nm)	Irradiance (mJ cm^{-2})	Time of UV-C exposure	Medium	Initial concentration	Reduction in viral concentration (log)	References
SARS-CoV-2	254	40.0	—	Liquid	250 μl	6	Patterson et al. (2020)
		20.0	—	Liquid	250 μl	3.9	Patterson et al. (2020)
		10.0	—	Liquid	250 μl	2.1	Patterson et al. (2020)
	280 ± 5	75.0	20 min	Liquid	150 μl	3.3	Inagaki et al. (2020)
		37.5	10 min	Liquid	150 μl	3.1	Inagaki et al. (2020)
		3.75	1 min	Liquid	150 μl	0.9	Inagaki et al. (2020)
	254	84.4	24 h	Liquid	976 μl	6	Bianco et al. (2020)
		16.9	48 h	Liquid	976 μl	6	Bianco et al. (2020)
		3.70	72 h	Liquid	976 μl	3	Bianco et al. (2020)
	254	2.14	72 h	Solid	—	1	Pendyala et al. (2020)
SARS-CoV-1	260	90.0	60 min	Solid	6 log$_{10}$ TCID$_{50}$	6	Duan et al. (2003)
	254	4016	6 min	—	5.5 log$_{10}$ TCID$_{50}$	4	Darnell et al. (2004)
		134	15 min	—	7.5 log$_{10}$ TCID$_{50}$	5.3	Kariwa et al. (2006)
		134	60 min	—	7.5 log$_{10}$ TCID$_{50}$	6.3	Kariwa et al. (2006)

SARS-CoV-2, Severe Acute Respiratory Syndrome Coronavirus-2; SARS-CoV-1, Severe Acute Respiratory Syndrome Coronavirus-1; TCID, Tissue Culture Infectious Dosage.

References

Askari, S.G., Khatbasreh, M., Ehrampoush, M.H. et al. (2018). The relationship between environmental exposures and hormonal abnormalities in pregnant women: an epidemiological study in Yazd, Iran. *Women and Birth* 31: e204–e209. https://doi.org/10.1016/j.wombi.2017.09.002.

Barratt, R., Shaban, R.Z., and Gilbert, G.L. (2019). Clinician perceptions of respiratory infection risk; a rationale for research into mask use in routine practice. *Infect. Dis. Heal.* 24: 169–176. https://doi.org/10.1016/j.idh.2019.01.003.

Bhattacharjee, S. (2020). Statistical investigation of relationship between spread of coronavirus disease (COVID-19) and environmental factors based on study of four mostly affected places of China and five mostly affected places of Italy. arXiv:200311277.

Bianco, A., Biasin, M., Pareschi, G. et al. (2020). UV-C irradiation is highly effective in inactivating and inhibiting SARS-CoV-2 replication. medRxiv 2020.06.05.20123463. https://doi.org/10.1101/2020.06.05.20123463.

Bin, S.Y., Heo, J.Y., Song, M.-S. et al. (2016). Environmental contamination and viral shedding in MERS patients during MERS-CoV outbreak in South Korea. *Clin. Infect. Dis.* 62: 755–760. https://doi.org/10.1093/cid/civ1020.

Bowdle, A. and Munoz-Price, L.S. (2020). Preventing infection of patients and healthcare workers should be the new normal in the era of novel coronavirus epidemics: reply. *Anesthesiology* 133: 463–464. https://doi.org/10.1097/ALN.0000000000003372.

Card, K.J., Crozier, D., Dhawan, A., Dinh, M., Dolson, E., Farrokhian, N., Gopalakrishnan, V., Ho, E., Jagdish, T., King, E.S., Krishnan, N., Kuzmin, G., Maltas, J., Mo, J., Pelesko, J., Scarborough, J.A., Scott, J.G., Sedor, G., Tian, E., Weaver, D.T., 2020. UV sterilization of personal protective equipment with idle laboratory biosafety cabinets during the Covid-19 pandemic. https://doi.org/10.1101/2020.03.25.20043489.

CDC (2020a). Infection control guidance for healthcare professionals about coronavirus (COVID-19). CDC [WWW Document]. https://www.cdc.gov/coronavirus/2019-ncov/hcp/infection-control.html?CDC_AA_refVal=https%3A%2F%2Fwww.cdc.gov%2Fcoronavirus%2F2019-ncov%2Finfection-control.html (accessed 10 October 2020).

CDC (2020b). How flu spreads. CDC [WWW Document]. https://www.cdc.gov/flu/about/disease/spread.htm (accessed 10 December 2020).

Chan, K.H., Peiris, J.S.M., Lam, S.Y. et al. (2011). The effects of temperature and relative humidity on the viability of the SARS coronavirus. *Adv. Virol.* 2011: 734690. https://doi.org/10.1155/2011/734690.

Chen, Y., Chen, L., Deng, Q. et al. (2020). The presence of SARS-CoV-2 RNA in the feces of COVID-19 patients. *J. Med. Virol.* 92: 833–840. https://doi.org/https://doi.org/10.1002/jmv.25825.

Chien, L.-C. and Chen, L.-W. (2020). Meteorological impacts on the incidence of COVID-19 in the U.S. *Stoch. Environ. Res. Risk Assess* 34: 1675–1680. https://doi.org/10.1007/s00477-020-01835-8.

Chin, A., Chu, J., Perera, M. et al. (2020). Stability of SARS-CoV-2 in different environmental conditions. *The Lancet Microbe* https://doi.org/10.1101/2020.03.15.20036673.

Chiyomaru, K. and Takemoto, K. (2020). Global COVID-19 transmission rate is influenced by precipitation seasonality and the speed of climate temperature warming. *medRxiv* https://doi.org/10.1101/2020.04.10.20060459.

Cramer, A., Tian, E., Yu, S.H., Galanek, M., Lamere, E., Li, J., Gupta, R., Short, M.P., 2020. Disposable N95 masks pass qualitative fit-test but have decreased filtration efficiency after cobalt-60 gamma irradiation. https://doi.org/10.1101/2020.03.28.20043471.

D'Amico, F., Baumgart, D.C., Danese, S., and Peyrin-Biroulet, L. (2020). Diarrhea during COVID-19 infection: pathogenesis, epidemiology, prevention, and management. *Clin. Gastroenterol. Hepatol.* 18: 1663–1672. https://doi.org/https://doi.org/10.1016/j.cgh.2020.04.001.

Darnell, M.E.R., Subbarao, K., Feinstone, S.M., and Taylor, D.R. (2004). Inactivation of the coronavirus that induces severe acute respiratory syndrome. *SARS-CoV. J. Virol. Methods* 121: 85–91. https://doi.org/10.1016/j.jviromet.2004.06.006.

Dehghani, R. and Kassiri, H. (2020). A brief review on the possible role of houseflies and cockroaches in the mechanical transmission of coronavirus disease 2019 (COVID-19). *Arch. Clin. Infect. Dis.* 15: https://doi.org/10.5812/archcid.102863.

Dey, A., Rao, P.K., and Rawtani, D. (2022). Risk management of COVID-19. In: *COVID-19 in the Environment*, 217–230. https://doi.org/10.1016/B978-0-323-90272-4.00018-X.

van Doremalen, N., Bushmaker, T., and Munster, V.J. (2013). Stability of middle east respiratory syndrome coronavirus (MERS-CoV) under different environmental conditions. *Eurosurveillance* 18: 20590. https://doi.org/10.2807/1560-7917.ES2013.18.38.20590.

van Doremalen, N., Bushmaker, T., Morris, D.H. et al. (2020). Aerosol and surface stability of SARS-CoV-2 as compared with SARS-CoV-1. *N. Engl. J. Med.* 382: 1564–1567. https://doi.org/10.1056/NEJMc2004973.

Duan, S.-M., Zhao, X.-S., Wen, R.-F. et al. (2003). Stability of SARS coronavirus in human specimens and environment and its sensitivity to heating and UV irradiation. *Biomed. Environ. Sci.* 16: 246–255.

Eggers, M., Eickmann, M., and Zorn, J. (2015). Rapid and effective virucidal activity of povidone-iodine products against middle east respiratory syndrome coronavirus (MERS-CoV) and modified vaccinia virus ankara (MVA). *Infect. Dis. Ther.* 4: 491–501. https://doi.org/10.1007/s40121-015-0091-9.

Eggers, M., Koburger-Janssen, T., Eickmann, M., and Zorn, J. (2018). In vitro bactericidal and virucidal efficacy of povidone-iodine gargle/mouthwash against respiratory and oral tract pathogens. *Infect. Dis. Ther.* 7: 249–259. https://doi.org/10.1007/s40121-018-0200-7.

Eslami, H. and Jalili, M. (2020). The role of environmental factors to transmission of SARS - CoV - 2 (COVID - 19). *AMB Express* https://doi.org/10.1186/s13568-020-01028-0.

Fears, A.C., Klimstra, W.B., Duprex, P. et al. (2020). Comparative dynamic aerosol efficiencies of three emergent coronaviruses and the unusual persistence of SARS-CoV-2 in aerosol suspensions. medRxiv 2020.04.13.20063784. https://doi.org/10.1101/2020.04.13.20063784.

Feldmann, F., Shupert, W.L., Haddock, E. et al. (2019). Gamma irradiation as an effective method for inactivation of emerging viral pathogens. *Am. J. Trop. Med. Hyg.* 100: 1275–1277. https://doi.org/10.4269/ajtmh.18-0937.

Frithiof, R., Bergqvist, A., Järhult, J.D. et al. (2020). Presence of SARS-CoV-2 in urine is rare and not associated with acute kidney injury in critically ill COVID-19 patients. *Crit. Care* 24: 587. https://doi.org/10.1186/s13054-020-03302-w.

Gorbalenya, A.E., Baker, S.C., Baric, R.S. et al. (2020). Severe acute respiratory syndrome-related coronavirus: the species and its viruses – a statement of the Coronavirus Study Group. *bioRxiv* https://doi.org/10.1101/2020.02.07.937862.

Graczyk, T.K., Knight, R., and Tamang, L. (2005). Mechanical transmission of human protozoan parasites by insects. *Clin. Microbiol. Rev.* 18: 128–132. https://doi.org/10.1128/CMR.18.1.128-132.2005.

Greenhalgh, T., Schmid, M.B., Czypionka, T. et al. (2020). Face masks for the public during the covid-19 crisis. *BMJ* 369: m1435. https://doi.org/10.1136/bmj.m1435.

Henwood, A.F. (2020). Coronavirus disinfection in histopathology. *J. Histotechnol.* 43: 102–104. https://doi.org/10.1080/01478885.2020.1734718.

Ijaz, M.K., Brunner, A.H., Sattar, S.A. et al. (1985). Survival characteristics of airborne human coronavirus 229E. *J. Gen. Virol.* 66 (Pt 12): 2743–2748. https://doi.org/10.1099/0022-1317-66-12-2743.

Inagaki, H., Saito, A., Sugiyama, H. et al. (2020). Rapid inactivation of SARS-CoV-2 with deep-UV LED irradiation. *Emerg. Microbes Infect.* 9: 1744–1747. https://doi.org/10.1080/22221751.2020.1796529.

Kampf, G., Todt, D., Pfaender, S., and Steinmann, E. (2020). Persistence of coronaviruses on inanimate surfaces and their inactivation with biocidal agents. *J. Hosp. Infect.* 104: 246–251. https://doi.org/10.1016/j.jhin.2020.01.022.

Kariwa, H., Fujii, N., and Takashima, I. (2006). Inactivation of SARS coronavirus by means of povidone-iodine, physical conditions and chemical reagents. *Dermatology* 212 (suppl): 119–123. https://doi.org/10.1159/000089211.

Kelly, N., Nic Íomhair, A., and McKenna, G. (2020). Can oral rinses play a role in preventing transmission of Covid 19 infection? *Evid. Based. Dent.* 21: 42–43. https://doi.org/10.1038/s41432-020-0099-1.

Kenney, P., Chan, B.K., Kortright, K., Cintron, M., Havill, N., Russi, M., Epright, J., Lee, L., Balcezak, T., Martinello, R., 2020. Hydrogen Peroxide Vapor sterilization of N95 respirators for reuse. https://doi.org/10.1101/2020.03.24.20041087.

Khatri, N., Tyagi, S., Tharmavaram, M., and Rawtani, D. (2020). Sewage water: from waste to resource – a review. 33: 108–135. https://doi.org/10.1080/10406026.2020.1822616.

Kobayashi, M., Agui, N., Sasaki, T. et al. (1999). Houseflies: not simple mechanical vectors of enterohemorrhagic Escherichia coli O157:H7. *Am. J. Trop. Med. Hyg.* 61: 625–629. https://doi.org/10.4269/ajtmh.1999.61.625.

Kowalski, W. (2009a). *UVGI Disinfection Theory BT - Ultraviolet Germicidal Irradiation Handbook: UVGI for Air and Surface Disinfection* (ed. W. Kowalski), 17–50. Berlin, Heidelberg: Springer https://doi.org/10.1007/978-3-642-01999-9_2.

Kowalski, W. (2009b). *Microbiological Testing BT - Ultraviolet Germicidal Irradiation Handbook: UVGI for Air and Surface Disinfection* (ed. W. Kowalski), 337–359. Berlin, Heidelberg: Springer https://doi.org/10.1007/978-3-642-01999-9_14.

van Kuijk, F.J. (1991). Effects of ultraviolet light on the eye: role of protective glasses. *Environ. Health Perspect.* 96: 177–184. https://doi.org/10.1289/ehp.9196177.

Lai, T.H.T., Tang, E.W.H., Chau, S.K.Y. et al. (2020). Stepping up infection control measures in ophthalmology during the novel coronavirus outbreak: an experience from Hong Kong. *Graefes Arch. Clin. Exp. Ophthalmol.* 258: 1049–1055. https://doi.org/10.1007/s00417-020-04641-8.

Li, X.-Y., Dai, W.-J., Wu, S.-N. et al. (2020). The occurrence of diarrhea in COVID-19 patients. *Clin. Res. Hepatol. Gastroenterol.* 44: 284–285. https://doi.org/10.1016/j.clinre.2020.03.017.

Lodder, W. and de Roda Husman, A.M. (2020). SARS-CoV-2 in wastewater: potential health risk, but also data source. lancet. *Gastroenterol. Hepatol.* 5: 533–534. https://doi.org/10.1016/S2468-1253(20)30087-X.

Loffredo, L., Pacella, F., Pacella, E. et al. (2020). Conjunctivitis and COVID-19: a meta-analysis. *J. Med. Virol.* 92: 1413–1414. https://doi.org/10.1002/jmv.25938.

Maleki, M., Mahmoudi, M.R., Heydari, M.H., and Pho, K.-H. (2020). Modeling and forecasting the spread and death rate of coronavirus (COVID-19) in the world using time series models. *Chaos, Solitons Fractals* 140: 110151. https://doi.org/10.1016/j.chaos.2020.110151.

Medema, G., Heijnen, L., Elsinga, G. et al. (2020). Presence of SARS-coronavirus-2 in sewage. *medRxiv.*

Naddeo, V. and Liu, H. (2020). Correction: editorial perspectives: 2019 novel coronavirus (SARS-CoV-2): what is its fate in urban water cycle and how can the water research community respond? *Environ. Sci. Water Res. Technol.* 6: 1939. https://doi.org/10.1039/d0ew90030c.

Omidbakhsh, N. and Sattar, S.A. (2006). Broad-spectrum microbicidal activity, toxicologic assessment, and materials compatibility of a new generation of accelerated hydrogen peroxide-based environmental surface disinfectant. *Am. J. Infect. Control* 34: 251–257. https://doi.org/10.1016/j.ajic.2005.06.002.

Ong, S.W.X., Tan, Y.K., Chia, P.Y. et al. (2020). Air, surface environmental, and personal protective equipment contamination by severe acute respiratory syndrome coronavirus 2 (SARS-CoV-2) from a symptomatic patient. *JAMA* 323: 1610–1612. https://doi.org/10.1001/jama.2020.3227.

Parry, J. (2004). WHO queries culling of civet cats. *BMJ* 328: 128. https://doi.org/10.1136/bmj.328.7432.128-b.

Patterson, E.I., Prince, T., Anderson, E.R. et al. (2020). Methods of inactivation of SARS-CoV-2 for downstream biological assays. bioRxiv 2020.05.21.108035. https://doi.org/10.1101/2020.05.21.108035.

Pendyala, B., Patras, A., and D'Souza, D. (2020). Genomic modeling as an approach to identify surrogates for use in experimental validation of SARS-CoV-2 and HuNoVs inactivation by UV-C treatment. bioRxiv 2020.06.14.151290. https://doi.org/10.1101/2020.06.14.151290.

Peng, J., Wu, X., Wang, R. et al. (2020). Medical waste management practice during the 2019-2020 novel coronavirus pandemic: experience in a general hospital. *Am. J. Infect. Control* 48: 918–921. https://doi.org/10.1016/j.ajic.2020.05.035.

Phua, J., Weng, L., Ling, L. et al. (2020). Intensive care management of coronavirus disease 2019 (COVID-19): challenges and recommendations. *Lancet Respir. Med.* 8: 506–517. https://doi.org/10.1016/S2213-2600(20)30161-2.

Pradhan, D., Biswasroy, P., Kumar Naik, P. et al. (2020). A review of current interventions for COVID-19 prevention. *Arch. Med. Res.* 51: 363–374. https://doi.org/10.1016/j.arcmed.2020.04.020.

Pratelli, A. (2008). Canine coronavirus inactivation with physical and chemical agents. *Vet. J.* 177: 71–79. https://doi.org/10.1016/j.tvjl.2007.03.019.

Purohit, S., Rao, P.K., and Rawtani, D. (2022). Sampling and analytical techniques for COVID-19. In: *COVID-19 in the Environment*, 75–94. https://doi.org/10.1016/B978-0-323-90272-4.00008-7.

Pyankov, O.V., Bodnev, S.A., Pyankova, O.G., and Agranovski, I.E. (2018). Survival of aerosolized coronavirus in the ambient air. *J. Aerosol Sci.* 115: 158–163. https://doi.org/10.1016/j.jaerosci.2017.09.009.

Qing, H., Li, Z., Yang, Z. et al. (2020). The possibility of COVID-19 transmission from eye to nose. *Acta Ophthalmol.* 98: e388–e388. https://doi.org/10.1111/aos.14412.

Qu, G., Li, X., Hu, L., and Jiang, G. (2020). An imperative need for research on the role of environmental factors in transmission of novel coronavirus (COVID-19). *Environ. Sci. Technol.* 54: 3730–3732. https://doi.org/10.1021/acs.est.0c01102.

Rabenau, H.F., Cinatl, J., Morgenstern, B. et al. (2005a). Stability and inactivation of SARS coronavirus. *Med. Microbiol. Immunol.* 194: 1–6. https://doi.org/10.1007/s00430-004-0219-0.

Rabenau, H.F., Kampf, G., Cinatl, J., and Doerr, H.W. (2005b). Efficacy of various disinfectants against SARS coronavirus. *J. Hosp. Infect.* 61: 107–111. https://doi.org/10.1016/j.jhin.2004.12.023.

Raeiszadeh, M. and Adeli, B. (2020). A critical review on ultraviolet disinfection systems against COVID-19 outbreak: applicability, validation, and safety considerations. *ACS Photonics* https://doi.org/10.1021/acsphotonics.0c01245.

Rao, P.K. and Rawtani, D. (2022). Modern digital techniques for monitoring and analysis. In: *COVID-19 in the Environment*, 115–130. https://doi.org/10.1016/B978-0-323-90272-4.00015-4.

Rizou, M., Galanakis, I.M., Aldawoud, T.M.S., and Galanakis, C.M. (2020). Safety of foods, food supply chain and environment within the COVID-19 pandemic. *Trends Food Sci. Technol.* 102: 293–299. https://doi.org/10.1016/j.tifs.2020.06.008.

Saadat, S., Rawtani, D., and Hussain, C.M. (2020). Environmental perspective of COVID-19. *Sci. Total Environ.* 728: 138870. https://doi.org/10.1016/j.scitotenv.2020.138870.

Saknimit, M., Inatsuki, I., Sugiyama, Y., and Yagami, K. (1988). Virucidal efficacy of physico-chemical treatments against coronaviruses and parvoviruses of laboratory animals. *Jikken Dobutsu* 37: 341–345. https://doi.org/10.1538/expanim1978.37.3_341.

Scheller, C., Krebs, F., Minkner, R. et al. (2020). Physicochemical properties of SARS-CoV-2 for drug targeting, virus inactivation and attenuation, vaccine formulation and quality control. *Electrophoresis* 41: 1137–1151. https://doi.org/10.1002/elps.202000121.

Schwartz, J., King, C.-C., and Yen, M.-Y. (2020). Protecting healthcare workers during the coronavirus disease 2019 (COVID-19) outbreak: lessons from Taiwan's severe acute respiratory syndrome response. *Clin. Infect. Dis.* 71: 858–860. https://doi.org/10.1093/cid/ciaa255.

Seymour, N., Yavelak, M., Christian, C. et al. (2020a). COVID-19 FAQ for food service: receiving and food packaging. EDIS 2020.

Seymour, N., Yavelak, M., Christian, C. et al. (2020b). COVID-19 preventative measures: Homemade hand sanitizer. EDIS 2020.

Shankar, A., Saini, D., Roy, S. et al. (2020). Cancer care delivery challenges amidst Coronavirus Disease - 19 (COVID-19) outbreak: specific precautions for cancer patients and cancer care providers to prevent spread. *Asian Pac. J. Cancer Prev.* 21: 569–573. https://doi.org/10.31557/APJCP.2020.21.3.569.

Siddharta, A., Pfaender, S., Vielle, N.J. et al. (2017). Virucidal activity of World Health Organization–recommended formulations against enveloped viruses, including Zika, Ebola, and emerging coronaviruses. *J. Infect. Dis.* 215: 902–906. https://doi.org/10.1093/infdis/jix046.

Sohrabi, C., Alsafi, Z., O'Neill, N. et al. (2020). Corrigendum to "World Health Organization declares global emergency: a review of the 2019 novel coronavirus (COVID-19)" [Int. J. Surg. 76 (2020) 71–76]. *Int. J. Surg.* 77: 217. https://doi.org/10.1016/j.ijsu.2020.03.036.

Sun, C.-B., Wang, Y.-Y., Liu, G.-H., and Liu, Z. (2020). Role of the eye in transmitting human coronavirus: what we know and what we do not know. *Front. Public Health* 8: 155. https://doi.org/10.3389/fpubh.2020.00155.

Swerdlow, D.L. and Finelli, L. (2020). Preparation for possible sustained transmission of 2019 novel coronavirus. *JAMA* 323: 1129. https://doi.org/10.1001/jama.2020.1960.

Tobías, A. and Molina, T. (2020). Is temperature reducing the transmission of COVID-19? *Environ. Res.* 186: 109553. https://doi.org/10.1016/j.envres.2020.109553.

Wang, J., Tang, K., Feng, K. et al. (2020a). High temperature and high humidity reduce the transmission of COVID-19. arXiv Popul. Evol.

Wang, M., Jiang, A., Gong, L., Luo, L., Guo, W., Li, Chuyi, Zheng, J., Li, Chaoyong, Yang, B., Zeng, J., Chen, Y., Zheng, K., Li, H., 2020b. Temperature significant change COVID-19 Transmission in 429 cities. https://doi.org/10.1101/2020.02.22.20025791.

Ward, M.P., Xiao, S., and Zhang, Z. (2020). Humidity is a consistent climatic factor contributing to SARS-CoV-2 transmission. *Transbound. Emerg. Dis.* https://doi.org/10.1111/tbed.13766.

Warnes, S.L., Little, Z.R., and Keevil, C.W. (2015). Human coronavirus 229E remains infectious on common touch surface materials. *MBio* 6: e01697–e01615. https://doi.org/10.1128/mBio.01697-15.

WHO (2020a). Report of the WHO-China Joint Mission on Coronavirus Disease 2019 (COVID-19). WHO-China Jt. Mission Coronavirus Dis. 2019 2019, 16–24.

WHO (2020b). Water, sanitation, hygiene and waste management for COVID-19: technical brief, 03 March 2020. World Health Organization, Geneva PP - Geneva.

WHO (2020c). COVID-19 and food safety: guidance for food businesses: interim guidance. COVID-19 Food Saf. Guid. food businesses Interim Guid. 1–6. https://doi.org/10.4060/ca8660en.

WHO (2020d). Water, sanitation, hygiene, and waste management for the COVID-19 virus: interim guidance, 23 April 2020. World Health Organization.

WHO (2020e). Laboratory biosafety guidance related to coronavirus disease (COVID-19). Interim Guid. 1–5.

Wood, A. and Payne, D. (1998). The action of three antiseptics/disinfectants against enveloped and non-enveloped viruses. *J. Hosp. Infect.* 38: 283–295. https://doi.org/10.1016/S0195-6701(98)90077-9.

Wu, Z. and McGoogan, J.M. (2020). Characteristics of and important lessons from the Coronavirus Disease 2019 (COVID-19) outbreak in China. *JAMA* 323: 1239. https://doi.org/10.1001/jama.2020.2648.

Xie, M. and Chen, Q. (2020). Insight into 2019 novel coronavirus an updated interim review and lessons from SARS-CoV and MERS-CoV. *Int. J. Infect. Dis.* 94: 119–124. https://doi.org/10.1016/j.ijid.2020.03.071.

Yang, C. (2020). Does hand hygiene reduce SARS-CoV-2 transmission? *Graefes Arch. Clin. Exp. Ophthalmol.* 258: 1133–1134. https://doi.org/10.1007/s00417-020-04652-5.

Yen, M.-Y., Schwartz, J., Hsueh, P.-R. et al. (2015). Traffic control bundling is essential for protecting healthcare workers and controlling the 2014 Ebola epidemic. *Clin. Infect. Dis.* 60: 823–825. https://doi.org/10.1093/cid/ciu978.

Yen, M.-Y., Schwartz, J., Chen, S.-Y. et al. (2020). Interrupting COVID-19 transmission by implementing enhanced traffic control bundling: implications for global prevention and control efforts. *J. Microbiol. Immunol. Infect.* 53: 377–380. https://doi.org/10.1016/j.jmii.2020.03.011.

Zhi, Z.Y.K.J. (2020). Suggestions from ophthalmic experts on eye protection during the novel coronavirus pneumonia epidemic. *Zhonghua. Yan Ke Za Zhi.* 56: E002. https://doi.org/10.3760/cma.j.issn.0412-4081.2020.0002.

4

Models and Strategies for Controlling the Transmission of COVID-19

Yiğitcan Sümbelli[1], Semra Köse[1], Rüstem Keçili[2], and Chaudhery Mustansar Hussain[3]

[1] Department of Chemistry, Eskişehir Tehnical University, Eskişehir, Turkey
[2] Department of Medical Services and Techniques, Anadolu University, Yunus Emre Vocational School of Health Services, Eskişehir, Turkey
[3] Department of Chemistry and Environmental Science, New Jersey Institute of Technology, Newark, NJ, USA

4.1   Introduction

When 2019 was coming to an end, a novel coronavirus disease (COVID-19) caused by severe acute respiratory syndrome coronavirus-2 (SARS-CoV-2) has started to spread, and the World Health Organization (WHO) has declared the disease a pandemic on 11 March 2020 (WHO 2020), which was arguably a late decision. The reason behind the critics for WHO's slow-acting was lying beneath the COVID-19's transmission ways. Globally, on 7 September 2021, there have been 221,134,742 confirmed COVID-19 cases and 4,574,089 deaths reported to WHO (2021).

Although most countries have taken domestic and international precautions since the outbreak's first signals, the transmission rate was much faster than to take it under control. The transmission dynamics for the COVID-19 were evaluated by researchers in many studies, and airborne spreading is pointed out as the major transmission model. In a recently reported study (Orenes-Piñero et al. 2021), real-world data about the air transmission dynamics of COVID-19 were presented. The achieved data exhibited that the virus could transmit through several surfaces, although the air of the room was completely renewed 50–60 times per hour. This was a shred of direct evidence for the air transmittance of the virus since the incubated patients have not spread the virus in their study.

This chapter focuses on the transmission models and control strategies for the transmission of COVID-19. The chapter starts with the description of the various routes for the transmission of COVID-19. Then, different models for the transmission of COVID-19 are presented, and finally, various strategies for the transmission control of COVID-19 are provided and discussed.

4.2 Routes for the Transmission of COVID-19

Various routes for the transmission of COVID-19 have been proposed as schematically demonstrated in Figure 4.1. These routes include surface contamination, aerosol, and the fecal-oral routes.

The direct route of transmission can be through aerosols generated from respiratory droplets of patients infected with COVID-19 during different processes including surgery and dental treatments. The other routes of direct transmission are secretions from a person infected with COVID-19, such as saliva, tears, semen, urine, and fecal matter. The transmission of virus from mother to newborn is also a direct mode of transmission. Indirect mode of transmission includes surfaces of furniture and fixtures came in immediate contact of the infected person or the objects used by the patient.

There are some reported studies recommending the duration of viability of the COVID-19 virus on different surfaces. For example, Stanam and colleagues reported that the virus is viable on the surfaces of plastic and stainless steel-based materials for three days. It was also reported that the virus is stable in the fecal matter for a couple of days at room temperature. However, a temperature of more than 55 °C lead to degradation of COVID-19 virus structure (Pawar et al. 2020). In addition, the COVID-19 virus can also be controlled through ultraviolet radiations, and therefore this process can be successfully applied for sterilization purpose.

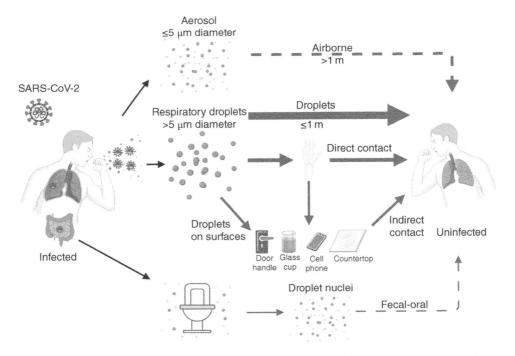

Figure 4.1 The proposed various routes for the transmission of COVID-19. *Source:* Reproduced with permission from Harrison et al. (2020).

There are a number of published reports that indicate the transmission of COVID-19 virus through fecal-oral transmission since COVID-19 virus was detected in the sewage samples and stools (Heller et al. 2020). The transmission of COVID-19 virus may also occur via eyes. There are less reported studies on this issue. However, the COVID-19 virus is tested through the teas and other conjunctival emissions. The COVID-19 virus may spread during treatment of eyes, and thus there were special guidelines for the ophthalmic diagnosis to follow while the procedures opted (Sun et al. 2020). In a study carried out by Repici and colleagues, it was highlighted that various treatments including endoscopy may also result in transmission of the virus due to very less distance between the health personnel and the infected patient. Even asymptomatic patients can be a risk for the person executing endoscopy (Repici et al. 2020).

The quarantine period optimal for controlling the COVID-19 is 14 days as the incubation period of the virus is 14 days, approximately. The COVID-19 virus may spread from pregnant woman to infant. The first such case was reported in Shenzhen, and there after many such cases were reported. However, the fatality or mortality is negligible (Jiang et al. 2020).

In another report published by Chen and co-worker, a case study of four newborns born to infected mothers at initial stage of the pregnancy was presented. The infected mothers exhibited the typical symptoms of COVID-19 such as cough, fever, and body ache; however, the level of lymphocytes was found to be less than the normal values at the time of hospitalization. The newborns tested negative, and the four mothers recovered from the disease after few days. So, it showed that the virus did not spread from the mothers to the newborns (Chen et al. 2020). On the other hand, Liu and colleagues recommended their immunological point of view for the reason of more susceptibility of pregnant women to COVID-19 (Liu et al. 2020).

4.3   Models for the Transmission of COVID-19

Ying and O'Clery used an agent-based model for COVID-19 spreading in supermarkets (Ying and O'Clery 2021). They ignored the fomite and airborne transmission in their model due to short exposure time and considered respiratory droplet transmission, which is the main reason according to WHO (n.d.). There are two components in their model: customer mobility and viral spreading, which are people's and viruses' movement in the store, respectively. According to their model, when a customer spends 5.97 minutes in the store with an average of 14.96 customers present in the store at the same time, the potential infection rate is found to be 17.69%, when every customer is exposed to an infected person for 0.26 minutes in average.

In a study which was conducted by Chang et al., researchers modeled the transmission in a larger area than Ying and O'Clery's study. They used Australia as their network and applied their model to compare different control mechanisms for the transmission of COVID-19. According to their data, while school closures are not very effective to prevent the spreading, social distancing is found as the most effective method.

Nouvellet et al.'s study also supports the same finding as Chang et al.'s study. According to their data which was obtained by comparing 52 countries' data, social distancing and the reduction of mobility have a significant effect on the transmission of the disease (Nouvellet et al. 2021).

In a more clustered study conducted by Azimi et al., they modeled a transmission model on a cruise ship, Diamond Princess specifically (Azimi et al. 2021). According to their model, it was stated that more than half of the transmission was caused by ineffective social distancing, thus airborne spread. Even with high ventilation rates in a closed network such as a cruise ship, their findings support the airborne spread by small aerosols is the dominant transmission model.

Lastly, Ndaïrou et al. used mathematical modeling for the transmission dynamics of COVID-19 by using a case study in Wuhan in their study (Ndaïrou et al. 2020). According to their study, researchers were able to predict the number of confirmed cases in a more approximate way than the other modeling studies, which was due to taking super-spreaders into account by using their approach.

4.4 Strategies for the Transmission Control of COVID-19

Different control measures are recommended by the researchers for the transmission control of COVID-19. On social front, the countries impacted by diseases, initially, planned and executed some well-organized policies that provided the control of the pandemic. The countries issued measures taken by government and quickly disseminated the information that helped to get full compliance and public support. For example, in Africa, various strategies such as education awareness campaigns, testing for those who appeared to be infected with some other contacts were planned in order to efficient control of the pandemic. The measures were to put a hold on the flourishing of the COVID-19 virus and therefore its harmful impacts on humans (Fanidi et al. 2020). One of the most severely impacted countries was Switzerland, which reported a huge number of cases per capita. Salathé and colleagues reported the importance of testing and contact tracing and isolation in the country. Contact tracing and isolation are common intrusion to careful control of the transmission of COVID-19. Testing may not directly stop the spread of virus; however, the spread can be controlled by detecting the people with infections even for clinical disease compatible with COVID-19. The testing is a very crucial part of measure to control the disease as rapid diagnosis. Therefore, instant isolation of the people infected with COVID-19 may help to combat the disease. In their study, the authors concluded that the testing is a tool to strengthen the measures to control the diseases (Salathé et al. 2020).

The drug therapy against COVID-19 is still in the trial phase. However, there are various drugs which are used for the treatment of people infected with COVID-19 virus based on the extensive research on the virology studies on COVID-19 virus. For example, as reported by Sanders and coworkers in a review paper, Remdesivir is one the most promising drug in use against COVID-19 virus since it exhibited appreciable in vitro activity toward the virus. However, it has not been approved by FDA. The other drugs such as Oseltamivir and corticosteroids were not recommended for the treatment of COVID-19 (Sanders et al. 2020).

On the other hand, in a study reported by Mamo (2020), a Susceptible-Stay-at-Home-Exposed-Infected-Quarantine-Recovery-Death (SHEIQRD) model was used to investigate the spread dynamics of COVID-19 with public health intervention The findings of the research stated that negative effects on the socioeconomic situation can be prevented by applying useful control measures by public health intervention. Forgoston and Thorne's study (Forgoston and Thorne 2020) had also used the same modeling approach and found that early lockdown and relaxation programs as a public intervention strategy will not have long-lasting positive effects on the spread control. Their suggestions pointed out the immense effects of test, trace, and isolation program in combination with public intervention such as lockdown strategies as stated earlier.

Another study considering the transmission in the United States was interested in 15 states in the country. Li et al. studied the transmission kinetics in their study (Li et al. 2020), and their findings support the airborne spread mechanisms, the social distancing, and face covering's importance in preventing the transmission. According to their data, approximately 17% of the total infections in the United States were prevented by face covering in seven states, even though only one-third of the country mandated face covering.

One of the most applicable transmission control strategies is suggested as wearing a face mask by most of the authorities, and Rader et al. pointed out the importance of it in their study (Rader et al. 2021). According to that, high mask-wearing ratios in communities have a positive effect on the control of the transmission, and a 10% increase in mask-wearing resulted in an increase in transmission control probability. Clapham and Cook were also supporting these findings in their study with a note stating that mask use is a non-targeted control strategy (Clapham and Cook 2021).

In a study where Law et al. used a time-varying Susceptible-Infectious-Removed (SIR) model, researchers found that lockdown and movement restrictions have a positive effect on the transmission control (Law et al. 2020), which was also supported by Sanyaolu et al.'s study (2020). In another study using the Susceptible-Exposed-Infectious-Recovered (SEIR) model to discuss the effect of control strategies in South Korea, it was found that school closure and social distancing are effective only when the timing of implementation and the levels of transmission were considered. Lee et al. also stated that quarantine and isolation have a sensible effect on the number of cases in their study (Lee et al. 2021).

Li et al. also used the same modeling approach in their study to discuss the transmission control effectiveness in Wenzhou, China (Li et al. 2021). The achieved results confirmed the applied SEIR model can efficiently simulate the spread of COVID-19 in Wenzhou, China. The lockdown in Wuhan cut-off the major transmission routes of imported cases. Therefore, the number of imported cases decreased quite rapidly (<10 cases/day). However, before that, 175 cases had entered the region and lead to significant increase in the transmissions.

The research carried out by Zhang et al. on the control measures in China showed drugs that had the low early report rate was one of the main reasons for the rapid spread (Zhang et al. 2020). Their statement on the undetected cases explains most of the transmissibility of the disease for the initial stages of the pandemic in China.

On the other hand, in a very short time (less than one year) just after the beginning of the COVID-19 pandemic, a number of researchers started to design and develop effective COVID-19 vaccines using various technologies such as mRNA, viral vector, and conventional inactive vaccines (Sharma et al. 2021). The mRNA vaccine designed and developed by Pfizer and BioNTech was the first COVID-19 vaccine approved by the WHO and FDA (FDA 2021; WHO 2021) and the others such as Moderna, Sputnik V, AstraZeneca and Coronovac, and Johnson & Johnson's Janssen vaccines were produced by different companies. Then, a massive vaccine campaign was started in a number of countries with these vaccines (Mathieu et al. 2021).

4.5 Conclusions

When all the studies and data have been evaluated since the beginning of the pandemic, an approximation for the transmission dynamic can be made. Viruses transmitted through small aerosols are seemed to be the main reason for the airborne spread of COVID-19 up to date, and most of the precautions are taken by considering that. Wearing face masks is the proven self-caution in the personal level and self-quarantining, social distancing, and reducing the number of social gatherings are the following precautions. Official control strategies such as travel restrictions and decreasing the crowds in every aspect of life (such as mandatory working-from-home regulations) are the other part of the transmission control. Various studies showed that rapid testing, tracing, and isolation programs are some of the key elements combined with well-programmed lockdown strategies to control the transmission of the disease.

References

P. Azimi, Z. Keshavarz, J.G. Cedeno Laurent, B. Stephens, J.G. Allen, Mechanistic transmission modeling of COVID-19 on the Diamond Princess cruise ship demonstrates the importance of aerosol transmission, *Proc. Natl. Acad. Sci. U. S. A.* 118 (2021). doi:https://doi.org/10.1073/pnas.2015482118.

Chen, Y., Peng, H., Wang, L. et al. (2020). Infants born to mothers with a new coronavirus (COVID-19). *Front. Pediatr.* 8: 104.

H.E. Clapham, A.R. Cook, Face masks help control transmission of COVID-19, *Lancet Digit. Heal.* 3 (2021) e136–e137. doi:https://doi.org/10.1016/S2589-7500(21)00003-0.

Fanidi, A., Jouven, X., and Gaye, B. (2020). Strategies to control COVID-19 and future pandemics in Africa and around the globe. *Eur. Heart J.* 41 (41): 3973–3975.

FDA (2021). Pfizer-BioNTech COVID-19 Vaccine. https://www.fda.gov/emergency-preparedness-and-response/coronavirus-disease-2019-covid-19/pfizer-biontech-covid-19-vaccine (accessed 8 September 2021).

Forgoston, E. and Thorne, M. (2020). Strategies for controlling the spread of COVID-19. *MedRxiv* https://doi.org/10.1101/2020.06.24.20139014.

Harrison, A.G., Lin, T., and Wang, P. (2020). Mechanisms of SARS-CoV-2 transmission and pathogenesis. *Trends Immunol.* 41 (12): 1100–1115.

Heller, L., Mota, C.R., and Greco, D.B. (2020). COVID-19 faecal-oral transmission: are we asking the right questions? *Sci. Total Environ.* 729: 138919.

Jiang, X., Niu, Y., Li, X. et al. (2020). Is a 14-day quarantine period optimal for effectively controlling coronavirus disease 2019 (COVID-19)? *medRxiv* https://doi.org/10.1101/2020.03.15.20036533.

K.B. Law, K.M. Peariasamy, B.S. Gill, S. Singh, B.M. Sundram, K. Rajendran, S.C. Dass, Y.L. Lee, P.P. Goh, H. Ibrahim, N.H. Abdullah, Tracking the early depleting transmission dynamics of COVID-19 with a time-varying SIR model, *Sci. Rep.* 10 (2020) 1–11. doi:https://doi.org/10.1038/s41598-020-78739-8.

T. Lee, H.D. Kwon, J. Lee, The effect of control measures on COVID-19 transmission in South Korea, *PLoS One* 16 (2021) e0249262. doi:https://doi.org/10.1371/journal.pone.0249262.

Y. Li, R. Zhang, J. Zhao, M.J. Molina, Understanding transmission and intervention for the COVID-19 pandemic in the United States, *Sci. Total Environ.* 748 (2020) 141560. doi: https://doi.org/10.1016/j.scitotenv.2020.141560.

W. Li, J. Gong, J. Zhou, L. Zhang, D. Wang, J. Li, C. Shi, H. Fan, An evaluation of COVID-19 transmission control in Wenzhou using a modified SEIR model, *Epidemiol. Infect.* 149 (2021). doi:https://doi.org/10.1017/S0950268820003064.

Liu, H., Wang, L.-L., Zhao, S.-J. et al. (2020). Why are pregnant women susceptible to viral infection: an immunological viewpoint? *J. Reprod. Immunol.* 139: 103122.

D.K. Mamo, Model the transmission dynamics of COVID-19 propagation with public health intervention, *Results Appl. Math.* 7 (2020) 100123. doi:https://doi.org/10.1016/j.rinam. 2020.100123.

Mathieu, E., Ritchie, H., Ortiz-Ospina, E. et al. (2021). A global database of COVID-19 vaccinations. *Nat. Hum. Behav.* https://doi.org/10.1038/s41562-021-01122-8.

F. Ndaïrou, I. Area, J.J. Nieto, D.F.M. Torres, Mathematical modeling of COVID-19 transmission dynamics with a case study of Wuhan, *Chaos, Solitons Fractals* 135 (2020) 109846. doi:https://doi.org/10.1016/j.chaos.2020.109846.

P. Nouvellet, S. Bhatia, A. Cori, K.E.C. Ainslie, M. Baguelin, S. Bhatt, A. Boonyasiri, N.F. Brazeau, L. Cattarino, L. V. Cooper, H. Coupland, Z.M. Cucunuba, G. Cuomo-Dannenburg, A. Dighe, B.A. Djaafara, I. Dorigatti, O.D. Eales, S.L. van Elsland, F.F. Nascimento, R.G. FitzJohn, K.A.M. Gaythorpe, L. Geidelberg, W.D. Green, A. Hamlet, K. Hauck, W. Hinsley, N. Imai, B. Jeffrey, E. Knock, D.J. Laydon, J.A. Lees, T. Mangal, T.A. Mellan, G. Nedjati-Gilani, K. V. Parag, M. Pons-Salort, M. Ragonnet-Cronin, S. Riley, H.J.T. Unwin, R. Verity, M.A.C. Vollmer, E. Volz, P.G.T. Walker, C.E. Walters, H. Wang, O.J. Watson, C. Whittaker, L.K. Whittles, X. Xi, N.M. Ferguson, C.A. Donnelly, Reduction in mobility and COVID-19 transmission, *Nat. Commun.* 12 (2021) 1–9. doi:https://doi.org/10.1038/s41467-021-21358-2.

E. Orenes-Piñero, F. Baño, D. Navas-Carrillo, A. Moreno-Docón, J.M. Marín, R. Misiego, P. Ramírez, Evidences of SARS-CoV-2 virus air transmission indoors using several untouched surfaces: a pilot study, *Sci. Total Environ.* 751 (2021) 142317. doi:https://doi.org/10.1016/j.scitotenv.2020.142317.

B. Rader, L.F. White, M.R. Burns, J. Chen, J. Brilliant, J. Cohen, J. Shaman, L. Brilliant, M.U.G. Kraemer, J.B. Hawkins, S. V Scarpino, C.M. Astley, J.S. Brownstein, Mask-wearing and control of SARS-CoV-2 transmission in the USA: a cross-sectional study, *Lancet Digit. Heal.* 3 (2021) e148–e157. doi:https://doi.org/10.1016/S2589-7500(20)30293-4.

Repici, A., Maselli, R., Colombo, M. et al. (2020). Coronavirus (COVID-19) outbreak: what the department of endoscopy should know. *Gastrointest. Endosc.* 92 (1): 192–197.

Salathé, M., Althaus, C.L., Neher, R. et al. (2020). COVID-19 epidemic in Switzerland: on the importance of testing, contact tracing and isolation. *Swiss Med. Wkly.* 150 (11–12): 20225.

Sanders, J.M., Monogue, M.L., Jodlowski, T.Z., and Cutrell, J.B. (2020). Pharmacologic treatments for Coronavirus Disease 2019 (COVID-19): a review. *JAMA* 323 (18): 1824–1836.

A. Sanyaolu, C. Okorie, S. Younis, H. Chan, N. Haider, A. F. Abbasi, O. Ayodele,. . ., S. Prakash and A. Marinkovic, Transmission and control efforts of COVID-19, *J. Infect. Dis. Epidemiol.* 6 (2020). doi:https://doi.org/10.23937/2474-3658/1510126.

Sharma, K., Koirala, A., Nicolopoulos, K. et al. (2021). Vaccines for COVID-19: where do we stand in 2021? *Paediatr. Respir. Rev.* 39: 22–31. https://doi.org/10.1016/j.prrv.2021.07.001.

Pawar, S., Stanam, A., Chaudhari, M., and Rayudu, D. (2020). Effects of temperature on COVID-19 transmission. *MedRxiv* https://doi.org/10.1101/2020.03.29.20044461.

Sun, C., Wang, Y.-Y., Liu, G.-H., and Liu, Z. (2020). Role of the eye in transmitting human coronavirus: what we know and what we do not know. *Front. Public Health* 8: 155.

WHO (2020). Director-General's opening remarks at the media briefing on COVID-19. https://www.who.int/director-general/speeches/detail/who-director-general-s-opening-remarks-at-the-media-briefing-on-covid-19---11-march-2020 (accessed 8 September 2021).

WHO (2021). WHO issues its first emergency use validation for a COVID-19 vaccine and emphasizes need for equitable global access. https://www.who.int/news/item/31-12-2020-who-issues-its-first-emergency-use-validation-for-a-covid-19-vaccine-and-emphasizes-need-for-equitable-global-access#:~:text=The%20WHO's%20Emergency%20Use%20Listing,distribution%20to%20countries%20in%20need (accessed 08 September 2021).

WHO (2021) Coronavirus disease (COVID-19): How is it transmitted?. https://www.who.int/news-room/q-a-detail/coronavirus-disease-covid-19-how-is-it-transmitted (accessed 28 December 2021).

World Health Organization (2021). WHO Coronavirus (COVID-19) Dashboard, Data as reported by 7 September 2021. https://covid19.who.int/ (accessed 7 September 2021).

F. Ying, N. O'Clery, Modelling COVID-19 transmission in supermarkets using an agent-based model, *PLoS One* 16 (2021) e0249821. doi:https://doi.org/10.1371/journal.pone.0249821.

X.-S. Zhang, E. Vynnycky, A. Charlett, D. De Angelis, Z. Chen, W. Liu, Transmission dynamics and control measures of COVID-19 outbreak in China: a modelling study *Sci. Rep.*, (2020). 11: 2652. doi:https://doi.org/10.1038/s41598-021-81985-z.

5

Traditional Analytical Techniques and Sampling of COVID-19

Aayush Dey[1], Piyush K. Rao[1], Pratik Kulkarni[1], and Deepak Rawtani[2]

[1] School of Doctoral Studies and Research, National Forensic Sciences University (Ministry of Home Affairs, GOI), Gandhinagar, Gujarat, India
[2] School of Pharmacy, National Forensic Sciences University (Ministry of Home Affairs, GOI), Gandhinagar, Gujarat, India

5.1 Introduction

The transmission of COVID-19 also known as the novel coronavirus caused due to the SARS-CoV-2, a novel betacoronavirus, has posed an unparalleled threat to public health. The rapid rates of disease transmission may be accredited to asymptomatic patients (Bai et al. 2020; Chan et al. 2020; Gudbjartsson et al. 2020). Infectious droplets and fluids from symptomatic patients are responsible for the spread of COVID-19 disease, which is an evident fact. Whereas the transmission of COVID-19 via asymptomatic patients may lead to transmission through the droplet route and indirect transmission if a healthy individual comes in contact with a contaminated environment. The major COVID-19 transmission events can directly be correlated to the massive increment in the number of cases which further complicates the transmission dynamics of COVID-19 (Frieden and Lee 2020; Liu et al. 2020). The basic reproductive number of SARS-CoV-2 (approximately –2.7) (Wu et al. 2020) was similar to that of SARS-CoV, which is markedly lower than that of airborne measles (Guerra et al. 2017), suggesting airborne transmission is not a major route of infection. However, there have been clinical and experimental investigations suggesting possible airborne transmission of SARS-CoV-2. In the experimental setting with the artificial generation of aerosol, SARS-CoV-2 remained detectable in aerosols for up to three hours. In the clinical setting, the collection of air samples in patients' rooms is the most direct approach to get a definitive answer but the findings were inconsistent. In an earlier Singapore study, SARS-CoV-2 RNA was not detected in the air samples collected adjacent to the patient's head. A subsequent study demonstrated SARS-CoV-2 RNA in 44% of air samples in an intensive care unit (ICU) in Wuhan, China, although the average viral load in the air samples was low (Guo et al. 2020).

It is an established fact that SARS-CoV-2 virus is mainly transmitted via infectious respiratory droplets. However, in cases regarding other viral strains of the coronavirus family

The Environmental Impact of COVID-19, First Edition. Edited by Deepak Rawtani and Chaudhery Mustansar Hussain.
© 2024 John Wiley & Sons Ltd. Published 2024 by John Wiley & Sons Ltd.

such as SARS and MERS, SARS-CoV-2 strain has been positively affirmed in stool samples from patients exhibiting symptoms of COVID-19 and also from patients exhibiting no symptoms of COVID-19, also known as asymptomatic patients. The duration of viral shedding has been observed to vary among patients with means of 14–21 days (Guerra et al. 2017) as well as the magnitude of shedding varies from 10^2 up to 10^8 RNA copies per gram. Infectious viruses derived from fecal and urine specimens have reportedly been cultured in Vero E6 cells. In addition, gastric, duodenal, and rectal epithelial cells are infected by SARS-CoV-2 and the release of the infectious virions to the gastrointestinal tract supports the possible fecal-oral transmission route. Even though the possibility of fecal-oral transmission has been hypothesized, the role of secretions in the spreading of the disease is not clarified yet. In the context of wastewater-based epidemiology, which is basically a pool for chemical and biological markers regarding human activity, viral diseases have been also charted by the detection of genetic material in wastewater as for enteric viruses. During the peak times of viral spread, several studies have been published that deal with the detection of SARS-CoV-2 in wastewater samples. Wastewater sample assessment has proved to be an essential and noninvasive early-warning tool for monitoring the status and trend of COVID-19 infection and as a tool for modifying public health response. In recent times, this environmental surveillance could be implemented in wastewater treatment plants as a primary strategy which will be designed to support appropriate authorities to device a fitting exit strategy to gradually lift the coronavirus lockdown (Parikh and Rawtani 2022).

5.2 Sample Collection from Patients

Patients with newly diagnosed COVID-19 who were hospitalized singly in Airborne Infection Isolation Room (AIIR) with separate toilet and shower facilities and consented to participate in air sample collection were recruited. To increase the proportion of exhaled air sampled and reduce the proportion of environmental air from the air conditioning system with 12 air changes per hour, an umbrella fitted with a transparent plastic curtain was used as an air shelter to cover patients during the collection. Air samples of patients put inside this air shelter were collected by the Sartorius MD8 airscan sampling device (Sartorius AG, Germany) with sterile gelatin filters (80 mm in diameter and 3 μm pore size) (type 17528-80-ACD) (Sartorius AG, Germany). Briefly, the air sampler was perpendicularly positioned at a distance of 10 cm away from the level of the patient's chin. One thousand liters of air at a rate of 50 l minute^{-1} were collected by each gelatin filter for 20 minutes while patients were with or without a surgical mask, which complies with the ASTM F2100 level 1 standard. Patients 1 to 6 were chosen as cases to detect whether SARS-CoV-2 RNA was present in the air. As positive controls, COVID-19 patients were instructed to sneeze directly and spit saliva droplets onto the gelatin filter used for the air sampler. Patients 7 to 10 were chosen as positive controls, while patient 6 served as both a case and his own control. After air sampling or collecting the positive controls, each gelatin filter was soaked into 5 ml of the viral transport medium (VTM) and incubated at 37 °C for 10 minutes. After the dissolution of the gelatin filter, 1 ml of the VTM was collected for nucleic acid extraction.

Swab samples from the patient's environment including bed rail, locker, bed table, toilet door handle, and patient's mobile phone were collected for SARS-CoV-2 viral load assay before daily environmental disinfection by sodium hypochlorite solution of 1000 ppm. Briefly, swab samples covering a mean surface area of $9\,cm^2$ ($3\,cm \times 3\,cm$) for bed rail, locker, and bed table, and the entire surfaces of toilet door handles and patients' mobile phones were collected. Swabs were then submerged into 2 ml VTM. Each swab sample in VTM was vortexed and centrifuged at $13\,000 \times g$ for one minute, and 1 ml of the supernatant was used for nucleic acid extraction. The nasopharyngeal (NP) flocked swab and deep throat saliva of patients were collected on the day of environmental sampling and subjected to viral load assay. If there were other clinical samples such as throat swab, sputum, and rectal swab collected, the results would be used to correlate with the results of environmental sampling. The clinical sample with the highest viral load from each patient was selected for correlation with the positivity rate of their own environmental samples (Parikh and Rawtani 2022).

5.2.1 Sample Acquisition from Nose

Nasal specimens were collected by mid-turbinate swabbing of both nares. Oropharyngeal (OP) specimens were collected by swabbing the posterior pharynx, avoiding the tongue. A flocked swab was utilized for the collection of all clinical samples and handled as recommended in international guidelines (CDC 2021). The presence of SAR-CoV-2 RNA in the samples was evaluated through quantitative reverse transcription-polymerase chain reaction (qRT-PCR), as described in international guidelines. The cycle threshold (CT) values of qRT-PCR are inversely related to the copy number of SARS-CoV-2 RNA and are commonly used as a proxy for viral loads. Therefore, CT values were used to compare viral loads in different clinical samples. If no increase in the intensity of the fluorescent signal was observed after 40 cycles, the sample was classified as negative (Palmas et al. 2020).

5.2.2 Sample Acquisition from Saliva

For the unsupervised self-collected oral fluid swab specimens, we provided written instructions with the testing kit, which included a sterile swab and a tube with an RNA preservative media. Participants were instructed to cough deeply three to five times collecting any phlegm or secretions in their mouth, rubbing the swab on both cheeks, above and below the tongue, both gums, and on the hard palate for a total of 20 seconds to ensure the swab was saturated with oral fluid. Following that, participants were instructed to place the swab into the tube, secure the lid, invert the tube three to five times, and place the capped tube into a collection bag. Unsupervised specimen collection was observed by a clinician but from a greater distance than the supervised collections, and the clinician did not provide any feedback to the participant. For the clinician-supervised self-collected oral fluid swab specimens, the same instructions were provided and a clinician provided real-time feedback. Without clinician feedback, some unsupervised patients did not cough before self-collecting their samples.

The samples were processed from the specimen collection tubes and further lysed and extracted RNA from samples using an automated instrument on a 96-well plate. A reverse transcription-quantitative PCR (RT-qPCR) assay was employed that utilized a single-color TaqMan probe with a modified version of the qualitative detection of SARS-CoV-2.

This sample analysis strategy was designed and validated by the Centers for Disease Control and Prevention (CDC). The CT values for tests were recorded. A human ribonuclease P RNA was detected with an additional single-color TaqMan assay, in a parallel reaction using an aliquot of the extracted participant specimen to serve as a control for specimen extraction, specimen adequacy, and RT-PCR inhibition. We ran samples on an RT-qPCR.

5.2.3 Stool Sample Acquisition

A convenience sample of remnant stool specimens submitted to the Clinical Microbiology Laboratory at Montefiore Medical Center for routine diagnostic testing was utilized. Stool specimens were collected between 21 April and 15 May 2020 and were tested for SARS-CoV-2 within seven days of collection. Stool specimens were stored at 2–8 °C prior to initial real-time RT-PCR testing, which was first performed using the Cepheid platform. A chart review of patients from whom stool was utilized was performed to identify all SARS-CoV-2 NP RT-PCR and serology results. Specimens for routine PCR testing during the study period consisted of combined NP/OP swabs transported in a universal transport medium or ESwab collection devices. Clinical testing of the swab PCR was performed using multiple platforms. Additional IgG serologic testing was performed using the Abbott SARS-CoV-2 immunoassay on the Architect i2000sr instrument (Szymczak et al. 2021).

The stool was tested by submerging a rayon-tipped swab into several areas of the specimen to obtain a coating of stool, followed by transfer into 1 ml of 0.85% normal saline. Real-time RT-PCR was then performed using the Hologic Panther Fusion assays following the package insert instructions for upper respiratory specimen testing. For the Cepheid assay, the GeneXpert Infinity instrument running software version 6.8 was utilized. The Cepheid assay detects the E and N2 gene of SARS-CoV-2 and contains a processing control to ensure extraction and amplification. The Hologic assay was performed on the Panther Fusion system. The Hologic assay detects two ORF1a regions of SARS-CoV-2 and also contains an internal control but utilizes only one fluorescent channel for reporting the ORF1a amplification product.

5.2.3.1 Sample Collection from Environmental Surfaces

The sample collection from different environmental surfaces is done for establishing the link between the location of the outbreak and its environment. It is also responsible for the identification of the risk factors associated with environmental contamination and for further transmission to other individuals (Dey et al. 2022). The data collected for the environmental samples provide supplementary information, which must be interpreted so that the origin of the outbreak can be established. The World Health Organization (WHO) has prescribed guidelines for the sampling of the virus from different environmental surfaces. The location of the sampling must be determined by the possible transmission route and by a literature review of the high touch surfaces. The outcome of the environmental samples can be influenced by different factors such as time and frequency of the sample collection. In the health care settings, multiple factors are responsible such as the type of disinfection activities, time and duration of the aerosol-generating procedures such as positive pressure ventilation, and continuous positive airway pressure, tracheostomy, and open airway suction, bronchoscopy must be indicated in the documentation (Purohit et al. 2022).

5.2.3.2 Timing of the Environmental Sample Collection

In an ideal situation, the sampling from the patient's room must be done daily, from the day patient was suspected or diagnosed with COVID-19 until seven days after the discharge of the patient or death of the patient. If aerosol-generating procedures are used, then the sampling of the room must be done before and after one hour of each procedure and for cross reference, another sample must be taken after 24 hours. A separate record must be kept for documenting the humidity and temperature of the sampled room. In case of an extensive outbreak, the samples must be collected from day 1 of sampling to every two to three days. The main priority for the collection of the samples must be the collection of high quality and frequency of samples from severe patients instead of the collection of samples of all patients involved in the outbreak. This approach would help in prioritizing the patients and planning the treatment of the patients according to the severity of the case.

5.2.3.3 Environmental Sampling Methods and Procedure

For the collection of environmental samples, a synthetic swab and a plastic shaft are used. The collected swabs are transferred to swab collection vials which contain 1–3 ml of VTM and neutralizing buffer. The contents of the transport medium include protein stabilizer, buffer solution, and antibiotics, and a neutralizing buffer is added to counteract the effect of any residual disinfectant. The isolation of the virus is done by virus isolation medium but the medium is effective for short-duration storage and transport because in the case of long-duration transport, the temperature and concentration of the viral media are very difficult to control. In case of long-term shipping, where the storage condition is not optimal, a chaotropic lysis buffer is used. This buffer stabilizes the viral genome load and is efficient for the storage of minute viral load. The sampling from the environmental surface involves a multistep procedure. This begins with the utilization of sterile, non-powdered nitrile or vinyl examination gloves over the gloves provided in the Personal Protective Kit. This is followed by the removal of the swab from the package and that swab is then dipped in the VTM. The wet swab is used for the collection of viruses from different surfaces. It must be ensured that at the time of collection, the swab should not get dry. The surface area for the collection of swabs should be around 25 cm^2 and pressure must be applied at the time of swabbing and the swab must be moved in at least two different directions with rotational motion. For enhancing the efficiency and positive predictive value of the environmental sampling process, multiple swabs must be taken from the sample. The samples must be labeled and placed in a self-sealing bag followed by the sanitization of the sealed bag with 60–80% ethanol, 80% of isopropyl alcohol, or 5% of hypochlorite solution (Kaushik and Rawtani 2022).

5.2.3.4 Transport and Storage of the Samples

The condition of the collected sample along with the location, time of sampling, and circumstances of storage of the samples along with the transportation medium must be enlisted with the sample. The WHO recommends that the samples must be stored in two different aliquots containing the VTM of which one aliquot must be stored at −70 °C or −80 °C at the earliest possible. This can be used as a reference sample for future use. After the collection of the sample from the environmental media, the sample must be transported to the lab within 72 hours. If that condition is not met, then the sample should be stored and shipped in dry ice. For the transportation of serum specimens, repeated freezing and thawing of the sample must be avoided as it may lead to spoilage of the sample.

5.2.3.5 Novel Sample Collection Technique

This technique was developed to prevent human-to-human interaction in the collection of the samples from suspected patients. The chamber was developed for the collection of the samples from the throat and NP tract. The device was named COVID Sample Collection Kiosk (COVSACK) and was developed by the Defence Research and Development Organisation (DRDO) of India (Tripathi 2020). The developed chamber utilized computational fluid dynamics for effective disinfection of the chamber. The motive behind innovation was to minimize the risk associated with manual sample collection. The additional benefits of the novel collection chamber include complete isolation of the suspected patients from medical personnel, which reduces fomite transmission of the virus. Along with that, disinfection of the chamber was done automatically without any human involvement. The disinfection process includes fumigation of the surfaces by sanitizers followed by complete sanitization by UV light. The chamber has an additional shield, which prevents the transmission of aerosol from infected patients to healthcare professionals. The use of Personal Protective Kits along with gloves, masks, and other protective equipment is also reduced because there is no human involvement. This led to a decreased generation of waste from hospitals and sample collection centers (Joshi 2020; PIB Delhi 2020; Tripathi 2020).

5.2.3.6 Current Diagnosis for COVID-19

Before lab analysis and within five to six days of the onset of symptoms, the COVID-19 patients show a higher number of viral loads in upper and lower respiratory tracts. Therefore, for early screening and diagnosis, an NP swab and/or an OP swab is suggested (Pan et al. 2020; Zhou et al. 2020). This type of sampling has proven to be well tolerated by the patient as well as safer to the operator. For quality control, it is crucial for the swab to reach the nasal cavity at the right spot in order to collect the sample. Initially, in China, OP swabs were more frequently collected and the detection rate was also low (32%) compared to NP swabs (63%) (Druce et al. 2012; To et al. 2020; Wang et al. 2020; Wölfel et al. 2020; Zou et al. 2020). For patients with pharyngitis, OP route can be more adequate for dominant initial screening. Theoretically, the collection of NP/OP swabs poses a threat of airborne infection to the operator. Many concurrent cases of viral infections have arisen from such situations, proving it to be risky for them. After the collection of swabs, they should be placed carefully in universal transport medium funder refrigeration for rapid delivery to clinical laboratories (Li et al. 2020; Tang et al. 2020; Wölfel et al. 2020). An alternative to this is to self-collect saliva and nasal wash specimens and submit them for screening. It must be noted that in some cases, when the specimens miss an early infection, recurrent testing or obtaining lower respiratory tract samples is required. Also, other viruses like influenza and respiratory syncytial viruses must be excluded.

In cases of late detection, sputum or bronchoalveolar lavage (BAL) fluid should be used for collecting lower respiratory tract samples because they yielded the highest quantity of viral loads. Patients with pneumonia have demonstrated high viral loads in fecal material. Patients with severe infections of the virus have shown enteric involvement with samples showing the presence of the virus in stool cultures and rectal swabs as well (WHO 2020; Yu et al. 2020).

Currently, nucleic acid-based testing and computed tomography (CT) scans are used for the diagnosis and screening of COVID-19. Molecular testing methods are more accurate for diagnosis than syndromic and CT scans as they can reveal the identity of specific pathogens (Uduguma et al. 2020). The development of a molecular method of diagnosis depends upon understanding the genetic composition of the virus and identifying changes in their gene/protein expression in the patient during and after infection. The genomic and proteomic compositions of the novel virus have been identified, but the host response to the virus is currently undergoing research. Genome sequencing is substantial for scientists in designing PCR primers and probe sequences and other nucleic acid-based tests (Lu et al. 2020; 20).

5.2.4 Nucleic Acid Testing

5.2.4.1 Reverse Transcription-Based Polymerase Chain Reaction (RT-PCR)

Nucleic acid-based testing is the prime method for the testing and diagnosis of COVID-19. For that purpose, numerous reverse transcription PCR (RT-PCR) kits have been developed for the genetic detection of the virus (Freeman et al. 1999). A general scheme of the process of RT-PCR involves the following steps: 1-reverse transcription of SARS-CoV-2 RNA into complementary DNA (cDNA) strands; 2-cDNA amplification (only specific regions). The designing process for kits involves the alignment of sequences and primer design followed by optimization of the assay and performing tests. Literature suggests three regions of interest that contain conserved sequences for designing primers: (i) RdRP gene (RNA-dependent RNA polymerase) in the open reading frame ORFlab region; (ii) the envelop protein gene, E and; (iii) the nucleocapsid protein gene, N. Sensitivity for both RdRP and E genes has shown high analytical sensitivity (3.6 and 3.9 copies per reaction, respectively) for detection compared to N gene (8.3 copies). A two-target system nucleic acid-based test can also be developed, where one primer could detect a large number of coronavirus including SARS-CoV-2, and a second primer to detect SARS-CoV-2 specifically. Optimization of the assay conditions, e.g. reagent conditions, temperatures, and incubation times should also be undertaken properly (Uduguma et al. 2020).

RT-PCR can be performed in either a one- or two-step method. In the one-step method, both reverse transcription and PCR amplification steps are completed as a single reaction. This method offers high throughput analysis as it provides rapid and reproducible results. However, the generation of enough target amplicon is often difficult as the reverse transcription and amplification reaction occur in tandem. Comparatively, in the two-step method, both the reactions are carried out in separate tubes and offer more sensitivity, but require optimization of additional parameters and are also time-consuming (Bustin et al. 2020; Wong and Medrano et al. 2020; Uduguma et al. 2020). Moreover, the selection of controls for the assay needs to be carefully done to ensure its reliability and to recognize experimental errors.

5.2.4.2 Real-Time RT-PCR (rRT-PCR)

In one-step real-time RT-PCR (rRT-PCR), as used by the US Centers for Disease Control and Prevention (CDC), a quantitative estimation of the viral load is achieved in order to detect the presence of the virus in the samples [21, Freeman et al. 2022]. In this method, the viral RNA is extracted and added to a master mix containing nuclease-free water, forward and reverse primers, a fluorescing-quencher probe and a reaction mix containing reverse transcriptase, polymerase, nucleotides, magnesium, and additives. The extracted viral RNA and the master mix are now added to the PCR thermocycler after setting the required incubation temperature to run the assay.

In rRT-PCR, cleaving of fluorophore quencher probe generates fluorescence, which is then detected by the thermocycler. Real-time recording and monitoring of progress in amplification are possible in this method. Some examples of the probe sequences under use are Fluorescein amidite (FAM, fluorophore) and Black Hole Quencher-1 (BHQ1, quencher). The reaction in rRT-PCR takes place in a 96-well plate reader and runs for approximately 45 minutes, with a different sample or control per well. For a correct interpretation of the result, both positive and negative controls must be present. In the case of SARS-CoV-2, CDC recommends the use of nCoVPC as the positive control sequence (Corman et al. 2020; Uduguma et al. 2020).

There is also a need to integrate the workflow of nucleic acid detection techniques for better clinical management. The RT-PCR method is implemented differently in various clinical settings. For instance, a three-step workflow method was proposed for the detection of the SARS-CoV-2 (Chu et al. 2020). The steps include first-line screening followed by confirmation and subsequent discriminatory assays. In the first step, all SARS-related viruses are identified by targeting different regions of the E-gene to maximize the number of patients found positive for the viral infection. If this test comes out as positive, then detection of the RdRP gene is proposed by using two different primers and probes (Chu et al. 2020). If this test also comes positive, then the discriminatory test is conducted with one of the two probe sequences. In other workflow conditions, the samples are screened by using the primers for the N-gene, which are used from the ORFlb gene for confirmation (Yang and Yan et al. 2020). A patient sample found positive for N-gene primer and negative for ORFlb gene deems to be inconclusive and hence in such cases, protein tests such as antibody tests or sequencing assays would be ideal to confirm the viral presence (Chu et al. 2020).

5.2.5 Computed Tomography

Initially, due to the dearth of the RT-PCR kits and false-negative rates in the detection, CT scans were used in Wuhan for clinical diagnosis of COVID-19 (Uduguma et al. 2020; Whiting et al. 2015). CT scans are noninvasive, which involve recording several X-ray measurements recorded at different angles across a patient's chest to obtain cross sectional images (Bernheim et al. 2020; Lee and Ng et al. 2020). These images are then analyzed by the radiologist to observe any abnormal features that could help in the diagnosis (Lee and Ng et al. 2020). The features in the X-ray images depend on the stage of infection following the onset of initial symptoms. Reports have revealed more or less normal CT findings in patients in the early stages of the infection with a significant peak in maximum lung involvement only after 10 days after the onset (Pan et al. 2020; Kobayashi et al. 2020). Common hallmark features in the images appear to be the presence of bilateral and peripheral ground-glass opacities and lung consolidation, which is characterized by presence of fluid or solid material in the compressible lung tissue. Reports indicating the presence of these opacities after four days have also been indicated. In the further stage of infection, along with the ground-glass opacities, a distinct crazy wave-like pattern is also visible, which is known as an irregularly shaped paved stone-like pattern and is usually followed by an increase in lung consolidation (Pan et al. 2020; Kobayashi et al. 2020; Fang et al. 2020). Retrospective studies based on these imaging features have revealed a greater sensitivity of this method (86–98%) and lesser false-negative compared to RT-PCR (Uduguma et al. 2020; Xie et al. 2020; Mahmoudi et al. 2020). But the issue of low specificity with CT scanning hinders its large-scale use as the morphological observations overlap with other viral pneumonia too.

The diagnosis of COVID-19 currently uses RT-PCR and CT scanning and each technique has its own drawbacks. For instance, the availability of RT-PCR kits has still not kept up with the growing demands. Also, lack of PCR infrastructure outside urban cities diminishes its high sample throughput. Moreover, RT-PCR relies on the presence of the virus in the collected sample, which makes the test unreliable in the case of an asymptomatic patient who has recovered since infection where some control measures would be necessary to enforce. Similarly, for CT scanning, expensive systems, the needs for technical expertise decrease their utilization on a large scale (Tang et al. 2020; Uduguma et al. 2020).

5.3 Conclusion

In the wake of the COVID-19 outbreak, it is important to resort to sampling and analytical techniques that are easy to perform and are rapid. There are several methods of sample collection from patients, who are confirmed with coronavirus infection. A swab from oral samples and nasal samples serves as the best method for sample collection techniques. Since several studies exhibit the presence of traces of the SARS-CoV-2 genome in stool samples, stool collection from infected patients has also gained emphasis. Environmental sampling has also been done keeping into consideration of the current situation of COVID-19. Animate and inanimate surfaces have been thoroughly inspected for traces of the novel coronavirus. According to the guidelines of the WHO, there are specific timing and storage conditions implied for the sampling of the environment and surroundings, especially that of an infected individual. Analytical techniques such as RT-PCR, although exhibit some degree of false positives, they serve as the gold standard for COVID-19 testing, while complicated techniques such as CT have also served in confirming the infection in an individual.

References

Bai, Y., Yao, L., Wei, T. et al. (2020). Presumed asymptomatic carrier transmission of COVID-19. *JAMA* 323: 1406–1407. https://doi.org/10.1001/jama.2020.2565.

Bernheim, A., Mei, X., Huang, M. et al. (2020). Chest CT findings in coronavirus disease-19 (COVID-19): relationship to duration of infection. *Radiology*, 295(3), 685–691.

Bustin et al. 2020, Bustin, S., Coward, A., Sadler, G., Teare, L., and Nolan, T. (2020). CoV2-ID, a MIQE-compliant sub-20-min 5-plex RT-PCR assay targeting SARS-CoV-2 for the diagnosis of COVID-19. *Scientific reports*, 10(1), 22214.

CDC (2021). Interim guidelines for clinical specimens for COVID-19. CDC [WWW Document]. https://www.cdc.gov/coronavirus/2019-nCoV/lab/guidelines-clinical-specimens.html (accessed 24 August 21).

Chan, J.F.-W., Yuan, S., Kok, K.-H. et al. (2020). A familial cluster of pneumonia associated with the 2019 novel coronavirus indicating person-to-person transmission: a study of a family cluster. *Lancet (London, England)* 395: 514–523. https://doi.org/10.1016/S0140-6736(20)30154-9.

Chu, D. K., Akl, E. A., Duda, S., et al. (2020). Physical distancing, face masks, and eye protection to prevent person-to-person transmission of SARS-CoV-2 and COVID-19: a systematic review and meta-analysis. *The lancet*, 395(10242), 1973–1987.

Corman, V. M., Landt, O., Kaiser, M., Molenkamp, R., Meijer., et al. (2020). Detection of 2019 novel coronavirus (2019-nCoV) by real-time RT-PCR. *Eurosurveillance*, 25(3), 2000045.

Dey, A., Rao, P. K., and Rawtani, D. (2022). Risk management of COVID-19. In COVID-19 in the Environment (pp. 217–230). Elsevier.

Druce, J., Garcia, K., Tran, T. et al. (2012). Evaluation of swabs, transport media, and specimen transport conditions for optimal detection of viruses by PCR. *J. Clin. Microbiol.* 50: 1064–1065. https://doi.org/10.1128/JCM.06551-11.

Fang, Y., Zhang, H., Xie, J. et al. (2020). Sensitivity of chest CT for COVID-19: comparison to RT-PCR. *Radiology*, 296(2), E115–E117.

Freeman, D., Waite, F., Rosebrock, L., Petit, A. et al. (2022). Coronavirus conspiracy beliefs, mistrust, and compliance with government guidelines in England. *Psychological medicine*, 52(2), 251–263.

Freeman, W. M., Walker, S. J., and Vrana, K. E. (1999). Quantitative RT-PCR: pitfalls and potential. *Biotechniques*, 26(1), 112–125.

Frieden, T. and Lee, C. (2020). Identifying and interrupting superspreading events— implications for control of severe acute respiratory syndrome coronavirus 2. *Emerg. Infect. Dis. J.* 26: 1059. https://doi.org/10.3201/eid2606.200495.

Gudbjartsson, D.F., Helgason, A., Jonsson, H. et al. (2020). Spread of SARS-CoV-2 in the icelandic population. *N. Engl. J. Med.* 382: 2302–2315. https://doi.org/10.1056/NEJMoa2006100.

Guerra, F.M., Bolotin, S., Lim, G. et al. (2017). The basic reproduction number (R_0) of measles: a systematic review. *Lancet Infect. Dis.* 17: e420–e428. https://doi.org/10.1016/S1473-3099(17)30307-9.

Guo, Z.-D., Wang, Z.-Y., Zhang, S.-F. et al. (2020). Aerosol and surface distribution of severe acute respiratory syndrome coronavirus 2 in hospital wards, Wuhan, China, 2020. *Emerg. Infect. Dis. J.* 26: 1583. https://doi.org/10.3201/eid2607.200885.

Joshi, J.R. (2020). COVSACK: an innovative portable isolated and safe COVID-19 sample collection kiosk with automatic disinfection. *Trans. Indian Natl. Acad. Eng.* 5: 269–275. https://doi.org/10.1007/s41403-020-00139-1.

Kaushik and Rawtani 2022, Kaushik, K., and Rawtani, D. (2022). Sensor-based techniques for detection of COVID-19. In COVID-19 in the Environment (pp. 95–114). Elsevier.

Kobayashi, Y., Tata, A., Konkimalla, A. et al. (2020). Persistence of a regeneration-associated, transitional alveolar epithelial cell state in pulmonary fibrosis. *Nature cell biology*, 22(8), 934–946.

Li, Q., Guan, X., Wu, P. et al. (2020). Early transmission dynamics in Wuhan, China, of novel coronavirus-infected pneumonia. *N. Engl. J. Med.* 382: 1199–1207. https://doi.org/10.1056/NEJMoa2001316.

Liu, Y., Eggo, R.M., and Kucharski, A.J. (2020). Secondary attack rate and superspreading events for SARS-CoV-2. *Lancet* 395: e47. https://doi.org/10.1016/S0140-6736(20)30462-1.

Lu, R., Zhao, X., Li, J. et. al (2020). Genomic characterisation and epidemiology of 2019 novel coronavirus: implications for virus origins and receptor binding. *The lancet*, 395(10224), 565–574.

Mahmoudi, S., Mehdizadeh, M., Shervin Badv, R., et al. (2020). The coronavirus disease 2019 (COVID-19) in children: a study in an Iranian Children's Referral Hospital. *Infection and drug resistance*, 2649–2655.

Medrano, M., Cadenas-Sanchez, C., Oses, M., Arenaza, L., Amasene, M., and Labayen, I. (2021). Changes in lifestyle behaviours during the COVID-19 confinement in Spanish children: A longitudinal analysis from the MUGI project. *Pediatric Obesity*, 16(4), e12731.

Ng, K., Poon, B. H., Kiat Puar, T. H. et al. (2020). COVID-19 and the risk to health care workers: a case report. *Annals of internal medicine*, 172(11), 766–767.

Palmas, G., Moriondo, M., Trapani, S. et al. (2020). Nasal swab as preferred clinical specimen for COVID-19 testing in children. *Pediatr. Infect. Dis. J.* 39: 267–270.

Pan, Y., Zhang, D., Yang, P. et al. (2020). Viral load of SARS-CoV-2 in clinical samples. *Lancet Infect. Dis.* https://doi.org/10.1016/S1473-3099(20)30113-4.

Parikh and Rawtani 2022, Parikh, G., and Rawtani, D. (2022). Environmental impact of COVID-19. In COVID-19 in the Environment (pp. 203–216). Elsevier.

PIB Delhi (2020). DRDO develops kiosk for COVID-19 sample collection.

Purohit, S., Rao, P. K., and Rawtani, D. (2022). Sampling and analytical techniques for COVID-19. In COVID-19 in the Environment (pp. 75–94). Elsevier.

Szymczak, W.A., Goldstein, D.Y., Orner, E.P. et al. (2021). Utility of stool PCR for the diagnosis of COVID-19: comparison of two commercial platforms. *J. Clin. Microbiol.* 58: e01369–e01320. https://doi.org/10.1128/JCM.01369-20.

Tang, Y.W., Schmitz, J.E., Persing, D.H., and Stratton, C.W. (2020). Laboratory diagnosis of COVID-19: Current issues and challenges. *J. Clin. Microbiol.* https://doi.org/10.1128/JCM.00512-20.

To, K.K.-W., Tsang, O.T.-Y., Leung, W.-S. et al. (2020). Temporal profiles of viral load in posterior oropharyngeal saliva samples and serum antibody responses during infection by SARS-CoV-2: an observational cohort study. *Lancet Infect. Dis.* 20: 565–574. https://doi.org/10.1016/S1473-3099(20)30196-1.

Tripathi, S. (2020). COVSACK: Kiosk for Covid-19 sample collection developed by DRDO.

Udugama, B., Kadhiresan, P., Kozlowski, H. N., Malekjahani, A., Osborne, M., Li, V. Y., Chan, W. C. et al. (2020). Diagnosing COVID-19: the disease and tools for detection. *ACS nano*, 14(4), 3822–3835.

Wang, W., Xu, Y., Gao, R. et al. (2020). Detection of SARS-CoV-2 in different types of clinical specimens. *JAMA* 323: 1843–1844. https://doi.org/10.1001/jama.2020.3786.

WHO (2020). Report of the WHO-China joint mission on coronavirus disease 2019 (COVID-19). WHO-China Jt. *Mission Coronavirus Dis*. 2019, 16–24.

Whiting, P., Singatullina, N., Rosser, J. H. et al. (2015). Computed tomography of the chest: I. Basic principles. *Bja Education*, 15(6), 299–304.

Wölfel, R., Corman, V.M., Guggemos, W. et al. (2020). Virological assessment of hospitalized patients with COVID-2019. *Nature* 581: 465–469. https://doi.org/10.1038/s41586-020-2196-x.

Wu, J.T., Leung, K., and Leung, G.M. (2020). Nowcasting and forecasting the potential domestic and international spread of the 2019-nCoV outbreak originating in Wuhan, China: a modelling study. *Lancet* 395: 689–697. https://doi.org/10.1016/S0140-6736(20)30260-9.

Xie, J., Ding, C., Li, J. et al. (2020). Characteristics of patients with coronavirus disease (COVID-19) confirmed using an IgM-IgG antibody test. *Journal of medical virology*, 92(10), 2004–2010.

Yan, R., Zhang, Y., Li, Y., et al. (2020). Structural basis for the recognition of SARS-CoV-2 by full-length human ACE2. *Science*, 367(6485), 1444–1448.

Yu, F., Yan, L., Wang, N. et al. (2020). Quantitative detection and viral load analysis of SARS-CoV-2 in infected patients. *Clin. Infect. Dis.* 71: 793–798. https://doi.org/10.1093/cid/ciaa345.

Zhou, P., Yang, X.L., Wang, X.G. et al. (2020). A pneumonia outbreak associated with a new coronavirus of probable bat origin. *Nature* 579: 270–273. https://doi.org/10.1038/s41586-020-2012-7.

Zou, L., Ruan, F., Huang, M. et al. (2020). SARS-CoV-2 viral load in upper respiratory specimens of infected patients. *N. Engl. J. Med.* 382: 1177–1179. https://doi.org/10.1056/NEJMc2001737.

6

Modern Sensor-Based Techniques for Identification of COVID-19

Pratik Kulkarni[1], Shyam Vasvani[2], Tejas D. Barot[1], Piyush K. Rao[1], and Aayush Dey[1]

[1] *School of Doctoral Studies & Research (SDSR), National Forensic Sciences University (Ministry of Home Affairs, GOI), Gandhinagar, Gujarat, India*
[2] *School of Pharmacy, National Forensic Sciences University (Ministry of Home Affairs, GOI), Gandhinagar, Gujarat, India*

6.1   Introduction: Current Diagnosis for COVID-19

The immunologically based detection kit along with RT-PCR has been mostly employed as a detection method for COVID-19. Such techniques require expertise and the training of professionals for optimal performance. Also, it requires up to 24 hours to get the PCR results. Similarly, immunology-based detection assays consist of complicated construction techniques for recombinant proteins and antibodies. Here though there is need to produce some innovative methods that are faster, have lower cost, and are more consistent in detecting SARS-CoV-2. This chapter discusses all the newer and emerging technologies for COVID-19 detection. Some methods are still under a nascent stage and have been recommended based on the probability of virus detection, as achieved previously with other categories of viruses. Several examples along with ongoing clinical studies have also been provided. Also, other methods which show initial promises need to be studied further with live samples in order to warrant their widespread use.

6.2   Newer and Emerging Technologies

The WHO has stated an immediate priority for the research in COVID-19 diagnosis for the Point Of Care (POC). Also, integration of these techniques into the multiplex panel has become a long-term priority. The addition of protein-based serological tests to nucleic acid tests is important to improve their surveillance. Unlike nucleic acid-based tests, these techniques provide viral detection following sample recovery, allowing efficient tracking of the sick and recovered patients by the researchers. This has helped in offering an improved projection of the SARS-CoV-2 epidemic. To diagnose patients outside

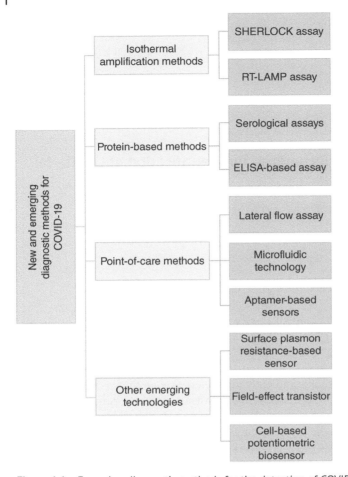

Figure 6.1 Emerging diagnostic methods for the detection of COVID-19.

integrated facilities, point-of-care tests that use easy-to-operate devices are cost-effective and helpful for reducing the workload of laboratories (Figure 6.1) (Craw and Balachandran 2012; Lu et al. 2020).

6.2.1 Isothermal Amplification Assays

Isothermal amplification is one of the latest technologies for the detection of SARS-CoV-2 and is based upon nucleic acid-based detection of the virus. Some examples of the technique are SHERLOCK assay, recombinase polymerase amplification (RPA), and loop-mediated isothermal amplification (LAMP) (Kang et al. 2020).

6.2.1.1 SHERLOCK Assay

The SHERLOCK (Specific High-sensitivity Enzymatic Reporter Unlocking) method based on CRISPR is a convenient and multiplexed method that allows ultrasensitive RNA or

DNA detection from clinical samples (Kellner et al. 2019). These assays are based on recombinase-mediated polymerase for pre-amplification of DNA or RNA with subsequent detection by colorimetry and fluorescence-assisted measurements, mediated by Cas13 or Cas12. These assays provide results within an hour and have a setup time of 15 minutes or less. Based on a sequence of the virus, 2 guide RNAs have been carefully designed by the researchers, one recognizing the S-gene of the novel virus and the other recognizing the ORF1ab-gene. Also, to maximize the exactness of recognition, the selection of specific sequences corresponding to the novel virus has been done. By doing this, interference from other respiratory viruses gets minimized. If the RNA corresponds to the novel virus in the sample, it can be easily recognized by the RNA guide to activate the binding of Cas13 to its surface. Cas13 is a unique enzyme, which, once activated, is known to cut any other RNA molecules it encounters. Therefore, to analyze whether the molecules get cut off, the existence of the novel virus in the initial sample can be easily identified. By using synthetic SARS-CoV-2 viral fragments, virus detection can be achieved with good consistency in the range of 20–200 aM (i.e. 10–100 copies μl^{-1} of input). This test can be read using a dipstick in less than an hour without the requirement of complex instruments; yet it needs to get confirmed with unknown samples (Kellner et al. 2019; Mori et al. 2001; Uduguma et al. 2017).

In a recent study, a novel CRISPR-based assay demonstrated robust detection of SARS-CoV-2 in a single reaction system (Chen et al. 2018; Ding et al. 2020). All the components to perform the assay were incubated in a specific reaction system for a rapid, highly sensitive, and specific detection of the nucleic acids without separate steps for doing pre-amplification. Upon the design of All-in-One Dual CRISPR-Cas12a (AIOD-CRISPR), the introduction of dual CRISPR RNAs (crRNAs) improved the sensitivity of detection signals owing to the high-concentration ssDNA-FQ reporters. The AIOD-CRISPR assay is also useful for POC identification in addition to real-time detection, as the results can be examined using fluorescence and color shift reactions. This proof-of-concept study has proved to be a good example of effective SARS-CoV-2 detection. Compared to other CRISPR-based nucleic acid detection assays, this method is more versatile and robust (Chen et al. 2018; Cong et al. 2013; Ding et al. 2020; Gootenberg et al. 2017; Li et al. 2019; Wang et al. 2019; Zhou et al. 2018). AIOD-CRISPR system is a one-of-its-kind true single reaction detection system and a true isothermal nucleic acid detection method. The study needs no preamplification of the target nucleic acids and all the components of the study are prepared prior to incubation. Also, physical separation of the Cas enzyme is not necessary, and the system is devoid of any specially designed reaction tubes or devices for reaction (Chen et al. 2018; Wang et al. 2019; Wu et al. 2020). AIOD-CRISPR is carried out at one temperature in a (one-step; one-pot) format. The need for an expensive thermocycler used in PCR methods and the initial denaturation of dsDNA targets in LAMP 8 and SDA methods is therefore removed by a single-step reaction (Walker et al. 1992). AIOD-CRISPR-based detection is rapid, extremely specific, and robust. A detection range as low as 1.2 and 4.6 copies of DNA and RNA targets, respectively after 35–40 minutes of incubation makes AIOD-CRISPR a very sensitive method. For emerging SARS-CoV-2 samples, along with high sensitivity, this novel system also performs high detection specificity. Also, AIOD-CRISPR allows one-step RNA detection based on CRISPR-Cas12a. This system can easily be developed as a one-step RT-AIOD-CRISPR to detect RNA targets such as SARS-CoV-2 RNAs by facilitating the supplementation of AMV reverse transcriptase, eliminating the need to prepare cDNA and facilitating the detection of RNA based on CRISPR-Cas12a (Chen et al. 2018; Wang et al. 2019; Wu et al. 2020).

6.2.1.2 RT-LAMP Assay

RT-LAMP, known as the loop-mediated isothermal amplification technique, is a nucleic acid-based test performed at a single temperature that prevents any specialized test center equipment from being used to provide PCR-like analytical results. For SARS-CoV-2 patients, many laboratories have produced and conducted clinical experiments. DNA polymerase and a total of 4–6 primers that can bind to separate regions of the target genome are used in this method. Therefore, RT-LAMP is a highly specific test due to the use of higher quantities of primers. It is a four-primer system that consists of two inner and outer primers (forward and reverse) (Kim et al. 2016). The process of RT-LAMP requires addition of sample collected from the patient to a tube where DNA amplification is done. The DNA amplification is the product of the reaction between the pH-sensitive dye and double-stranded DNA. The reaction is quantified by the measurement of turbidity (Elnifro et al. 2000). This reaction, maintained at 60–65 °C, takes less than an hour and has an empirical detection limit of 75 copies μl^{-1}. Due to the aforementioned reasons, RT-LAMP is an excellent approach because of its ease of handling, visual mode of detection, and less background signal without the utilization of thermocycler. Some drawbacks of this method involve the optimization of primers and reaction conditions (Kim et al. 2016).

During amplification or readout stages, isothermal amplification methods can be multiplexed. By using polymeric beads encoded with distinct optical properties such as organic fluorescent molecules, such multiplexing can be used for barcoding. It is possible to design barcodes with different biomarkers for multiple analyte detection, which are present in panels of a single patient sample in a reaction tube (Elnifro et al. 2000). Multiplexing thus improves the specificity and sensitivity of the detection as it collects a large quantity of information (Udugama et al. 2017). Encoding with agents that emit fluorescent signals can also be utilized. For instance, a positive detection in this test indicates the linking of a sequence or antigen from the patient's sample with the bead's capture molecule. This molecule has a fluorophore-labelled secondary probe that emits at a wavelength different from the beads (Elnifro et al. 2000).

Efforts to develop these systems for POC have been underway as of now. However, a difficulty in designing a readout device is a challenge (Elnifro et al. 2000). The barcode's signal is complex in nature as it stems out of organic molecules and thus needs a special instrument design to decipher the codes. Recently, smartphones have been paired with inorganic quantum dot barcodes and these are used for recording the emission and excitation signal with the help of a smartphone camera. These barcodes were used for the identification of hepatitis B patients with 95% sensitivity and 91% clinical specificity. Based on these models, barcode panels can be designed for the detection of SARS-CoV-2 (Elnifro et al. 2000; To et al. 2020).

6.2.2 Protein-Based Tests

Diagnosis of COVID-19 could be possible by using the antigens and antibodies of viral protein developed in answer to SARS-CoV-2 infection. Detection of the viral proteins can be difficult if the viral capacity changes over the course of infection. For example, after a week of infection, a recent study documented high viral loads in salivary samples that decreased with time (Lv et al. 2020). Contrastingly, antibodies produced in response to the virus may offer a larger period of the frame for indirect detection of the novel virus. Ab (Ab)-based tests can be predominantly useful for COVID-19 surveillance. Cross-reactivity of COVID-19 antibodies against those with other coronaviruses needs to be explored more for developing accurate serological tests (Zhang et al. 2020a).

Many serologic tests have been under development (Cai et al. 2020; Guan et al. 2020; Xiang et al. 2020). A recent report was successful in the detection of IgM and IgG immunoglobulins from the human serum of infected cases using enzyme-linked immunosorbent assay (ELISA) (Xiang et al. 2020). Due to 90% homology between SARS-CoV-2 Rp3 and other SARS-related viruses, nucleocapsid protein was used in the testing procedure. In the procedure, the surface of the 96-well plate is utilized for adsorption of the recombinant proteins on it, following which the remaining is washed away. To the wells, attenuated human serum is now added up for an hour and the plate is washed again. Now, horseradish peroxidase functionalized anti-human IgG is added to allow target binding. The ELISA plate is washed again after the addition of 3,3′,5,5′-tetramethylbenzidine. The change in color is initiated by the peroxidase reaction with the substrate and is detected by a plate reader. A positive signal will indicate its presence in the form of a sandwich between the adsorbed protein and the anti-human IgG test if the sample has anti-SARS-CoV-2 IgG. The IgM test has a similar approach, but the plate and a probe containing an anti-Rp3 nucleocapsid use an adsorbed antihuman IgM. These tests were done in 16 COVID-19 patients and the antibody levels in the patients were found to increase in the initial five days of symptom onset. The increase from 50 to 81% and 100% in the levels of IgG and IgM was observed in the patients from days zero to five, respectively. Antibodies were also found in respiratory, faecal, or blood samples (Xiang et al. 2020).

In a recently published work, the performance of the EUROIMMUN anti-SARS-CoV-2 ELISA test was evaluated for detecting IgA and IgG antibodies in the viral samples. For the study, samples were taken from patients after fourth day of getting infected and tested for the detection of antibodies. For the identification of IgA and IgG antigens from plasma and serum samples, S1 domain of the viral spike protein was utilized in the semiquantitative assay. The assay demonstrated good and excellent sensitivity as well as specificity for IgA as well as IgG detection, respectively (Beavis et al. 2020). The assay also showed no cross response with common human CoVs, except an average cross reactivity in 2 samples out of 28 samples.

Given the recent trend in developing newer assays, some other proteins or cellular markers might be used as a primary and potential selection tool for the detection of the novel viral load. In tests of infected patients, a new study has indicated the presence of C-reactive proteins, low levels of lymphocytes, D-dimers, leukocytes, and blood platelets. However, a big challenge for using these markers is their presence in other abnormal illnesses as well. Therefore, a novel test with both Ab and molecule markers leads to improvement in specificity (Huang et al. 2018).

6.2.3 Point-of-Care (POC) Testing

Point-of-care tests can be defined as ones which do not require sending the samples to clinical laboratories or centralized facilities. These tests enable affected people without having lab instruments (Cai et al. 2020). Lateral flow antigen detection assay is a type of POC test.

A paper-like membrane is coated with two different lines in a commercial lateral flow assay, one containing gold nanoparticles-Ab conjugates and another containing capture antibodies. When the patient's samples (blood or urine) are placed on the suggested strip area, the excipient moves throughout the strip by capillary action. A complex is formed when the antigen binds with the nanoparticle-Ab complex. This complex passes through the test line and then flows through the membrane. When the sample reaches the control line, the captured antibodies immobilize themselves on the complex and emit visible red and blue lines. Individually, gold nanoparticles appear to be red in color. However, a large cluster of such gold particles is blue in color due to plasmon band coupling.

The sensitivity, accuracy, and specificity of IgM and IgG in the assay were recorded at 57,69 and 100%, respectively. Yet, compared to RT-PCR, these tests are designed for single use and offer poor analytical sensitivity. On a hopeful note, combining two novel approaches may lead to better clinical efficiency for the diagnosis of the virus. For the detection of MERS-CoV detection, lateral flow assay was combined with the nucleic acid-based RT-LAMP technique (Cai et al. 2020; Spengler et al. 2015; Uduguma et al. 2017). Several studies have also cited the use of signal-amplifying techniques like temperature-sensitive imaging assembly to improve the readout signals of the lateral flow assay (Foudeh et al. 2012).

Microfluidic technology can be utilized as another POC approach for SARS-CoV-2 detection. Microfluidic devices are small palm-sized chips embedded with reaction chambers and micrometer-sized channels. The chip helps in mixing and separating the liquid samples by electrokinetic, vacuum, and capillary. The chips can be specially made of materials like glass, poly-dimethyl sulfoxide, cellulose, or simply paper. The benefits of using microfluidic devices are miniaturization due to less sample volume, rapid detection ability, and convenience (Zhou et al. 2020). A recent study reported the development of a smartphone-assisted Ab finding method against three sexually spread infections by a sequential movement of the reagents prestored on a cassette. This test showcased a clinical efficacy and specificity of 100 and 87%, respectively, for HIV on patients in Rwanda. This method can be adapted for detecting novel SARS-CoV-2 viral RNA or proteins as well.

In a recent example, microfluidic immunoassays were used for a precise and synchronized detection of the IgM/IgG/Antigen of SARS-CoV-2 in less than 20 minutes (Lin et al. 2020). The novel microfluidic device encompasses centrifugation, fluorescence detection, and display of the results for simultaneous detection of three samples and their fluorescence measurements. The results showed that detection using serum samples was more sensitive than the conventional pharyngeal swab samples as evident by their higher fluorescence values. With the whole assay taking only 15 minutes, this robust microfluidics-based immunoassay can become a handy tool for SARS-CoV-2 diagnosis in healthcare settings and a better tool for monitoring infected patients. Moreover, this novel system provides the enhancement of sensitivity and efficacy of viral load recognition (Table 6.1) (Lin et al. 2020).

6.2.4 Aptamer-Based Assay Techniques

Aptamers are termed simply as ssDNA or RNA molecules, which are able to form 3D structural motifs and bind to respective targets with good selectivity (Tuerk and Gold 1990). Monoclonal antibodies and aptamers are often compared with each other. Their properties are

Table 6.1 Definition of ASSURED diagnostics.

Inexpensive	Primarily used at risk of infection
Sensitive	Less to minimal false negatives
Specific	Less to minimal false positives
User-friendly	Easy to use with manual
Rapid and robust	Minimal requirement of time and storage
Apparatus-free	Minimal use of lab equipment
Distributed	To needful patients

however different from each other as they are completely a different class of biomolecules. The prime advantage of aptamers can be developed next to any target of interest, non-immunogenic site, toxic, or even small to single molecules, not applying to antibodies. Another advantage is their tendency for an easy and reversible nature when denaturized by heat or chemicals, owing to their strong phosphodiester backbone absent in antibodies. Moreover, their production is cheap, and has an extremely low manufacturing variation and extensive shelf life, compared to antibodies (Dhiman et al. 2017).

6.2.4.1 Rapid Lateral Flow Platforms Based on Aptamer Technology

As the total number of populations keeps increasing in the emerging countries, the demand for rapid testing has also improved substantially in many areas such as food safety testing, drug abuse testing, pregnancy testing, toxin analysis in the situation, and chiefly in clinical analysis, to attain quick results in minimal time. For the same purpose with this, lateral flow assays (LFAs) or immune-chromatographic assays (ICAs) have become hugely popular and important for such testing as they are very convenient, easy to use, and cheap. Along with increased test speeds, they are accurate and comprise disposable formats, which makes them adaptable further for efficient POC testing (Dzantiev et al. 2014; Bruno 2014). LFAs come in handy where the settings are predominantly resource-limited to provide both qualitative and semiquantitative disease checking (Chen and Yang 2015). In general, LFAs consist of an overlying sample and conjugate pads, a nitrocellulose analytical membrane (control and test line), and an absorbent pad placed on a sticky support sheet on a paper-like membrane strip format, as is evident in many reports such as sandwich assay, competitive assay (or inhibition) (Wong and Tse 2008), and multiplex detection formats (Sajid et al. 2015). In the sandwich-type format, enzymes or gold nanoparticles or fluorescence dyes-coated molecule recognition element (MRE) as reporter label is made to react with a target of interest in order to form a label-conjugated MRE – target analyte involved in the conjugate pad (Sajid et al. 2015). Capillary action is responsible for making the complex reach the test zone, which is then caught by another aptamer or Ab-like MRE, sandwiching the analyte between the two MREs. This reaction results in an immediately noticeable change in the test zone (usually a red line). All the additionally labelled MRE travel to the control line pad and get captured by an agent such as a complementary oligonucleotide to the aptamer or an anti-primary Ab. The total amount of target analyte present in the sample corresponds to the intensity of the test zone signal, which is easily visualized optically and computed through an optical strip reader (Sajid et al. 2015).

6.2.4.2 Aptamer-Based Diagnostics of COVID-19 in the Future

Aptamer use has some strong benefits in terms of development and ultra-high sensitivity and affinity, along with high error-less batch-to-batch reproducibility for highly accurate assays. However, unfamiliarity about its proper use and the ability to reduce the disadvantage of an immunological assay, which is already available in the market, may hinder its practical use in the commercial diagnostics market (Bruno 2015). To tackle this issue and increase their acceptability is to use them in highly popular "bind and detect" biosensor formats. The Abs either operate poorly or not at all in these formats. In both qualitative and quantitative methods, a "lights on" fluorescence detection serves as an example based on the use of aptamer beacons or the FRET-aptamer approach. Still, good-quality fluorometers can cost up to $2000 or more, which can limit their widespread use. However, visual detection by the naked eye using colorimetric techniques, where antibodies fail, can be used and act as a substitute for using expensive fluorometer in the detection of small molecular analytes (Sharma et al. 2014; Weerathunge et al. 2014). Also, as developing antibodies against small molecular targets (haptens) is challenging, the use of aptamers for that purpose and consistent success in demonstrating their efficiency as molecular recognition elements for detecting small molecules may bring them close to becoming a commercially viable technology. Furthermore, some interesting novel concepts of recent times have garnered much attention to make the use of aptamer technology widespread. Nanomaterials have a distinct enzyme-mimicking activity (nanozymes), and their combination with aptamer technology is a prominent example of recent technologies, which may help change the pattern of diagnosis and propel its widespread use (Carnovale et al. 2016). Another promising example of the "aptamers only" niche are electrochemical detectors, which possess huge commercial potential and cost around 500–600$ per unit. Enterprises such as ApolloDx, LLC is one such example which has started to market these handheld detectors. These can be regulated via smartphones and can utilize the ability of aptamers to go through drastic changes when bound to target moiety. This binding helps move aptamers attached to the methylene blue or ferrocene redox labels close to the electrode and enables electrical measurements in accordance with the Ohm law (Catanante et al. 2016). Antibodies can also function in such electrochemical systems wherein the electrodes consist of methylene blue coating (Veerapandian et al. 2016), but owing to their large size, less flexibility, and conductivity in comparison to aptamers, puts them at a significant disadvantage. As per a recent report, there is not a single Ab-based analogue yet to substitute for aptamers in the electrochemical format assay based on gold electrode-thiol-5-aptamer-3-methylene blue biosensor format (Catanante et al. 2016). Additionally, newer advances improve the electrode types or their sources using dyes (Hianik 2016), dendrimers, or more electrochemical- and redox-based coats in combination with aptamers and electrodes (Hianik et al. 2008; Miodek et al. 2014), which are increasing the sensitivity and utility of such sensors. If the aptamer-based assays exclude or dominate antibodies in these simpler ways, which are revolutionary, then aptamers may finally burst into the POC market and change the immunoassay standard and conventional scene as we know (Figure 6.2).

Detection of the COVID-19 virus from the surface of surgical masks and personal protective equipment is often overlooked. This aspect needs to be addressed by using optical techniques that can transform the diagnostic technique for the virus. Such a type of strategy can help people detect the viral infection and thereby it can prevent especially with very low

Figure 6.2 A schematic depicting the working of Aptamer-based detection of the virus.

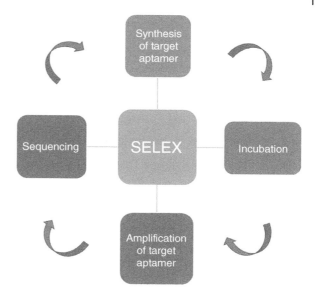

immune system from being infected. Currently, studies have been performed that utilize metal-organic frameworks (MOFs) as a coating material. These MOFs have high intact metal NPs like gold. When the coating comes in contact with the virus, the color of the surface changes from red to blue indicating the interaction of the virus with the surface. This technique can help detect even trace concentrations of the virus, which are based on the hypothesis that revealed the viral load of the coronavirus in the atmosphere for greater than three hours and its aerosol particles moved up to 8 m. For the synthesis of different MOFs, variations in the range of sizes, porosity, and interrelated volumes can be done. These MOFs possess the capacity to interact with active components of the novel virus on the surface being targeted, cysteine-sensitive molecules, along with the loading of distinct metals having several optical properties.

In a recent study, aptamers were used to detect the novel coronavirus in the early stages (Chen et al. 2020). Previously, researchers have demonstrated the binding of a single-stranded DNA aptamer to CoV19-N protein. The N protein (NP_828858.1) shares a ~90% sequence matching with the N protein of SARS-CoV-2 (YP_009724397.2). This finding was the basis behind the current aptamer-based detection assay (Cho et al. 2011). For the study, modification of the DNA aptamer was done to evaluate the binding capacity to the SARS-CoV-2-N protein. The enzyme-linked aptamer binding assay (ELAA) was employed to find out the binding efficiencies of the aptamers (1, 2, and 3). The results showed specific binding of all three aptamers to the N protein with comparable affinity. This affinity revealed that the presence of two-step loops in the aptamer is required for the binding of viral N proteins. There was no binding on the negative control aptamer with only one loop. The assay was able to detect a concentration as low as 10 ng ml^{-1}. In the same study, the viral N protein diluted in human sera samples collected from healthy donors was also measurable using the aptamers as probes. This finding indicates that viral protein detection in aptamer-laden human serum samples may be feasible for a rapid diagnosis of SARS-CoV-2 (Chen et al. 2020).

After the promising results, the binding efficiency of the aptamer was compared with that of a commercially available Ab (aptamer 2 or anti-N Ab) using western blot analysis. The immunoblotting analysis showed a dose-dependent increase in the signal similar to that of the commercial Ab sample. These results indicate the use of DNA aptamers as an alternative reagent for SARS-CoV-2 N protein detection in place of anti-N Ab (Chen et al. 2020).

6.2.5 Other Novel Technologies Developed for SARS-CoV-2 Detection

Biosensors are bioanalytical devices that possess the selectivity and sensitivity of a biomolecule and a physicochemical transducer, respectively (Kurbanoglu et al. 2020; Sheikhzadeh et al. 2020). For clinical diagnosis and real-time detection applications, and also for routine measurements, they can be a reliable and quick alternative (Wang et al. 2020). Many different types of biosensors have been utilized for diagnosing several infectious diseases (Sin et al. 2014).

6.2.5.1 Localized Surface Plasmon Resonance (LSPR) Sensor

When light waves trap conductive nanoparticles, an optical phenomenon occurs known as localized surface plasmon resonance (LSPR). This phenomenon occurs because the size of the nanoparticle is smaller than the wavelength of light. The interaction between the surface of electrons along with incident light in the conduction band gives rise to a phenomenon known as coherent localized plasmon oscillations. Any local changes such as refractive index variation and molecular binding make the resonance frequency vary (Petryayeva and Krull 2011). For the detection of viral sequences, a biosensor was developed, which utilized plasmonic photothermal effect and sensing transduction of LSPR. The developed biosensor was a dual functional plasmonic biosensor and was applied for the detection of viral sequences such as RdRP-COVID, E gene from SARS-CoV-2, and ORF lab COVID. Enhancement of RdRp in situ hybridization in SARS-CoV-2 and its complementary DNA were observed due to the conversion of PPT heat energy, as it was within the proximity of gold nanoislands, which helped it provide a stable heat source. The system without the photothermal effect had a lower slope than that of the photothermal-enhanced LSPR curve. Discrimination between SARS-CoV and SARS-CoV-2 viruses was found to be efficient. The RdRP-SARS sequence generates a false positive response if photothermal unit resistance is not available. The limit of detection for this signal was observed at 0.22 pM (Qiu et al. 2020). The induction of coherent oscillations in the free electrons present in the material is due to the oscillating electric field generated from the incident light. Compared to dielectric nanoparticles of similar size, this induced oscillating dipole significantly increases the scattering and absorption of its resonant wavelength, hence deeming it a superior label for use along with single-nanoparticle detection assays (Figure 6.3a).

6.2.5.2 Field-Effect Transistor (FET)

The field-effect transistor (FET) works on the variation of carrier mobility ions across due to electrostatic field application, the transducer contains a partial semiconductor. For selective target detection, the FET gate surface is covered with a biomolecule layer (Ahmad et al. 2018). For detection of spike protein S1 of the virus graphene-based FET was fabricated. The FET had graphene coating, which was immobilized with S1 subunit protein and

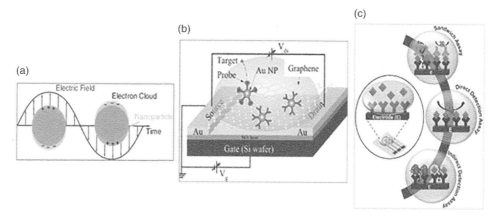

Figure 6.3 Novel diagnostic technologies for COVID-19 detection. (a) Localized surface plasmon resonance (LSPR) sensor. (b) Field-effect transistor (FET). (c) Cell-based potentiometric biosensor.

angiotensin-converting enzyme-2 (ACE-2). The detection was based on a change in graphene-FET conductance/resistance after binding the slightly positively charged S1 protein to the graphene surface with the presence of CSAb/ACE2 receptors. Due to the higher Ab affinity, used with an LOD of 0.2 pM, this CSAb-modified graphene-FET showed better sensitivity in detection (Zhang et al. 2020b). The principle behind the FET system for SARS-CoV-2 detection is the change in channel surface potential and its immediate effect on the electrical response. The S protein being a major transmembrane protein of the virus is also an excellent antigen showing a great amount of diversity in the amino acid sequence amongst other coronaviruses. In PBS and clinical samples, the level of FET sensor detection was down to 1 and 100 fg ml^{-1}, respectively. In addition, an LOD of 1.6*101 pfu ml^{-1} in culture medium and 2.42*102 pfu ml^{-1} in clinical samples for SARS-CoV-2 detection was shown by the FET sensor. The biosensor also discriminated between the SARS-CoV-2 antigen protein and the MERS-CoV protein indicating good selectivity of the platform (Seo et al. 2020). A handheld rapid COVID-19 diagnosis and testing device was developed by the Pritzker School of Molecular Engineering and Department of Pathology. This device enabled point-of-care diagnosis at home for the cost of $10 and for the development of this device, the researchers received a BIG grant [Figure 6.3b].

6.2.5.3 Cell-Based Potentiometric Biosensor
In a recent study, detection of SARS-CoV-2 S1 antigen was done using a membrane-engineered kidney cell after its modification with the relevant SARS-CoV-2 Spike S1 Ab using the electro-insertion method. The interaction between the target protein and Ab initiates a change in the membrane potential. The fabricated device had gold screen-printed electrodes coated with polydimethylsiloxane (PDMS). Eight screen-printed electrodes had the same number of wells. The modified membrane suspension was added well to the PDMS and the protein solution was subsequently added using a potentiometer to measure the signal. The developed sensor exhibited an excellent detection limit of 1 fg ml^{-1} with a wide linear range of 1 µg ml^{-1} to 10 fg. (Mavrikou et al. 2020) (Figure 6.3c).

6.3 Conclusion

With more technologies coming out for the detection of viruses, it is expected that in future, easier and more established molecular-based diagnostic systems like LAMP, CRISPR, microfluidics, and integration of several different methods and biosensor platforms will eventually replace the conventional detection techniques like RT-PCR. In order to achieve good sensitivity, specificity, accuracy, reliability, and robustness of the test, its comparison must be done with each other and the older methods to ascertain their widespread use. In addition, sample analysis from developed techniques and various routes should be combined with oral swab detection methods for the proper validation of the results to make an informed decision on whether to discharge people from hospitals or suggest home quarantine. Instead of nasopharyngeal samples, sputum, saliva, amd posterior oropharyngeal fluids could act as potential replacements as they are less invasive and dangerous for the healthcare staff. The current tests, despite many advances, are not sufficient enough to distinguish the infected in public areas. Therefore, new POC devices that can provide on-site detection without the need for professionally trained staff are still urgently needed. We need to create new nanosystems to prevent, diagnose, treat, and reduce the spread of the virus, with the pandemic spreading exponentially and affecting millions. A well-coordinated, fast, timely, and efficient response is the need for the hour in order to deal with the current situation.

References

Ahmad, R., Mahmoudi, T., Ahn, M.S., and Hahn, Y.B. (2018). Recent advances in nanowires-based field-effect transistors for biological sensor applications. *Biosensors and Bioelectronics* 100: 312–325.

Beavis, K.G., Matushek, S.M., Abeleda, A.P.F. et al. (2020). Evaluation of the EUROIMMUN Anti-SARS-CoV-2 ELISA assay for detection of IgA and IgG antibodies. *Journal of Clinical Virology* 129: 104468.

Bruno, J.G. (2014). Application of DNA aptamers and quantum dots to lateral flow test strips for detection of foodborne pathogens with improved sensitivity versus colloidal gold. *Pathogens* 3 (2): 341–355.

Bruno, J.G. (2015). Predicting the uncertain future of aptamer-based diagnostics and therapeutics. *Molecules* 20 (4): 6866–6887.

Cai, X., Chen, J., Hu, J. et al. (2020). A peptide-based magnetic chemiluminescence enzyme immunoassay for serological diagnosis of Corona Virus Disease 2019 (COVID-19). *medRxiv* 129: 104468.

Carnovale, C., Bryant, G., Shukla, R., and Bansal, V. (2016). Size, shape and surface chemistry of nano-gold dictate its cellular interactions, uptake and toxicity. *Progress in Materials Science* 83: 152–190.

Catanante, G., Mishra, R.K., Hayat, A., and Marty, J.L. (2016). Sensitive analytical performance of folding based biosensor using methylene blue tagged aptamers. *Talanta* 153: 138–144.

Chen, A. and Yang, S. (2015). Replacing antibodies with aptamers in lateral flow immunoassay. *Biosensors and Bioelectronics* 71: 230–242.

Chen, J.S., Ma, E., Harrington, L.B. et al. (2018). CRISPR-Cas12a target binding unleashes indiscriminate single-stranded DNase activity. *Science* 360 (6387): 436–439.

Chen, Z., Wu, Q., Chen, J. et al. (2020). A DNA aptamer based method for detection of SARS-CoV-2 nucleocapsid protein. *Virologica Sinica* 71: 1.

Cho, S.J., Woo, H.M., Kim, K.S. et al. (2011). Novel system for detecting SARS coronavirus nucleocapsid protein using an ssDNA aptamer. *Journal of Bioscience and Bioengineering* 112 (6): 535–540.

Cong, L., Ran, F.A., Cox, D. et al. (2013). Multiplex genome engineering using CRISPR/Cas systems. *Science* 339 (6121): 819–823.

Craw, P. and Balachandran, W. (2012). Isothermal nucleic acid amplification technologies for point-of-care diagnostics: a critical review. *Lab on a Chip* 12 (14): 2469–2486.

Dhiman, A., Kalra, P., Bansal, V. et al. (2017). Aptamer-based point-of-care diagnostic platforms. *Sensors and Actuators B: Chemical* 246: 535–553.

Ding, X., Yin, K., Li, Z., and Liu, C. (2020). All-in-one dual CRISPR-cas12a (AIOD-CRISPR) assay: a case for rapid, ultrasensitive and visual detection of novel coronavirus SARS-CoV-2 and HIV virus. *bioRxiv* [Preprint]. 2020.03.19.998724. doi: 10.1101/2020.03.19.998724. Update in: Nature Communication. 2020 Sep 18;11(1):4711. PMID: 32511323; PMCID: PMC7239053.

Dzantiev, B.B., Byzova, N.A., Urusov, A.E., and Zherdev, A.V. (2014). Immunochromatographic methods in food analysis. *TrAC Trends in Analytical Chemistry* 55: 81–93.

Elnifro, E.M., Ashshi, A.M., Cooper, R.J., and Klapper, P.E. (2000). Multiplex PCR: optimization and application in diagnostic virology. *Clinical Microbiology Reviews* 13 (4): 559–570.

Foudeh, A.M., Didar, T.F., Veres, T., and Tabrizian, M. (2012). Microfluidic designs and techniques using lab-on-a-chip devices for pathogen detection for point-of-care diagnostics. *Lab on a Chip* 12 (18): 3249–3266.

Gootenberg, J.S., Abudayyeh, O.O., Lee, J.W. et al. (2017). Nucleic acid detection with CRISPR-Cas13a/C2c2. *Science* 356 (6336): 438–442.

Guan, W.J., Ni, Z.Y., Hu, Y. et al. (2020). Clinical characteristics of coronavirus disease 2019 in China. *New England Journal of Medicine* 382 (18): 1708–1720.

Hianik, T. (2016). Affinity biosensors for detection immunoglobulin E and cellular prions. Antibodies vs. DNA aptamers. *Electroanalysis* 28 (8): 1764–1776.

Hianik, T., Porfireva, A., Grman, I., and Evtugyn, G. (2008). Aptabodies-new type of artificial receptors for detection proteins. *Protein and Peptide Letters* 15 (8): 799–805.

Huang, P., Wang, H., Cao, Z. et al. (2018). A rapid and specific assay for the detection of MERS-CoV. *Frontiers in Microbiology* 9: 1101.

Kang, S., Peng, W., Zhu, Y. et al. (2020). Recent Progress in understanding 2019 novel coronavirus associated with human respiratory disease: detection, mechanism and treatment. *International Journal of Antimicrobial Agents* 55 (5): 105950.

Kellner, M.J., Koob, J.G., Gootenberg, J.S. et al. (2019). SHERLOCK: nucleic acid detection with CRISPR nucleases. *Nature Protocols* 14 (10): 2986–3012.

Kim, J., Biondi, M.J., Feld, J.J., and Chan, W.C. (2016). Clinical validation of quantum dot barcode diagnostic technology. *ACS Nano* 10 (4): 4742–4753.

Kurbanoglu, S., Erkmen, C., and Uslu, B. (2020). Frontiers in electrochemical enzyme based biosensors for food and drug analysis. *TrAC Trends in Analytical Chemistry* 124: 115809.

Li, L., Li, S., Wu, N. et al. (2019). HOLMESv2: a CRISPR-Cas12b-assisted platform for nucleic acid detection and DNA methylation quantitation. *ACS Synthetic Biology* 8 (10): 2228–2237.

Lin, Q., Wen, D., Wu, J. et al. (2020). Microfluidic immunoassays for sensitive and simultaneous detection of IgG/IgM/Antigen of SARS-CoV-2 within 15 min. *Analytical Chemistry* 92 (14): 9454–9458.

Lu, R., Zhao, X., Li, J. et al. (2020). Genomic characterisation and epidemiology of 2019 novel coronavirus: implications for virus origins and receptor binding. *The Lancet* 395 (10224): 565–574.

Lv, H., Wu, N.C., Tsang, O.T.Y. et al. (2020). Cross-reactive Ab response between SARS-CoV-2 and SARS-CoV infections. *Cell Reports* 31 (31): 107725.

Mavrikou, S., Moschopoulou, G., Tsekouras, V., and Kintzios, S. (2020). Development of a portable, ultra-rapid and ultra-sensitive cell-based biosensor for the direct detection of the SARS-CoV-2 S1 spike protein antigen. *Sensors* 20 (11): 3121.

Miodek, A., Castillo, G., Hianik, T., and Korri-Youssoufi, H. (2014). Electrochemical aptasensor of cellular prion protein based on modified polypyrrole with redox dendrimers. *Biosensors and Bioelectronics* 56: 104–111.

Mori, Y., Nagamine, K., Tomita, N., and Notomi, T. (2001). Detection of loop-mediated isothermal amplification reaction by turbidity derived from magnesium pyrophosphate formation. *Biochemical and Biophysical Research Communications* 289 (1): 150–154.

Petryayeva, E. and Krull, U.J. (2011). Localized surface plasmon resonance: nanostructures, bioassays and biosensing—a review. *Analytica Chimica Acta* 706 (1): 8–24.

Qiu, G., Gai, Z., Tao, Y. et al. (2020). Dual-functional plasmonic photothermal biosensors for highly accurate severe acute respiratory syndrome coronavirus 2 detection. *ACS Nano* 14 (5): 5268–5277.

Sajid, M., Kawde, A.N., and Daud, M. (2015). Designs, formats and applications of lateral flow assay: a literature review. *Journal of Saudi Chemical Society* 19 (6): 689–705.

Seo, G., Lee, G., Kim, M.J. et al. (2020). Rapid detection of COVID-19 causative virus (SARS-CoV-2) in human nasopharyngeal swab specimens using field-effect transistor-based biosensor. *ACS Nano* 14 (4): 5135–5142.

Sharma, T.K., Ramanathan, R., Weerathunge, P. et al. (2014). Aptamer-mediated 'turn-off/turn-on' nanozyme activity of gold nanoparticles for kanamycin detection. *Chemical Communications* 50 (100): 15856–15859.

Sheikhzadeh, E., Eissa, S., Ismail, A., and Zourob, M. (2020). Diagnostic techniques for COVID-19 and new developments. *Talanta* 220: 121392.

Sin, M.L., Mach, K.E., Wong, P.K., and Liao, J.C. (2014). Advances and challenges in biosensor-based diagnosis of infectious diseases. *Expert Review of Molecular Diagnostics* 14 (2): 225–244.

Spengler, M., Adler, M., and Niemeyer, C.M. (2015). Highly sensitive ligand-binding assays in pre-clinical and clinical applications: immuno-PCR and other emerging techniques. *Analyst* 140 (18): 6175–6194.

To, K.K.W., Tsang, O.T.Y., Leung, W.S. et al. (2020). Temporal profiles of viral load in posterior oropharyngeal saliva samples and serum Ab responses during infection by SARS-CoV-2: an observational cohort study. *The Lancet Infectious Diseases* 20: 565–574.

Tuerk, C. and Gold, L. (1990). Systematic evolution of ligands by exponential enrichment: RNA ligands to bacteriophage T4 DNA polymerase. *Science* 249 (4968): 505–510.

Udugama, B., Kadhiresan, P., Samarakoon, A., and Chan, W.C. (2017). Simplifying assays by tableting reagents. *Journal of the American Chemical Society* 139 (48): 17341–17349.

Veerapandian, M., Hunter, R., and Neethirajan, S. (2016). Dual immunosensor based on methylene blue-electroadsorbed graphene oxide for rapid detection of the influenza A virus antigen. *Talanta* 155: 250–257.

Walker, G.T., Fraiser, M.S., Schram, J.L. et al. (1992). Strand displacement amplification—an isothermal, in vitro DNA amplification technique. *Nucleic Acids Research* 20 (7): 1691–1696.

Wang, B., Wang, R., Wang, D. et al. (2019). Cas12aVDet: a CRISPR/Cas12a-based platform for rapid and visual nucleic acid detection. *Analytical Chemistry* 91 (19): 12156–12161.

Wang, M., Fu, A., Hu, B. et al. (2020). Nanopore targeted sequencing for the accurate and comprehensive detection of SARS-CoV-2 and other respiratory viruses. *Small* 16 (32): 2002169.

Weerathunge, P., Ramanathan, R., Shukla, R. et al. (2014). Aptamer-controlled reversible inhibition of gold nanozyme activity for pesticide sensing. *Analytical Chemistry* 86 (24): 11937–11941.

Wong, R. and Tse, H. (ed.) (2008). *Lateral Flow Immunoassay*. Springer Science & Business Media.

Wu, H., He, J.S., Zhang, F. et al. (2020). Contamination-free visual detection of CaMV35S promoter amplicon using CRISPR/Cas12a coupled with a designed reaction vessel: rapid, specific and sensitive. *Analytica Chimica Acta* 1096: 130–137.

Xiang, J., Yan, M., Li, H. et al. (2020). Evaluation of enzyme-linked immunoassay and colloidal gold-immunochromatographic assay kit for detection of novel coronavirus (SARS-Cov-2) causing an outbreak of pneumonia (COVID-19). *MedRxiv*.

Zhang, W., Du, R.H., Li, B. et al. (2020a). Molecular and serological investigation of 2019-nCoV infected patients: implication of multiple shedding routes. *Emerging Microbes and Infections* 9 (1): 386–389.

Zhang, X., Qi, Q., Jing, Q., et al. (2020b). Electrical probing of COVID-19 spike protein receptor binding domain via a graphene field-effect transistor. arXiv preprint arXiv:2003.12529.

Zhou, W., Hu, L., Ying, L. et al. (2018). A CRISPR–Cas9-triggered strand displacement amplification method for ultrasensitive DNA detection. *Nature Communications* 9 (1): 1–11.

Zhou, P., Yang, X.L., Wang, X.G. et al. (2020). A pneumonia outbreak associated with a new coronavirus of probable bat origin. *Nature* 579 (7798): 270–273.

7

Advanced Digital Tools for Tracing and Analysis of COVID-19

Archana Singh[1], Aayush Dey[2], and Deepak Rawtani[3]

[1] *School of Engineering and Technology, National Forensic Sciences University (Ministry of Home Affairs, GOI), Gandhinagar, Gujarat, India*
[2] *School of Doctoral Studies and Research, National Forensic Sciences University (Ministry of Home Affairs, GOI), Gandhinagar, Gujarat, India*
[3] *School of Pharmacy, National Forensic Sciences University (Ministry of Home Affairs, GOI), Gandhinagar, Gujarat, India*

7.1   Introduction

The novel coronavirus disease 2019 (COVID-19) is an incessant disease that was first discerned in December 2019, which is a menace to global health (Fauci et al. 2020). The SARS-CoV-2 virus is responsible for the high mortality rates, which are evident in the human population. Several nations across the globe have utilized different resources at their disposal for the mitigation of COVID-19, among which strategies such as digital tools play a vital role (Gasser et al. 2020). The WHO declared the novel coronavirus disease a pandemic on 30 January 2020 (Roser et al. 2020). Since then, digital tools have been utilized for the tracing and analysis of COVID-19. There have been plenty of developments in the digital strategies required for the tracing and monitoring of the novel coronavirus disease. The incubation period for the SARS-CoV-2 virus extends from 12–14 days (Oran and Topol 2020). During this period, a person may or may not experience symptoms, and this fact requires the deployment of digital tools for COVID-19 tracing and analysis. Digital tools for tracing and analysis of the novel coronavirus have been categorized on the basis of technologies used in different mobile software applications. Tools such as flow modeling, quarantine compliance, COVID-19 symptom checkers, and contact tracing have been used extensively for curbing the spread of COVID-19.

Flow modeling tools, also known as mobility reporting tools, are used to evaluate the movement of a user. These tools are helpful in mapping whether an individual is coming in contact with COVID-19 high-risk areas. Quarantine compliance tools are used to ensure that an infected individual is under self-isolation or quarantine in order to stop the transmission of the COVID-19 disease. Proximity-tracing tools in the context of COVID-19 are used to detect different users and the infected individuals who might be present in their vicinity. Similar to other tools as aforementioned, contact tracing tools also use Bluetooth,

GPS, and WiFi technologies that are used to differentiate between healthy and infected individuals. These digital tools along with artificial intelligence (AI) are the recent developments in tracing and analysis of COVID-19. The applications of AI lie beyond subjects such as computing, robotics, and automobiles. AI in the context of COVID-19 has aided frontline workers such as doctors and surgeons in predicting the transmission of the disease.

This chapter aims to educate its readers about the novel developments in the strategies that have been used to mitigate the transmission of COVID-19. Mobile-based digital tools and AI all together have overcome the traditional methods of tracking down individuals with probable infections. The advantages of digital tools have also been dealt with in detail in this chapter. This chapter also emphasizes AI, which has been used for the development of vaccines and drugs, which will be further discussed in this chapter.

7.2   Developments in Digital Strategies for COVID-19

The deployment of mobile software and applications for detecting and analysis of COVID-19 is evident. Previously, mobile software technology has been developed by governments for the analysis and tracing of different viral outbreaks. One of the most established examples of the aforementioned statement is the use of an application called the "Flu Phone." This application was developed by a panel of scientific researchers in the United Kingdom in the year 2010 and is based on Bluetooth and Global Positioning System (GPS). The data collected by this application aided in predicting patterns of influenza virus transmission (Computer Laboratory Systems Research Group 2020). The infrastructure of digital techniques for tracing and analysis of COVID-19 incorporates the utility of Bluetooth, application programming interfaces (APIs), and GPS technology. These technologies are provided by major tech giants, mainly Google, Apple, and Microsoft (Owusu 2020). Interaction between smartphones, tablets, and personal digital assistants in close vicinity is facilitated via the usage of technologies such as Bluetooth, API, and GPS. Communication via the aforementioned technologies is a part of all iOS and Android-enabled devices. When an individual accesses such technologies in the advent of any pandemic, in this case, COVID-19, an anonymous identification code is generated for the userbase linked to that particular individual (Owusu 2020). If any person exhibits symptoms of COVID-19 or tests positive for COVID-19, the application accesses the database of those identification codes generated earlier for reference to the public health authority. The concerned authority, in turn, notifies the close contacts of the infected individual in an effort to mitigate SARS-COV-2 transmission (Owusu 2020).

7.2.1   Monitoring of COVID-19 Infection

Iceland has a unique technique for tracing and analysis of individuals who are infected with COVID-19 but do not exhibit any evident symptoms of the disease. Such individuals are also known as asymptomatic individuals (USA Today 2020). This initiative by the country named Iceland gathers data on symptoms that are reported by patients and this data is further combined with other data sets such as clinical and genomic sequencing data. As a result, vital information regarding the pathology and the transmission of the SARS-COV-2 virus is discovered. This particular strategy applied by the country has given a greater insight into the prevalence of the novel coronavirus (USA Today 2020). Also, this strategy incorporated by Iceland has resulted in the lowest mortality rate due to COVID-19 and the highest per-capita testing (USA Today 2020). South Korea and Germany are other countries that offer a similar kind of testing strategy that has helped in mitigating the spread of the novel coronavirus (Reuters 2020; The New York Times 2020).

A strategy in the United States of America has been developed to detect acute fever using digital thermometers (Miller et al. 2018). Another mobile software application has been developed to monitor the heart rate of an individual (Topol 2020). The data collected from these applications are useful to track down emergent COVID-19 outbreaks. These techniques are in the developmental phase and have not been strategized.

Screening technologies adopted by countries like Germany, Iceland, South Korea, and the United States of America are expensive and they require a professional to operate (Rauhala 2020). These aspects limit the incorporation of monitoring strategies in many developing or underdeveloped countries. Other disadvantages of monitoring strategies include their ineffectiveness in capturing the infection in asymptomatic individuals and vital science or self-reporting of symptoms (Rauhala 2020; Topol 2020).

7.2.2   Digital Techniques in Tracing and Analysis

Amidst the novel coronavirus pandemic, the capabilities of digital techniques have been put to use in a novel way for the tracing and analysis of COVID-19. These digital techniques have been put to use in correspondence to public health responses. The spectrum of applications of digital tools for public welfare (Figure 7.1) is broad. Communities with a high risk of COVID-19 transmission can be surveyed via such digital tools. Prior identification of individuals with the risk of COVID-19 infection can be done via digital tools. Although

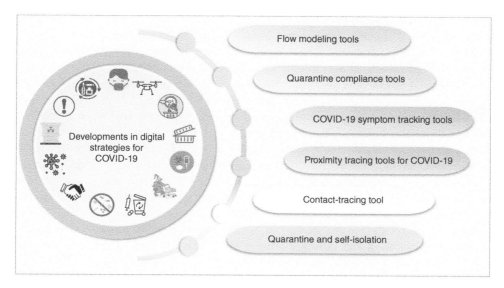

Figure 7.1   Digital tools for tracing and analysis of COVID-19.

the benefits of such digital tools are many, some issues regarding the legal, ethical, and privacy concerns over digital techniques do arise. The use of digital techniques in the domain of public health in the future and its use will further be continued for probable outbreaks or pandemics (Gasser et al. 2020).

7.2.2.1 Flow Modeling Tools

Such tools are also known as mobility reports, which are used to enumerate and map the movement of a community population in a particular topographical location of interest. The data aggregated from this modeling tool depends solely upon the topographical location of the user. Flow modeling tools can be utilized to map the efficiency of measures, for example, physical distancing and self-quarantine, that have been employed for combatting COVID-19 (Guevara 2019). Flow modeling tools incorporate anonymized and combined data to monitor the tendencies in population movement in accordance with topography. The data collected from such tools can be utilized to analyze how crowded a particular location is. Policies framed for people going to offices including work from home or staying at home are intended at curbing the COVID-19 growth curve, and the effectiveness of such policies can be mapped via the flow modeling tools (Dwork et al. 2006). The flow modeling tools or community mobility reports can be used to map any geographical location such as workplaces and corporate offices, retail sites, grocery and supermarket shops, residential localities, transit stations, etc. The time range in data acquired from flow modeling tools can vary from 48 hours to several weeks (Google 2020).

7.2.2.2 Quarantine Compliance Tools

The quarantine compliance tools are employed to monitor symptomatic or asymptomatic individuals, whether they are complying with the rules of self- or home quarantine (Gasser et al. 2020). The quarantine compliance tools have a particular workflow that can be divided into three parts. The first step involves the identification of individuals with symptoms of COVID-19. The identification of individuals can be done via Bluetooth, GPS, and quick response (QR) codes. Bluetooth-compatible devices are used by almost everyone, which can be used to deduce digital handshakes (Kleinman and Merkel 2020) occurring between two individuals. Bluetooth-enabled devices can also be used for mapping the proximity between a healthy and an infected individual. GPS in combination with Bluetooth-enabled devices can also be used to generate precise coordinates of an individual, which would help generate warnings or notifications if a person is in close proximity to COVID-19 hotspots. Generally, Bluetooth-based applications are more respectful of the privacy of an individual. QR codes if scanned by an individual can be used to maintain a digitized log of the places that a person has visited. These logs generated are stored in the device of a user, which are further used by the concerned health authorities in case a person tests positive for COVID-19. There are several other tools that invade the privacy of a person and include the utilization of credit card transactions, closed-circuit television (CCTV) cameras, and mobile network details (Lin and Hou 2020). Such strategies could be utilized to triangulate an individual's location and infringes privacy. Such tools can be utilized to identify the probable extent of COVID-19 transmission (WHO 2020a).

Once identification of probable sources of infection in the context of COVID-19 has been done, quarantine compliance tools can be utilized for issuing a targeted notification or issuing a general notification to the public. Notifications to the general public regarding high-risk areas or hotspots can also be issued using quarantine compliance tools (WHO 2020b). The last phase of the compliance tools is the quarantine phase in which people with confirmed COVID-19 infection are kept in an isolation ward or are adviced home quarantine (Abeler et al. 2020).

7.2.2.3 COVID-19 Symptom Tracking Tools

Symptom tracking tools for COVID-19 have been useful in scenarios where an individual self-reports his conditions and adequate steps are taken by the concerned authorities to diagnose those symptoms. One such example of a COVID-19 symptom tracking tool is "COVID Near You," which was designed by epidemiologists and software developers at the Innovation and Digital Health Accelerator at Boston Children's Hospital. The team that developed this software holds prior expertise in disease outbreak surveillance. This team of developers was also capable of creating visualization-based tools for public health and well-being. The "COVID Near You" app targets to back up surveillance regarding COVID-19 symptom tracking using self-reported data. This strategy would aid in a better understanding and prediction of COVID-19 transmission (Moss et al. 2020). Another similar strategy involves the utilization of the "How We Feel" mobile software application. This application requires the self-reporting of symptoms that an individual may experience (Moss et al. 2020).

7.2.2.4 Proximity Tracing Tools for COVID-19

Such tools are used to evaluate the spatial proximity among individuals in order to map the interaction between them. Proximity tracing tools in coordination with patient history reports and other non-digital techniques have been utilized for tracing COVID-19-infected patients (WHO 2020c). GPS and Bluetooth technologies have been incorporated into proximity-tracing utilities to evaluate the vicinity of two individuals. An app used in Singapore known as "TraceTogether" emphasizes Bluetooth connection technology that notifies an individual who has been close to an infected individual (Babones 2020).

7.2.2.5 Contact Tracing Tool

Amongst the most vital policies for mitigating the novel coronavirus disease is contact tracing. On a global scale, different nations have introduced mobile software applications to notify individuals who have been exposed to the coronavirus. The risk of getting infected with coronavirus disease increases when the individual is in close contact with the infected person. These individuals can also act as a medium to infect other healthy individuals. Prior to knowing about the strategies involved in contact tracing, it would be feasible to know what contact tracing is. Basically in the advent of COVID-19 caused by the novel coronavirus strain SARS-CoV-2, the technique for monitoring people who have been exposed to this virus is known as contact tracing. Contact tracing-based strategies have also been employed for monitoring individuals who act as the potential transmission of COVID-19. Contact tracing is a tedious process that is carried out by a specialized team that carries out interviews across a community to find out potentially infected individuals (WHO 2020d). Further, the team notifies the people associated with the infected persons and identifies them as contacts. The investigated process of contact tracing is challenging.

Contact tracing is a strategy that has been utilized in accordance with public health and a major effort to control the transmission of the SARS-CoV-2 (WHO 2020e) can be further categorized into three basic steps, which have been further described in Section 7.2.2.5.1.

7.2.2.5.1 *Traditional Form of Contact Tracing*

Contact tracing corresponding to COVID-19 has played the role of a vital strategy in minimizing COVID-19 transmission and also mitigating the mortality rates due to COVID-19. In the advent of the novel coronavirus pandemic, it is an important step to recognize chains of COVID-19 transmission and the primary hotspots and sources of COVID-19 exposures. The traditional form of contact tracing (Figure 7.2) can be categorized into three steps – the first step is termed contact identification, the second step is known as a listing of contacts, and the third step involves following up on those potential contacts (Owusu 2020).

Identification of contacts: A contact can be defined as an individual who has been in direct proximal contact with an infected individual or has been in contact with an individual without the utilization of recommended personal protective equipment (PPE). In this step of identification of contacts, infected individuals are interviewed about their whereabouts and actions since the onset of symptoms of COVID-19 (WHO 2020d).

Listing of contacts: There must be some scenarios in which it is not feasible to identify, prioritize, and assess each contact. Therefore, the priority of listing must be given to contacts who are at a higher risk of COVID-19 infection depending on their extent of exposure. This would be helpful in dismantling chains of COVID-19 transmission. The priority of listing must also be given to those contacts who can develop severe COVID-19 disease to provide them adequate healthcare (WHO 2020d).

Following up of contacts: Every individual that has been identified as a contact must be provided with a set of information that includes the methodology and the objective for contact tracing. Each contact must be educated regarding the specific symptoms to look out

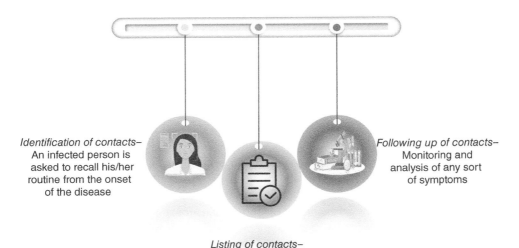

Identification of contacts–
An infected person is
asked to recall his/her
routine from the onset
of the disease

Following up of contacts–
Monitoring and
analysis of any sort
of symptoms

Listing of contacts–
Infected individual provides
the concerned authority

Figure 7.2 Steps of conventional contact tracing.

for during the screening period and what steps to follow if the symptoms of COVID-19 become evident. An individual must inform the concerned authority regarding their health condition and must practice self-isolation and treatment in-home quarantine if they are diagnosed with a positive COVID-19 infection. Also, personal queries raised by the individual to the concerned authority must be cleared out by the concerned authorities (WHO 2020d).

7.2.2.5.2 Recent Developments in Contact Tracing

Countries such as South Korea, India, China, Iran, Israel, and the USA have implemented novel strategies for contact tracing and launched mobile software applications as depicted in Table 7.1. These strategies have immensely helped in the early tracing of COVID-19 hotspots. A belligerent strategy for contact tracing of individuals infected with COVID-19 has been utilized by the government of South Korea. In this strategy, CCTV camera tape, facial biometrics technology, and GPS data from vehicles and mobile phones were accumulated to obtain real-time data on transport and travel. These data are further analyzed and details specific to COVID-19 cases and risks of possible transmission are mapped. The population of South Korea is then notified about these mapped specifics regarding COVID-19. This contact tracing tool also notifies an individual who could have been in possible contact with an infected individual and directs the person to report to the COVID-19-testing center and to isolate themselves. Such measures employed by South Korea have helped them achieve the lowest per-capita mortality rate in the world (The New York Times 2020).

The government of India (GoI) launched a mobile software application known as "Aarogya Setu." The only prerequisite for registering in this application is the mobile contact number of the user. This application incorporates Bluetooth technology for contact tracing. Supplementary information such as age, the gender of the user, countries, or the number of cities the user has visited is also required to completely access the application. Further, the GoI claims that the information collected from the user will be stored locally on the individual's smartphone and further it could be uploaded to the government servers. The basic working principle of the application is that when a user or an individual registers into the application, a unique identification number is generated, which is further utilized to trace all of the contacts in the close vicinity of an individual infected with COVID-19. A benefit of using this application is that a user can delete the account created by them, and it has been

Table 7.1 Nations and their initiatives in digital technologies for contact tracing (Shukla et al. 2020).

S. No.	Country	Digital tool application	Integrated technology
1.	South Korea	Kakao Map	GPS
2.	India	Aarogya Setu	Bluetooth, GPS
3.	China	Alipay, WeChat	Bluetooth, GPS
4.	Iran	AC19	GPS, WiFi
5.	Israel	Hamagen	GPS
6.	USA	Safe Paths	Bluetooth, GPS, WiFi SSID

assured by the government that the data collected from the user end will be eliminated from the government database after 30 days of account deactivation (Gupta et al. 2020).

The country where the pandemic of COVID-19 originated, i.e. China has utilized mobile software applications such as "Alipay" and "WeChat." These mobile applications rely on data accumulated by self-reporting by the user. Data such as help status, travel log, and government records are used to assign specific color codes, namely green, yellow, and red. These color codes have a special meaning that denotes the health status of the user. The color green denotes that the user is healthy, the color yellow signifies that the user is suspected of probable infection, and the color red signifies that the user is COVID-19 positive (Davidson 2020). This system of color coding is aggressive as the color is denoted to a user who decides the freedom of movement. Any violations done by a user are threatened with gruesome punishments. In terms of privacy and user safety, the system of contact tracing utilized by China is very invasive. The usage of this application is mandatory by the people of China, and this fact alone makes the people of China vulnerable to the misuse of digital data. These applications necessitate user identity, user address, and travel logs, which is a complete breach of the privacy of an individual. Additionally, the color codes assigned by these applications can be used as a tool for surveillance of the people living in China (Knight 2020).

The contact-tracing application "AC19" launched by the government of Iran has a prerequisite of a mobile phone number which is used to register in the mobile software application. This contact-tracing application employs an unencrypted GPS technology that is used to triangulate the user's precise coordinates (Chrysaidos 2020). Additionally, this application identifies the user activity which is a concern regarding user privacy. Security experts have found a loophole in the coding of this mobile software application used for contact tracing in Iran in which the user's personal information such as name, height, weight, and gender is stored in a different server that belongs to the developer (Cimpanu 2020).

Israel has launched a contact-tracing application named the "Hamagen." When a user registers into this contact-tracing application, real-time data about the precise location of the user is accumulated in the background. A significant data about the most probable hotspots in Israel has been collected which is further compared to the travel history of the user, and if the user has come in contact with an infected individual within the proximity of these locations, a targeted notification is issued to the users, which consists of additional precautionary measurements. One of the primary benefits of using this application is that no user data is collected by the government of Israel (Winer 2020).

One of the most prestigious institutions in the USA, i.e. the Massachusetts Institute of Technology (MIT) has introduced a contact-tracing application named "Safe Paths." This method of contact tracing is incorporated with technology such as Bluetooth, GPS, and WiFi SSID for absolute tracking of individuals and users with the probable risk of the COVID-19 infection (Berke et al. 2020).

7.2.2.5.3 Advantages of COVID-19 Contact Tracing

One of the primary advantages of contact-tracing applications is that it acknowledges user willingness via features such as account creation and account deletion that give the user complete freedom to participate in the application. Another advantage of digital technology is that it abolishes the need for self-reporting. One of the most important advantages of digital tracing tools is that it eliminates the need of face-to-face interviews with the official contact-tracing investigation team (Owusu 2020).

Some pioneers in global health subjects have cherished the usage of digital technology against COVID-19. They believe that the usage of digital technology has set up a new standard in the implementation of mass interventions. Some digital techniques such as the Internet of Healthcare Things (IoHT), big data, and machine learning have played a vital role in mitigating COVID-19 transmission besides contract tracing (Kumar et al. 2020; Vaishya et al. 2020). In the future, the scope of these contact-tracing applications will be widened to the development of therapeutic treatments for patients infected with COVID-19, drug and vaccine formulations for COVID-19, and mapping real-time data to predict future outbreaks.

7.2.2.6 Quarantine and Self-Isolation

The immediate lockdowns on the global scale have left a great impact on the socioeconomic aspects. Digital technology can be used to impose isolation and quarantine protocols on individuals infected with the novel coronavirus. A QR code system employed by China mandates individuals to fill out a survey in which the temperature of the individual is measured, which, in turn, authorizes concerned personnel to monitor the health and movement of the user (Liu 2020). This QR code system in China acts as a travel pass and health status certificate. International travelers were quarantined in hotels on arrival in Australia and travelers from Wuhan were quarantined far away from the Australian mainland. According to the rules set by the Australian government individuals who would be found violating quarantine rules would be forced to wear tracking devices, additionally, hefty fines would be imposed upon quarantine rule violaters (Pannett and Cherney 2020). Taiwan has come up with another novel strategy for quarantine rules. In this strategy, mobile phones have been issued by the government, which are tracked by GPS technology. In any scenario, where an individual breaks quarantine rules, a digital fence generates warnings, and fines are imposed (Wang et al. 2020). In South Korea, people were asked to download a mobile application whose sole purpose is to notify concerned authorities if those individuals leave their place of self-quarantine (The New York Times 2020). Hong Kong is another city that incorporates the use of a wristband that is linked to cloud technology and, in return, it alerts concerned authorities if the quarantine regulations are violated (Liu 2020). In Iceland, a mobile software application has been launched that monitors infected individuals to ensure that they remain in self-isolation (Homeland Security Today 2020).

7.3 Artificial Intelligence in Curbing COVID-19

Any study or computer program that emulates human intelligence is known as AI. The scope of applications of AI is broad enough and not just limited to computing, robotics, or automobiles. The applications of AI can be extended to areas such as disease diagnosis, prediction, tracking and treatment, patient monitoring, drug and vaccine formulations, prediction of future outbreaks, predicting mortality rates associated with COVID-19, etc. (Arora et al. 2020; Tayarani 2021). The applications of AI (Figure 7.3) are described as follows.

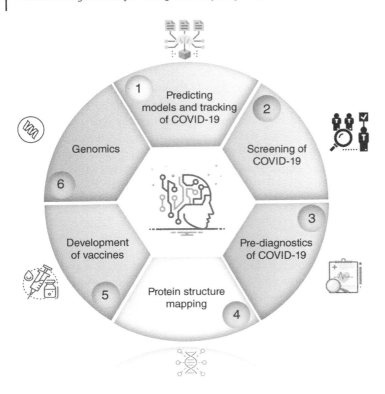

Figure 7.3   Artificial Intelligence (AI) in curbing of COVID-19.

7.3.1   Predictive Models and Tracking of COVID-19 via AI

Social media platforms, news channels, and websites provide much information about areas with high contamination risks. These data can be segregated and accumulated with the aid of AI to predict the morbidity and mortality of that particular area. An outbreak response software is known as the "Bluedot" aided in the identification of a cluster of pneumonia cases. Further, this information helped in the identification of the geographical location from where the outbreak of COVID-19 could have occurred. "HealthMap" is another AI-based software that collects publicly available information about COVID-19 and is used for the effective tracking of its transmission (Santosh 2020).

7.3.2   AI in the Screening of COVID-19 Cases

The screening of COVID-19 infected individuals in clinical settings can be carried out through AI. Prediction of a pathway to the treatment of COVID-19-infected individuals can also be done with the help of AI. Vital statistics and clinical factors are the two aspects from which vital data regarding resource allocation can be done. This is primarily assisted by an AI. Decision-making by listing the requirement of ventilators and respiratory supports in ICU is also assisted by an AI (Rahmatizadeh et al. 2020). Recovery and mortality rate prediction, the prevalence of the virus and screening of transmission of SARS-CoV-2, and predicting the course of treatment can also be done by AI (Arora et al. 2020).

7.3.3 Pre-Diagnostics of COVID-19 and AI

Chest X-ray images and computerized tomographic (CT) scanned images can be used for the detection and quantification of COVID-19. "COVnet," an AI-based platform, has been created to differentiate between pneumonia and COVID-19. This differentiation was created on the basis of 2D and 3D structures extracted from volumetric chest CT scans (Gozes et al. 2020; Sethy et al. 2020). Multi-objective differential evolution in association with convolutional neural networks has been used for the detection of COVID-19 using a CT scan of the chest (Singh et al. 2020).

7.3.4 AI in Protein Structure Mapping

Protein structures that may be crucial regarding viral entry and replication can be mapped through AI. In order to counter the viral entry, the drug structure can also be mapped in a short time through AI. "ResNets," also known as Google Deep mind-deep residual networks (DRNs) and AlphaFold algorithms, were used together to map the protein structures of the membrane protein of SARS-CoV-2. Proteins 3a, nsp2, nsp4, nsp6, and papain-like C-terminal were predicted through AI (Senior et al. 2020). The protein complex structure of SARS-CoV-2 from high-resolution cryoelectron microscopy density maps was predicted through AI (Pfab et al. 2020).

7.3.5 AI and Development of Vaccines

Since the onset of the novel coronavirus, there have been innumerable attempts for the development of COVID-19 vaccines. AI can accelerate the development of COVID-19 vaccine production. A probable vaccine contender was predicted via the utilization of the Vaxign reverse vaccinology-machine learning platform (Ong et al. 2020).

7.3.6 AI in Genomics

A rapid strategy for the precise categorization of the available SARS-CoV-2 genome was devised via the application of machine learning on already recognized genomic signatures (Randhawa et al. 2020). Ontology-based side effect prediction framework and artificial neural network have been utilized in unison to enumerate the side effects of conventional Chinese medicines for the treatment of SARS-CoV-2 (Wang et al. 2021).

7.4 Conclusion

Due to the onset of the novel coronavirus pandemic, every resource at its disposal is vital for its mitigation. Digital technologies along with AI have been used to a great extent to curb the transmission of COVID-19. These digital technologies and AI-based platforms strengthen the global health initiatives launched across the world against COVID-19. Different nations have welcomed and supported the use of digital tools and AI for rapid contact tracing. These tools have also been used to alert the general public about the transmission patterns of the novel coronavirus. One of the greatest benefits of digital tools and AI is that, at a particular time, notifications issued by the government can reach a huge user base. Experts in epidemic studies and behavioral studies have recognized the potential of data accumulated from these tracing and analysis tools. The data collected in real-time finds its applications in predicting future viral outbreaks too. Conventional tracing strategies are potentially augmented when modern digital techniques along with AI are combined and are helpful in the successful implementation of health policies. However, there are some loopholes in the usage of such strategies. Privacy breaches and personal information misuse and misconduct are some of the downsides that have been reported due to the use of such tools. Assurance regarding the safety of personal information given by the general public must be given, which would therefore dominate the benefits of using such tools. Further, freedom of choice must be awarded to the general public regarding the usage of such technologies. In order to overcome such shortcomings, a legal framework must be formed that would ensure transparency between the user base and technology developers.

References

Abeler, J., Bäcker, M., Buermeyer, U., and Zillessen, H. (2020). COVID-19 contact tracing and data protection can go together. *JMIR mHealth uHealth* 8: e19359–e19359. https://doi.org/10.2196/19359.

Arora, N., Banerjee, A.K., and Narasu, M.L. (2020). The role of artificial intelligence in tackling COVID-19. *Future Virol.* 15: 717–724. https://doi.org/10.2217/fvl-2020-0130.

Babones, S. (2020). Coronavirus tracking apps won't work, as South Korea, Singapore, and Australia show. Foreign Policy. https://foreignpolicy.com/2020/05/12/coronavirus-tracking-tracing-apps-cant-work-south-korea-singapore-australia/ (accessed 12 March 2021).

Berke, A., Bakker, M., Vepakomma, P., et al. (2020). Assessing disease exposure risk with location data: A proposal for cryptographic preservation of privacy. arXiv Prepr. arXiv2003.14412 8. https://arxiv.org/abs/2003.14412#:~:text=We%20offer%20an%20alternative%20approach,with%20a%20semi%2Dtrusted%20authority (accessed 12 March 2021)

Chrysaidos, N. (2020). Iranian coronavirus app collecting sensitive information. Avast. https://blog.avast.com/iranian-coronavirus-app-collecting-sensitive-information-avast (accessed 12 March 2021).

Cimpanu, C. (2020). Spying concerns raised over Iran's official COVID-19 detection app | ZDNet. https://www.zdnet.com/article/spying-concerns-raised-over-irans-official-covid-19-detection-app/ (accessed 12 March 2021).

Computer Laboratory Systems Research Group (2020). FluPhone project: Understanding spread of infectious disease and behavioural responses. https://www.cl.cam.ac.uk/research/srg/netos/projects/archive/fluphone2/ (accessed 11 MArch 2022).

Davidson, H. (2020). China's coronavirus health code apps raise concerns over privacy | China | The Guardian [WWW Document]. Guard.

Dwork, C., McSherry, F., Nissim, K., and Smith, A. (2006). Calibrating noise to sensitivity in private data analysis BT. In: *Theory of Cryptography* (ed. S. Halevi and T. Rabin), 265–284. Berlin, Heidelberg: Springer.

Fauci, A.S., Lane, H.C., and Redfield, R.R. (2020). Covid-19 — navigating the uncharted. *N. Engl. J. Med.* 382: 1268–1269. https://doi.org/10.1056/nejme2002387.

Gasser, U., Ienca, M., Scheibner, J., et al. (2020). Digital tools against COVID-19: Framing the ethical challenges and how to address them.

Google (2020). Manage your location history - Google account help. https://support.google.com/accounts/answer/3118687?hl=en (accessed 12 March 2021).

Gozes, O., Frid-Adar, M., Sagie, N., et al. (2020). Coronavirus detection and analysis on chest ct with deep learning. arXiv Prepr. arXiv2004.02640.

Guevara, M. (2019). Google developers blog: Enabling developers and organizations to use differential privacy. https://developers.googleblog.com/2019/09/enabling-developers-and-organizations.html (accessed 12 March 2021).

Gupta, R., Bedi, M., Goyal, P. et al. (2020). Analysis of COVID-19 tracking tool in India: case study of *Aarogya Setu* mobile application. *Digit. Gov. Res. Pr.* 1: https://doi.org/10.1145/3416088.

Homeland Security Today (2020). Iceland has tested more of its population for coronavirus than anywhere else: Here's what it learned – homeland security today. https://www.hstoday.us/subject-matter-areas/pandemic-biohazard/iceland-has-tested-more-of-its-population-for-coronavirus-than-anywhere-else-heres-what-it-learned/ (accessed 12 March 2021).

Kleinman, R.A. and Merkel, C. (2020). Digital contact tracing for COVID-19. *Can. Med. Assoc. J.* 192: E653–E656. https://doi.org/10.1503/cmaj.200922.

Knight, W. (2020). Phones could track the spread of Covid-19. Is it a good idea? | WIRED. https://www.wired.com/story/phones-track-spread-covid19-good-idea/ (accessed 12 March 2021).

Kumar, A., Gupta, P.K., and Srivastava, A. (2020). A review of modern technologies for tackling COVID-19 pandemic. *Diabetes Metab. Syndr. Clin. Res. Rev.* 14: 569–573.

Lin, L. and Hou, Z. (2020). Combat COVID-19 with artificial intelligence and big data. *J. Travel Med.* 27: https://doi.org/10.1093/jtm/taaa080.

Liu, J. (2020). Deployment of health IT in China's fight against the COVID-19 pandemic | Imaging Technology News [WWW Document]. Imaging Technol. News.

Miller, A.C., Singh, I., Koehler, E., and Polgreen, P.M. (2018). A smartphone-driven thermometer application for real-time population- and individual-level influenza surveillance. *Clin. Infect. Dis.* an Off. Publ. Infect. Dis. Soc. Am. 67: 388–397. https://doi.org/10.1093/cid/ciy073.

Moss, A., Spelliscy, C., and Borthwick, J. (2020). Demonstrating 15 contact tracing and other tools built to mitigate the impact of COVID-19. TechCrunch. https://techcrunch.com/2020/06/05/demonstrating-15-contact-tracing-and-other-tools-built-to-mitigate-the-impact-of-covid-19/ (accessed 12 March 2021).

Ong, E., Wong, M.U., Huffman, A., and He, Y. (2020). COVID-19 coronavirus vaccine design using reverse vaccinology and machine learning. *Front. Immunol.* 11: 1581.

Oran, D.P. and Topol, E.J. (2020). Prevalence of asymptomatic SARS-CoV-2 infection: a narrative review. *Ann. Intern. Med.* https://doi.org/10.7326/M20-3012.

Owusu, P.N. (2020). Digital technology applications for contact tracing: the new promise for COVID-19 and beyond? *Glob. Heal. Res. Policy* 5: 36. https://doi.org/10.1186/s41256-020-00164-1.

Pannett, R. and Cherney, M. (2020). Australia's coronavirus evacuation plan: A tiny island 1,000 miles away. Wall Str. J. https://www.wsj.com/articles/australias-coronavirus-evacuation-plan-a-tiny-island-1-000-miles-away-11580295354 (accessed 12 March 2021).

Pfab, J., Phan, N.M., and Si, D. (2020). DeepTracer: Automated protein complex structure prediction from CoV-related Cryo-EM density maps. bioRxiv.

Rahmatizadeh, S., Valizadeh-Haghi, S., and Dabbagh, A. (2020). The role of artificial intelligence in management of critical COVID-19 patients. *J. Cell. Mol. Anesth.* 5: 16–22.

Randhawa, G.S., Soltysiak, M.P.M., El Roz, H. et al. (2020). Machine learning using intrinsic genomic signatures for rapid classification of novel pathogens: COVID-19 case study. *PLoS One* 15: e0232391.

Rauhala, E. (2020). Some countries use temperature checks for coronavirus. Others don't bother. Here's why. - The Washington Post [WWW Document]. Washington Post.

Reuters (2020). Germany launches smartwatch app to monitor coronavirus spread. Reuters. https://www.reuters.com/article/us-health-coronavirus-germany-tech/germany-launches-smartwatch-app-to-monitor-coronavirus-spread-idUSKBN21P1SS (accessed 12 March 2021).

Roser, M., Ritchie, H., Ortiz-Ospina, E., and Hasell, J. (2020). Coronavirus Pandemic (COVID-19). Our World Data.

Santosh, K.C. (2020). AI-driven tools for coronavirus outbreak: need of active learning and cross-population train/test models on multitudinal/multimodal data. *J. Med. Syst.* 44: 1–5.

Senior, A.W., Evans, R., Jumper, J. et al. (2020). Improved protein structure prediction using potentials from deep learning. *Nature* 577: 706–710.

Sethy, P.K., Behera, S.K., Ratha, P.K., and Biswas, P. (2020). Detection of coronavirus disease (COVID-19) based on deep features and support vector machine. https://www.preprints.org/manuscript/202003.0300/v1 (accessed 12 March 2021).

Shukla, M., Rajan, M. A., Lodha, S., Shroff, G., Raskar, R. (2020). Privacy Guidelines for Contact Tracing Applications.

Singh, D., Kumar, V., and Kaur, M. (2020). Classification of COVID-19 patients from chest CT images using multi-objective differential evolution–based convolutional neural networks. *Eur. J. Clin. Microbiol. Infect. Dis.* 39: 1379–1389.

Tayarani, N.M.-H. (2021). Applications of artificial intelligence in battling against covid-19: a literature review. *Chaos. Solitons. Fractals* 142: 110338. https://doi.org/10.1016/j.chaos.2020.110338.

The New York Times (2020). How South Korea flattened the coronavirus curve. The New York Times. https://www.nytimes.com/2020/03/23/world/asia/coronavirus-south-korea-flatten-curve.html (accessed 12 March 2021).

Topol, E. (2020). Opinion | how digital data collection can help track covid-19 cases in real time. The Washington Post. Washington Post. https://www.washingtonpost.com/opinions/2020/04/10/how-digital-data-collection-can-help-track-covid-19-cases-real-time/ (accessed 12 March 2021).

USA Today (2020). Coronavirus: tiny Iceland has a lot of big COVID-19 data. https://www.usatoday.com/story/news/world/2020/04/10/coronavirus-covid-19-small-nations-iceland-big-data/2959797001/ (accessed 12 March 2021).

Vaishya, R., Javaid, M., Khan, I.H., and Haleem, A. (2020). Artificial Intelligence (AI) applications for COVID-19 pandemic. *Diabetes Metab. Syndr. Clin. Res. Rev.* 14: 337–339.

Wang, C.J., Ng, C.Y., and Brook, R.H. (2020). Response to COVID-19 in Taiwan: big data analytics, new technology, and proactive testing. *JAMA* 323: 1341–1342. https://doi.org/10.1001/jama.2020.3151.

Wang, Z., Li, L., Song, M. et al. (2021). Evaluating the traditional chinese medicine (TCM) officially recommended in China for COVID-19 using ontology-based side-effect prediction framework (OSPF) and deep learning. *J. Ethnopharmacol.* 272x: 113957.

WHO (2020a). Technical guidance on contact tracing for COVID-19 in the World Health Organization (WHO) African region. WHO | Regional Office for Africa. https://www.afro.who.int/publications/technical-guidance-contact-tracing-covid-19-world-health-organization-who-african (accessed 12 March 2021).

WHO (2020b). Selecting digital contact tracing and quarantine tools for COVID-19: guiding principles and considerations for a stepwise approach.

WHO (2020c). Ethical considerations to guide the use of digital proximity tracking technologies for COVID-19 contact tracing. [WWW Document].

WHO (2020d). Contact tracing in the context of COVID-19. [WWW Document].

WHO (2020e). Digital tools for COVID-19 contact tracing. [WWW Document].

Winer, S. (2020). Health Ministry launches phone app to help prevent spread of coronavirus. The Times of Israel [WWW Document]. Times Isr.

8

Challenges and Preventive Interventions in COVID-19 Transmission through Domestic Chemistry Hygiene: A Critical Assessment

Kanika Sharma[1], Payal Kesharwani[1,5], Ankit Jain[2], Nishi Mody[3], Gunjan Sharma[4], Swapnil Sharma[5], and Chaudhery Mustansar Hussain[6]

[1] Department of Pharmacy, Ram-Eesh Institute of Vocational and Technical Education, Greater Noida, Uttar Pradesh, India
[2] Department of Materials Engineering, Indian Institute of Science, Bangalore, Karnataka, India
[3] Department of Pharmaceutical Sciences, Dr. Hari Singh Gour Central University, Sagar, Madhya Pradesh, India
[4] Department of Pharmacology, Amity Institute of Pharmacy, Amity University, Noida, Uttar Pradesh, India
[5] Department of Pharmacy, Banasthali Vidyapith, Banasthali, Rajasthan, India
[6] Department of Chemistry and EVSC, New Jersey Institute of Technology, Newark, NJ, USA

8.1   Introduction

COVID-19 emanated from Wuhan, China in December 2019 which causes severe acute respiratory syndrome coronavirus 2 (SARS-CoV-2) and has affected more than 200 countries in the world. The previous pandemic caused by the virus of the same family has hit the world before. SARS (Severe Acute Respiratory Syndrome) and MERS (Middle East respiratory syndrome-2012) outbreaks recognized fecal shedding as one of the media of transmission and raised concerns toward community spread. Such infection is mostly seen in common toilets and public washrooms (Li et al. 2020). Centers for Disease Control and Prevention (CDC) indicates that approximately 25% of infected patients are asymptomatic (no symptoms) but can spread the virus by using the common toilet and infecting the surrounding area (Cheng et al. 2018; Petersen et al. 2015). Governments all around the world have adopted different policies to decrease transmission such as holding the population under lockdowns, but since the lifting of these extreme steps, people have regained their access to public places, which has further raised the risk of transmission (Chen et al. 2020; Dey et al. 2022). The use of the same toilet by multiple users has further increased the risk (Lai et al. 2018). This increased transmission is a major risk because of the process called bioaerosolization, which occurs when flushing the toilet (Li et al. 2020). This expels the virus present in the toilet bowl into the surrounding environment. Van Doremalen et al. confirmed the existence of SARS-CoV-2 in aerosols for approximately three hours at room temperature (Van Doremalen et al. 2020). This is the possible mechanism of transmission followed by touching contaminated hands to the eyes, nose, or mouth that results in self-inoculation of the virus (Gerba et al. 1975). Major steps need to be taken to stop the transmission of the microbiome through the use of toilets. The comprehensive knowledge about occurrence and transmission helps overcome outbreaks and prevents their catastrophic effect (Petersen et al. 2015). Recently, many strategies have been developed to avoid contamination and propagation of infection on surfaces. The self-disinfecting and antiadhesive surfaces are efficient and cheap approaches that can be utilized to control the infection (Querido et al. 2019). The material having intrinsic antimicrobial characteristics such as silver, zinc, copper, or chitosan can be applied on steel surfaces and ceramic bowls with a special polymer that diminishes the transmission of microbes. The aviation industry has harnessed advancement in technology by utilizing sensor-based approaches such as set-in motion high-efficiency particulate absorbing (HEPA) filters combined with the exhaust in the lavatory that would help in controlling the airborne microbial load. Furthermore, lavatories are introduced with UV-light disinfectants offering an option of handheld UV-diode as a portable disinfectant. Moreover, to diminish the overall contact area flushing, soap dispensing and doorknob handling have been based on smart sensors (Purohit et al. 2022). For personal washrooms, some inexpensive methods can be harnessed such as the use of separate slippers, closing the lid before flushing, and disinfecting the toilet as often as possible.

This chapter focuses on a possible mode of transference of COVID-19 through toilet bioaerosolization. It also presents a perspective of various approaches and techniques to reduce the viral growth, and hence transmission from the toilet bowl and lavatory area. Various precautions that can be implemented in public toilets have also been discussed.

8.2 Bioaerosolization: Ground for Transmission of SARS-CoV-2

The bioaerosol contamination caused by various microorganisms such as bacteria, fungi, and viruses makes the air contaminated and endangers human safety, especially for patients. Exposure to such contamination daily increases the morbidity and mortality rates by the transmission of infectious diseases, toxic effects, and respiratory syndrome.

Bioaerosol is a droplet nucleus consisting of airborne particles of biological origin such as bacteria, fungi, archaea, virus, pollen, and their by-products such as DNA, endotoxin, and mycotoxins. The particles (solid and liquid) found suspended in the air with a size of $0.3–100\,\mu m$ in diameter infected with a microorganism (Zhao et al. 2020). The virus and its remanent have affected the air not only outside the house but also the space present inside. Even the toilets used in the house have a high risk of spreading viruses infecting the surrounding area in the bathroom and also can spread outside through the exhaust fan and central ventilation system (Nissen et al. 2020). Any individual inhaling or swallowing the infected air marks the entry of the virus into the body followed by its inoculation and can spread it to other family members by a direct surface-hand-mouth pathway.

Several studies support the spread of viruses through the toilet. Lelieveld et al. studied the presence of the virus in four rooms where 25 healthy subjects and a COVID-19 patient were left for two days (six hours per day). SARS-CoV-2 was detected ($5\,\mu m$ in diameter) infecting the healthy individual in the room by aerosol (Lelieveld et al. 2020). Letizia et al. studied a similar case where SARS-CoV-2 was transmitted among the marine recruits during quarantine resulting due to airborne infection (Letizia et al. 2020). These studies suggest that the SAR-CoV-2 has become airborne and infects the person inhaling the contaminated air. The aerosol is generated in the air due to droplets released by an infected person through sneezing or coughing and also due to the use of the toilet by an infected person.

Studies reflect that the flow of fluid and movement of aerosol particles experience an upward velocity of almost $5\,\mathrm{m\,s^{-1}}$ during flushing, which expels the aerosol particles out of the toilet bowl with a height of 106.5 cm (Li et al. 2020; Ong et al. 2020b). The flush energy produced by the degree of agitation of the bowl after flushing water determines the droplet production. Different characteristics such as airflow, negative air pressure, ventilation, and stability of the virus determine its capacity to spread infection (Ong et al. 2020b). The large droplet settles on the toilet seat and bathroom area making it a medium of transmission or fomite for other users. The transmission may occur either by contact with the infected area or by drawing droplet nuclei into the respiratory tract. Studies conducted by (Smither et al. 2020; Van Doremalen et al. 2020) showed the viability of viruses in aerosols and on other surfaces. It was concluded that the virus can stay viable in aerosols for up to three hours, the half-life of the virus is between 1.1 and 1.2 hours, and the range is within 0.2–3 hours (Van Doremalen et al. 2020). Studies support that a biological film is formed in a bowl due to flushing after defecation by an infected person. A single flush does not mark the removal of the film, which makes it a medium of infection to the next person using the same seat. This is a major cause of infection in a family using the same toilet or in a public place (Barker and Jones 2005; Johnson et al. 2017).

The previous pandemic also points to the spread of infection through the toilet. During the SARS outbreak in 2003, aerosol was the presumed route of transmission adversely affecting the residents at the Amoy Gardens complex in Hong Kong leading to 300 cases and 42 deaths. The reports confirmed the spread of virus RNA through flushing, which prevailed out through winds by the exhaust fan. The increased concentration of virus load was also found in aerosol in building sewer plumbing systems. This shows that surveillance for wastewater-based epidemiology could be an important point in the case of SARS-CoV-2 (Yu et al. 2004). Similarly, the spread of H1N1 and MERS marked its spread (Nghiem et al. 2020). The present scenario also confirms the presence of SARS-CoV-2 in air samples and surrounding areas of the toilet, but no study as of yet, to the best of our knowledge, has shown virus viability by isolating the virus in virus cultures. Identification of viable viruses from toilets and surrounding areas would provide a better stand on this transmission hypothesis.

8.3 Fomites: Role in the Transmission of COVID-19

The production of bioaerosol during flushing was first reported by Jessen in 1950, when several types of the toilet were seeded with Serratia marcescens and measured bioaerosol produced during flushing. The microbial presence was detected using an agar-filled settle plate and impactor air collector (Jessen 1955). The toilet when used by the infected person has become the source of bioaerosolization acting as a fomite for the next user. This phenomenon settles the virus on the surface throughout the toilet such as the flush handle, bathroom floor, and other nearby areas (Gibbens 2020).

Darlow and Bale studied the washdown-type toilet seeded with *S. marcescens* and collected the air above the toilet with liquid impingers and a bourdillon impactor. It was found that the washdown type of toilet consists of an S-shaped exit trap way detecting the presence of bioaerosol even after five to seven minutes of flushing (Darlow and Bale 1959). Bound and Atkinson found that the siphonic type of toilet produces bioaerosol at much high energy for the same flush volume (Bound and Atkinson 1966). Barker and Bloomfield (2000) also studied the bowl water after 12 days and the waterline after 50 days of seeding the toilet with salmonella where they found that bowl water is the reservoir of pathogenic organisms spreading while flushing (Barker and Bloomfield 2000). Gerba et al. conducted a similar type of study where they observed the incomplete clearance of microorganisms succeeding seven flushings (Gerba et al. 1975). Johnson et al. examined the common toilet in homes, infected by a family member who suffered an attack of salmonellosis. The bacteria were found to exist as a biofilm on the porcelain surface and bowl rim infecting the four members among six present in the house (Johnson et al. 2017). Many studies have reported that the vomit and feces of an infected person contain a very high percentage of pathogen concentration, e.g. 105–109 Shigella (Thomson 1955), 104–108 Salmonella (Thomson 1955), and 108–109 noroviruses (Atmar et al. 2008) per gram of stool and at least 106 noroviruses per milliliter of vomit (Caul 1994). The bowl water, rim, and sidewalls of the toilet seat are directly exposed with fecal matter acting as a reservoir of viral RNA due to absorption on the porcelain surface and continual flushing does not remove its persistent fraction which increases the chance of infection (Ong et al. 2020a). The toilet lid (no or raised lid) is another area for a colony of virus RNA as it comes in direct contact with flushing and aerosolization (Barker and Jones 2005). Other areas such as toilet and sink handles, countertops, soap and towel dispensers, doorknobs, hand dryers, and toothbrushes, etc., also pose a greater risk for transmission (Greed 2006; Pearson 2020). This explains the fast transmission of SAR-CoV-2 in a society where flushing, ventilation, and building drainage act as a reservoir for virus-RNA (Lin et al. 2021). A survey conducted in 2018 found that almost 80 and 69% of men and women use their cell phones, newspaper, laptops, novels, etc., while on a toilet (Panigrahi et al. 2020). They can be contaminated by unhygienic hands, which makes them a carrier of the infection (Bernstein et al. 2020). Moreover, another concern is oral sex and other non-natural types as pointed out in various guidelines, should be avoided to get accidental infections originating from toilets and toiletries (Kowalik et al. 2019). Another important and ignored medium are the clothes which one wears while on a toilet. The usual practice is to wipe the bottom with toilet paper or via water and then pull up the undergarments followed by other clothes and that is generally done before washing hands. After using the toilet, one washes the hands but not the clothes, which ultimately act as a carrier for the infection (Bae et al. 2020). Figure 8.1 represents the major areas which can act as a medium for the spread of COVID-19.

8.4 Vulnerable Places for COVID-19

The opening of public spaces such as restaurants, malls, and bars has raised the concern of more speedy transmission of COVID-19. With this comes the inevitable utilization of public toilets. The stranger with unknown background uses the same sanitary facilities, which

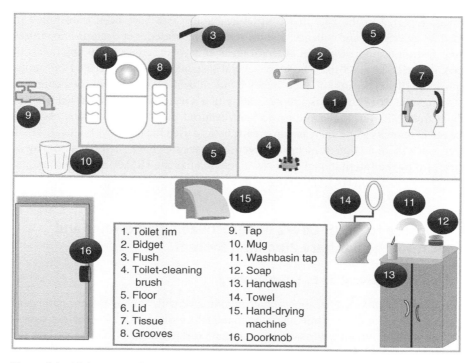

Figure 8.1 Major areas of concern in a toilet acting as a medium of spread.

generate the threat of exchange of bodily fluids, contamination, and transmission of micro-organisms. The small cubicle designed with a toilet seat, sanitary disposal bin, and a toilet roller placed in the same area could act as fomites owing to the phenomenon of bioaero-solization. A study revealed that 25–85% of women hover over the seat while using a toilet in a public area (Kowalik et al. 2019), which enhances the probability of transmission to others. Sitting down on the toilet seat increases the contact area as well as the chances of transmission (Greed 2006). A study from the New England Journal of Medicines states that the virus remains viable on steel and plastic surfaces for up to two to three days, which only lifts the odds of transference of infection to a healthy person coming in contact with these fomites (Pearson 2020; Van Doremalen et al. 2020). The same is the case involving shared toilet facilities in a hospital environment (Parikh and Rawtani 2022). Several reports stating the presence of SARS-CoV-2 in infected patients' toilets have been discussed before. A strict protocol has to be followed while considering the cleaning and ventilation system used in the toilets, as any carelessness will raise the peril to its use. A similar carefulness has to be observed in COVID-19 hospitals, as well as apartment buildings where patients are living and using community toilets. Furthermore, since the lockdown has lifted in most countries, there have been guidelines to reopen schools, daycare centers, and universities. The children who are at a smaller age cannot be trusted enough to maintain hygiene. It will lead to the propagation of accidental contamination/infection to other children, staff, parents, etc.

It has been reported in the past that communicable diseases have been transmitted in schools, daycare centers, and colleges. A study reflects the presence of bacteria and viruses including gastrointestinal viruses in different areas at daycare centers including toilets in Denmark (Querido et al. 2019). There are several instances where variegated infections have spread on flights because of a few infected individuals following usage of a common toilet (Cheng et al. 2018). There is a report stating that a woman passenger tested positive on a flight from Milan to Korea and it was later deduced that the transmission occurred because of her toilet usage after an asymptomatic patient used the lavatory (Bae et al. 2020). However, since then, a large number of preventive measures have been put into play as recommended by the International Civil Aviation Organization (ICAO) and International Air Transport Association (IATA) (Guidance 2020).

8.5 Exposure to SARS-CoV-2 in Aerosolized Wastewater and Dynamic from the Sanitary Plumbing System

8.5.1 Bioaerosol Generation by Toilet Flushing

The toilet used by an infected person is often contaminated with disease-causing pathogens acting as a reservoir for the transmission. The contagious viruses such as norovirus, rotavirus, rhinovirus and now coronavirus can contaminate surfaces such as toilet seats, lids, the rims of toilet seats, doorknobs, flush handles, taps, sinks, hand-drying machines, etc., acting as the major areas of contact when one uses the toilet (Verani et al. 2014). In a study, 22 samples were collected from different areas of a regularly disinfected hospital. Among them, two samples were found SARS-CoV-2 positive, which were collected from the toilet washbasin and flush button of the toilet bowl (Ge et al. 2021). Many similar studies have been conducted since the start of the ongoing pandemic. The majority of these studies show the presence of SARS-CoV-2 in, on, and around the toilet environment (Ding et al. 2021).

8.5.2 Bioaerosol Produced During Wastewater Treatment

The sewage wastewater is highly contagious to spread the virus in the air. The wastewater treatment leads to the aerosolization of viruses contaminating the nearby community. The report from past pandemics has suggested that virus RNA was found in air samples near wastewater. The risk of spread of SARS-CoV-2 through aerosolization is extremely high under wastewater treatment. Many studies are suggesting the presence of SARS-CoV-2 in the toilet so the virus load can be found in the aerobic tank and activated sludge process. It can also subsequently flow through the drainage network to many places infecting the whole building and the nearby community.

8.5.3 Bioaerosol Produced During Irrigation

In many countries, wastewater is used for sprinkle/spray irrigation. This process can aerosolize the virus into urban green space and vegetation soil. This cause of transmission was first identified in France where about 15% of the virus was found on soil and about 89%

were aerosolized in the air. The underdeveloped countries possess a high chance of transmission where is no proper mechanism for the treatment of wastewater (Usman et al. 2021).

8.6 Scientific and Technological Solution for the Hygiene of Toilet Area to Curb COVID-19 and Other Infections

With the existence of the virus still in the community, governments across different countries have adopted different technologies to reduce the prevalence of the virus and its transmission. The primary way to stop the spread of transmission is by regular sanitization, practicing social distancing, and wearing masks (Tang et al. 2020). The toileting habits of a person and the people in contact should be monitored deeply to diminish transmission of infection. Following are the few interventions that can be put in place to ameliorate transmission: Lavatory equipped with HEPA and ultra-low particulate air (ULPA) filters and disinfection by UV light, and antiadhesive/antimicrobial coating of surfaces that frequently come in contact. Sensor-based technology should be employed in making the whole process as contactless as possible and avoiding the use of phones in the washroom.

8.6.1 Maintaining Hygiene and Sanitation of Bathroom by Physical and Chemical Disinfection

The WHO has recommended many physical and chemical disinfectants such as sodium hypochlorite, hydrogen peroxide (Bogler et al. 2020), alcohol, soaps (dissolve the lipid membrane) (Gordon et al. 2010), sanitizer, UV rays (prevent from replicating), and light-emitting diode (LED) (kill virus) (Dhas et al. 2015), etc. to fight against SAR-CoV-2. A scientist has demonstrated the virucidal efficacy of hydrogen peroxide against SAR-CoV-2 (Bogler et al. 2020). The device used for UV disinfection consists of a mercury-based source or pulsed xenon bulb for generating UV rays. Many studies have reported that a dose ranging from 3.7 to 10.6 mJ cm^{-2} helps inactivate the virus in five minutes with 4.2 $\log_{10}$ reductions on hard surfaces and 4.79 $\log_{10}$ reductions on N95 respirators. The survival rate of the virus depends upon the wavelength, dose, distance, and duration of UV radiation (Simmons et al. 2021). Choi et al. investigated the use of an ultraviolet LED (UV-LED) robot for disinfecting the rooms of patients suffering from coronavirus disease. The study found it to be effective in cleaning the place from the virus (Choi et al. 2021). The UV light helps reduce the indoor pathogen (SAR-CoV-2) by passing through the stratum corneum and producing a cytotoxic effect by the destruction of the DNA of a virus (Jaglarz 2020). The application of this system into the toilet seats would help reduce the virus transmission and also kill the virus generated by aerosolization. This would prove beneficial in cases of sharing toilets in hospital facilities (Dhas et al. 2015). Lai and Nunayon performed a study where UVC-LED irradiation was fixed in a toilet seat for disinfecting and making it free from pathogens. It showed a promising result in disinfecting a toilet seat with 17% efficacy for airborne disinfection (Lai and Nunayon 2021). The UV disinfection devices were used in Middle East respiratory syndrome coronavirus (MERS-CoV) where it was proved to be effective in killing the virus in five minutes (Bedell et al. 2016). Thus, UV technology can be a very effective approach to kill the SAR-CoV-2 virus also. Air filtration systems like HEPA and ULPA can capture and filter droplets of size 5 μ or larger which can be employed in a closed environment near the infected patients to decrease the viral load. A fluid droplet originated from sneezing generally ranges up to 3 μ. However, if the virus is not attached to the droplet, then its size is approximately 0.12 μ, which the ULPA filter can capture efficiently, given that these viruses/droplets reach the filter (Elias and Bar-Yam 2020). Parameters like air flow rate, the extent of negative pressure created by the exhaust, technical design, and the appropriate location for their installation are needed to be further analyzed (Sportelli et al. 2020).

8.6.2 Antimicrobial Surface

Antimicrobial coatings have been in the markets for a long time. Many industries have introduced toilets that have been coated with special chemicals preventing the attachment of microbes to the surfaces. Many materials possess a natural tendency to eliminate microbes from their surface such as silver, zinc, copper, and polymer such as chitosan, thus, acting as an antimicrobial surface that would help kill the microbes. This effect can be generated with physical (photoactivated surfaces) or chemical (antibiotics or biocides) modification. Silver is known to kill microbes by attachment of its atoms with the thiol (SH) and disulfide (S-S) group of protein present in microbes (Gordon et al. 2010). The technological development leads to the enforcement of various silver materials such as silver nanoparticles (Dhas et al. 2015), glass incorporating silver ions, the silver coating on various steel or metal surfaces, and silver-embedded textile material (Schweizer and Kolar 2012; Querido et al. 2019), which would help destroy the microbes. One such coating was introduced by Pennsylvania State University in November 2019. The ceramic surface of the toilet would be coated twice, first with the hair-like polymer composed of a polydimethylsiloxane-grafted layer, whose diameter would be 100,0000 times smaller than a human hair, followed by a second coat of lubricant, which helps in creating a super slippery surface. The engineers introduced this coating as a liquid-entrenched smooth surface (LESS). This coating would not allow any fecal matter to get stuck on the surface of the toilet. It was introduced to reduce water consumption while flushing, but now this can also be repurposed as a glaze to prevent transmission, as all the fecal matter would get slipped off, thereby inhibiting microbes from the fecal matter to act as a fomite (Wang et al. 2019). Researchers at the University of Birmingham introduced and patented an antimicrobial-resistant coating specifically for steel surfaces – NitroPep. The major areas of contact after using the toilets include taps, doorknobs, and handles which are specifically made of steel. This type of coating is made of titanium dioxide and zirconium, which is proved to be effective in healthcare and industrial setting as most of the bed rails, medical equipment, handrails, some types of toilets, handles for flushes, etc., are made up of steel (Riordan et al. 2019).

Natural compounds from soda-lime to glaze possess an antimicrobial property that can be used as a coating on the walls of the washroom. Soda-lime has been in the construction business for at least 10000 years possessing both antimicrobial and antiviral properties (Carran et al. 2012). Patents have been granted for the activity of soda-lime against the virus by exposing them to biocidal surfaces and by inhibiting the entry of the virus into the cell. Soda-lime can either be painted on the walls or can be adhered to as wallpaper.

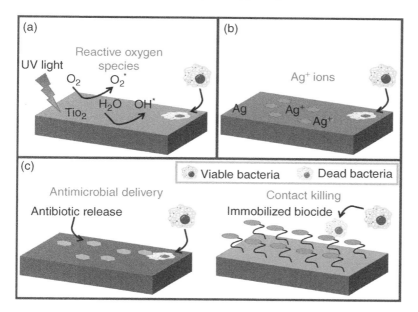

Figure 8.2 Various antimicrobial surfaces resistant to microbes: (a) Photoactivated, (b) Intrinsically active antimicrobial materials, and (c) Coating. *Source:* Querido et al. (2019)/with permission of Elsevier.

Graphene derivatives have been reported to be used as antimicrobial composites with different metals (Ag, Fe, Cu, Zn, etc.) and photocatalysts (TiO_2, CdS, MnS_2, etc.). In principle reported in some papers, the presence of metal ions could reduce (or set to zero) the viability of SARS-CoV-2 on these substrates, which can be considered as simple carrier interfaces for the infection spread (Sportelli et al. 2020). Figure 8.2 depicts various antimicrobial coatings showing resistance to microbial growth.

8.6.3 Anti-adhesive Surface

The micro-/nanostructured surface having an anti-adhesive property is studied, which prevents the attachment of cells, particles, or microorganisms on the material surface. The various self-assembled monomers and polymers with chemical or physical modification are mobilized to achieve anti-adhesive properties (Gao et al. 2011). The chemical modifications such as the use of functional groups, positively or negatively charged particles, and zwitterionic material (viz. carboxy betaine, sulfobetaine, phosphobetaine, etc.) help possess antifouling properties on the material surface (Kwon et al. 2017). One such study was conducted by Kwon et al. in which tyramine-conjugated sulfobetaine polymer was conjugated with polyurethane resulting in a decrease in *S. aureus* adhesion on a surface. The surface can be physically modified by superficial nanostructures such as nanoparticles, nanofibers, or nanotubes, which reduce the attachment of microbes to the surface by reducing the area in contact. The sharkskin topography can also be utilized which declines the microorganism adhesion and also the biofilm formation (Querido et al. 2019). Thus, an antiadhesive surface can be a boom to stop the spread of the SAR-CoV-2 virus.

8.6.4 No-Contact Use for the Operation of Sanitary Facility: Sensor Technology

The sensors, actuators, and interactive display equipped in the bathroom area are an innovative approach to maintain hygiene. The electronic and automatic devices controlled by a photocell help minimize the touch by multiple users. The use of such an approach is increased since the prevalence of pandemics. Following are some of the sensor-based technologies used in the bathroom:

- The weight sensor used for flushing that sets off the flush when the user gets up from the seat.
- Automatic sensor-based flushing system without touching with hands.
- Automatic and contactless opening and closing of the door using a weight sensor.
- The automatic tap and soap dispenser triggering the release due to the smart sensor attached.
- Automatic control of lights turned on/off, dimmed, and directed upward or downward with simple gesture control, making them touchless and intuitive.
- Automatic tissue dispenser.

These smart sensors are linked with biomarkers present in the toilet bowl that could collect the data from the urine and feces, feed that data back to the iPhones and laptops, and even share it with the physician. Such technology provides fast and accurate data of urine and feces analysis (Kristoff 2020). Airplanes have come with a self-cleaning lavatory system in which the motorized toilet seat moves in an upright position to expose it to the UV light, which would flood and sanitize the whole lavatory. Furthermore, all the controls would be sensor-based and touchless, and the use of HEPA filters has also been introduced (Wash 2020). The major obstacle in producing these types of toilets is the economic challenge. The toilets, which are in public spaces, offices, movie theaters, and hospitals can however utilize this approach, whereas toilets in homes and personal spaces can opt for inexpensive methods to retard transmission.

8.6.5 Inexpensive Preventive Approaches Used at Home

Transmission can be reduced by proper cleaning of the area that is often in contact by using disinfectants after every use. The hygienic and sanitary conditions can be maintained by creating a microclimate in the bathroom space. This includes maintaining proper air quality by effective heating, ventilation, air conditioning, and, if possible, natural ventilation through a window (Jaglarz 2020). The practice of adjusting clothes without washing hands can be corrected by installing a washbasin, or a sanitizer dispenser close to the toilets, so that users can wash their hands after anal washing or using toilet paper/bidet and before wearing clothes (Zhuang et al. 2021). The use of toilet paper is also a common practice in the western world. These papers can be lined with an antimicrobial coat to decrease the chances of infection. Used toilet paper can also act as fomite if not disposed of properly. The dustbin wherein these toilet papers are disposed of should be kept close all the time, preferably with the help of a lid (WebStockReview 2020). Moreover, the habit of using mobile phones while using the toilets should be avoided by simply not taking these gadgets to washrooms in the first place. However, if one requires, and has psychological issues

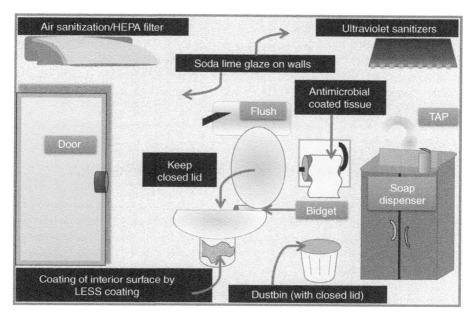

Figure 8.3 Schematic diagram representing interventions that can be employed to decrease transmission.

preventing them from defecating/urinating without phones, then they can opt for a coating made up of silver and titanium dioxide, which are known to have antibacterial and antiviral properties (NBIC 2020). These are some inexpensive methods that can be utilized in-home/personal settings to reduce transmission. Figure 8.3 summarizes the interventions that can be employed to decrease transmission (WebStockReview 2020).

8.6.6 Technology to Detect Virus

The technology to detect the virus in the surrounding area is now being updated into smartphones. Virus particles can be detected with the help of nanoparticles and a deep neural network inserted in a smartphone. The microchip captures the virus and labels it using a platinum nanoprobe, which produces a gas bubble in presence of hydrogen peroxide. The convolutional network helps detect viral load using a distinct pattern formed through bubbles. This technology is efficiently used in cases of hepatitis B virus (HBV), hepatitis C virus (HCV), and Zika virus (ZIKV) (Draz et al. 2020). This technology could also be helpful in the case of COVID-19 to detect the viral load in the surrounding area. The smartphone can also be used for alternative and quantitative saliva tests for detecting COVID-19 in a patient within 15 minutes. The technology involves CRISPR/Cas12a activity, which enhances the signal obtained from viral RNA. The signals are integrated into a smartphone using a laser diode-based fluorescence microscope readout device. The smartphone gives the data related to the viral load (Ning et al. 2021).

8.6.7 Steps for Wastewater Management

Studies report that treating the feces of SARS-CoV-2-positive individuals before flushing them out saves further contamination as well as managing wastewater and sewages would decrease the channeling of COVID-19, as SARS-CoV-2 genomic RNA was recently found in wastewater in the Netherlands (Letizia et al. 2020; Lodder and de Roda Husman 2020). Reports have it that the immunity acquired by getting infected or the herd immunity would not last longer than six months (Niclas 2020).

8.7 Conclusive Remarks and Prospects for Future Research

The various aspects mentioned in the review indicate the fecal-oral route is turning to be a major key factor for transmission of SARS-CoV-2 among the community through infected individuals' feces and urine. The aerosolization generated during flushing contaminates the surface and its droplet as it enters the respiratory tract of the user. The surface contamination needs to be paid urgent attention to by the authorities to introduce suitable guidelines for use of toilets, especially in the public places as toileting habits of the previous user are unknown and could contribute to channeling COVID-19 further into the community. People carrying mobile phones and laptops to the toilet should be discouraged as they can act as fomites and would further fuel the transmission. The various antimicrobial/anti-adhesive coatings made of silver and titanium dioxide discussed in the review help overcome the issues of surface contamination and show long-term efficacy. The use of sensor-based devices such as weight sensors for flushing, soap dispenser, tap, and motorized toilet seat will give a boon to the public toilets' safety. The UV light scanner and HEPA filter help harness the airborne transmission at bay. These suggestions would help break the chain of COVID-19, leading to lower chances of infection and reinfection by mutated viruses. In underdeveloped countries, due to inadequate sewage systems, coronavirus is found to spread at a much greater rate. A gap is found regarding the detection of SAR-CoV-2 in wastewater. A proper and safe technique is to be determined by expertise in wastewater science and technology to make wastewater free from viruses. Research is also needed for the rapid characterization of aerosols, measurement of SARS-CoV-2 in wastewater aerosols, and their risk assessment.

Acknowledgments

Dr. A. J. gratefully acknowledges the financial support as C. V. Raman postdoctoral fellowship under the Institution of Eminence (IoE) scheme at the Indian Institute of Science, Bengaluru (Karnataka), India.

Conflict of Interest

The authors report no conflict of interest.

References

Atmar, R.L., Opekun, A.R., Gilger, M.A. et al. (2008). Norwalk virus shedding after experimental human infection. *Emerging Infectious Diseases* 14 (10): 1553.

Bae, S.H., Shin, H., Koo, H.Y. et al. (2020). Asymptomatic transmission of SARS-CoV-2 on evacuation flight. *Emerging Infectious Diseases* 26 (11): 2705.

Barker, J. and Bloomfield, S.F. (2000). Survival of Salmonella in bathrooms and toilets in domestic homes following salmonellosis. *Journal of Applied Microbiology* 89 (1): 137–144.

Barker, J. and Jones, M.V. (2005). The potential spread of infection caused by aerosol contamination of surfaces after flushing a domestic toilet. *Journal of Applied Microbiology* 99 (2): 339–347.

Bedell, K., Buchaklian, A.H., and Perlman, S. (2016). Efficacy of an automated multiple emitter whole-room ultraviolet-C disinfection system against coronaviruses MHV and MERS-CoV. *Infection Control and Hospital Epidemiology* 37 (5): 598–599.

Bernstein, L., Johnson, C.Y., Kaplan, S., and McGinley, L. (2020). Coronavirus destroys lungs. But doctors are finding its damage in kidneys, hearts and elsewhere. https://www.washingtonpost.com/health/coronavirus-destroys-lungs-but-doctors-are-finding-its-damage-in-kidneys-hearts-and-elsewhere/2020/04/14/7ff71ee0-7db1-11ea-a3ee-13e1ae0a3571_story.html, 2020 (accessed 22 August 2020).

Bogler, A., Packman, A., Furman, A. et al. (2020). Rethinking wastewater risks and monitoring in light of the COVID-19 pandemic. *Nature Sustainability* 3 (12): 981–990.

Bound, W. and Atkinson, R. (1966). Bacterial aerosol from water closets. A comparison of two types of pan and two types of coyer. *Lancet* 1369–1370.

Carran, D., Hughes, J., Leslie, A., and Kennedy, C. (2012). A short history of the use of lime as a building material beyond Europe and North America. *International Journal of Architectural Heritage* 6 (2): 117–146.

Caul, E.O. (1994). Small round structured viruses: airborne transmission and hospital control. *The Lancet* 343 (8908): 1241–1243.

Chen, S., Jones, P.B., Underwood, B.R. et al. (2020). The early impact of COVID-19 on mental health and community physical health services and their patients' mortality in Cambridgeshire and Peterborough, UK. *Journal of Psychiatric Research* 131: 244–254.

Cheng, S., Li, Z., Uddin, S.M. et al. (2018). Toilet revolution in China. *Journal of Environmental Management* 216: 347–356.

Choi, H.K., Cui, C., Seok, H. et al. (2021). Feasibility of ultraviolet light-emitting diode irradiation robot for terminal decontamination of coronavirus disease 2019 (COVID-19) patient rooms. *Infection Control and Hospital Epidemiology* 43 (2): 232–237.

Darlow, H.M. and Bale, W.R. (1959). Infective hazards of water-closets. *Lancet* 1196–1200.

Dey, D., Srinivas, D., Panda, B. et al. (2022). Use of industrial waste materials for 3D printing of sustainable concrete: a review. *Journal of Cleaner Production.* 130749.

Dhas, S.P., Anbarasan, S., Mukherjee, A. et al. (2015). Biobased silver nanocolloid coating on silk fibers for prevention of post-surgical wound infections. *International Journal of Nanomedicine* 10 (Suppl 1): 159.

Ding, Z., Qian, H., Xu, B. et al. (2021). Toilets dominate environmental detection of severe acute respiratory syndrome coronavirus 2 in a hospital. *Science of the Total Environment* 753: 141710.

Draz, M.S., Vasan, A., Muthupandian, A. et al. (2020). Virus detection using nanoparticles and deep neural network–enabled smartphone system. *Science Advances* 6 (51): eabd5354.

Elias, B. and Bar-Yam, Y. (2020). Could air filtration reduce COVID-19 severity and spread. *New England Complex Systems Institute* 9: 1–2.

Gao, G., Yu, K., Kindrachuk, J. et al. (2011). Antibacterial surfaces based on polymer brushes: investigation on the influence of brush properties on antimicrobial peptide immobilization and antimicrobial activity. *Biomacromolecules* 12 (10): 3715–3727.

Ge, T., Lu, Y., Zheng, S. et al. (2021). Evaluation of disinfection procedures in a designated hospital for COVID-19. *American Journal of Infection Control* 49 (4): 447–451.

Gerba, C.P., Wallis, C., and Melnick, J.L. (1975). Microbiological hazards of household toilets: droplet production and the fate of residual organisms. *Applied Microbiology* 30 (2): 229–237.

Gibbens, S. (2020). In public toilets, flushing isn't the only COVID-19 risk.

Gordon, O., Vig Slenters, T., Brunetto, P.S. et al. (2010). Silver coordination polymers for prevention of implant infection: thiol interaction, impact on respiratory chain enzymes, and hydroxyl radical induction. *Antimicrobial Agents and Chemotherapy* 54 (10): 4208–4218.

Greed, C. (2006). The role of the public toilet: pathogen transmitter or health facilitator? *Building Services Engineering Research and Technology* 27 (2): 127–139.

Guidance, T. C. T. -o (2020) Guidance for air travel through the COVID-19 public health crisis. https://www.icao.int/covid/cart/Pages/CART-Take-off.aspx

Jaglarz, A. (2020). Ergonomic criteria for bathroom and toilet design with consideration to potential health and hygiene hazards for users. *Technical Transactions* 117: e2020041.

Jessen, C.U. (1955). *Airborne Microorganisms: Occurrance and Control*. Copenhagen: GEC Gad Forlag.

Johnson, D.L., Lynch, R.A., Villanella, S.M. et al. (2017). Persistence of bowl water contamination during sequential flushes of contaminated toilets. *Journal of Environmental Health* 80 (3): 34.

Kowalik, C.G., Daily, A., Delpe, S. et al. (2019). Toileting behaviors of women—what is healthy? *The Journal of Urology* 201 (1): 129–134.

Kristoff, A. (2020). Intelligent toilet to flush out healthcare issues. https://www.businessweekly.co.uk/news/academia-research/intelligent-toilet-flush-out-real-healthcare-issues.

Kwon, H.J., Lee, Y., Seon, G.M. et al. (2017). Zwitterionic sulfobetaine polymer-immobilized surface by simple tyrosinase-mediated grafting for enhanced antifouling property. *Acta Biomaterialia* 61: 169–179.

Lai, A.C.K. and Nunayon, S.S. (2021). A new UVC-LED system for disinfection of pathogens generated by toilet flushing. *Indoor Air* 31 (2): 324–334.

Lai, A.C.K., Tan, T.F., Li, W.S. et al. (2018). Emission strength of airborne pathogens during toilet flushing. *Indoor Air* 28 (1): 73–79.

Lelieveld, J., Helleis, F., Borrmann, S. et al. (2020). Model calculations of aerosol transmission and infection risk of COVID-19 in indoor environments. *International Journal of Environmental Research and Public Health* 17 (21): 8114.

Letizia, A.G., Ramos, I., Obla, A. et al. (2020). SARS-CoV-2 transmission among marine recruits during quarantine. *New England Journal of Medicine* 383 (25): 2407–2416.

Li, Y., Wang, J.-X., and Chen, X. (2020). Can a toilet promote virus transmission? From a fluid dynamics perspective. *Physics of Fluids* 32 (6): 65107.

Lin, G., Zhang, S., Zhong, Y. et al. (2021). Community evidence of severe acute respiratory syndrome coronavirus 2 (SARS-CoV-2) transmission through air. *Atmospheric Environment* 246: 118083.

Lodder, W. and de Roda Husman, A.M. (2020). SARS-CoV-2 in wastewater: potential health risk, but also data source. *The Lancet Gastroenterology & Hepatology* 5 (6): 533–534.

NBIC (2020). Your phone is dirtier than a toilet seat! here is nanotechnology's solution.

Nghiem, L.D., Zhang, S., Zhong, Y. et al. (2020). The COVID-19 pandemic: considerations for the waste and wastewater services sector. *Case Studies in Chemical and Environmental Engineering* 1: 100006.

Niclas, C.M.F.R. (2020) Covid antibodies fade rapidly, may not offer lasting immunity: report.

Ning, B., Yu, T., Zhang, S. et al. (2021). A smartphone-read ultrasensitive and quantitative saliva test for COVID-19. *Science Advances* 7 (2): eabe3703.

Nissen, K., Krambrich, J., Akaberi, D. et al. (2020). Longdistance airborne dispersal of SARS-CoV-2 in COVID-19 wards. *Scientific Reports* 10: 19589.

Ong, S.W.X., Tan, Y.K., Chia, P.Y. et al. (2020a). Air, surface environmental, and personal protective equipment contamination by severe acute respiratory syndrome coronavirus 2 (SARS-CoV-2) from a symptomatic patient. *Jama* 323 (16): 1610–1612.

Ong, S.W.X., Coleman, K.K., Chia, P.Y. et al. (2020b). Transmission modes of severe acute respiratory syndrome coronavirus 2 and implications on infection control: a review. *Singapore Medical Journal* 1: 21.

Panigrahi, S.K., Toedesbusch, C.D., McLeland, J.S. et al. (2020). Diurnal patterns for cortisol, cortisone and agouti-related protein in human cerebrospinal fluid and blood. *The Journal of Clinical Endocrinology & Metabolism* 105 (4): e1584–e1592.

Parikh, G. and Rawtani, D. (2022). Environmental impact of COVID-19. In *COVID-19 in the Environment* (1 January 2022). Elsevier, pp. 203–216.

Pearson, E. (2020). How risky is using a public restroom during the COVID-19 pandemic? Minnesota experts weigh in.

Petersen, T.N., Rasmussen, S., Hasman, H. et al. (2015). Meta-genomic analysis of toilet waste from long distance flights; a step towards global surveillance of infectious diseases and antimicrobial resistance. *Scientific Reports* 5 (1): 1–9.

Purohit, K., Kesarwani, A., Ranjan Kisku, D., and Dalui, M. (2022). Covid-19 detection on chest x-ray and ct scan images using multi-image augmented deep learning model. In: *Proceedings of the Seventh International Conference on Mathematics and Computing*, 395–413. Singapore: Springer.

Querido, M.M., Aguiar, L., Neves, P. et al. (2019). Self-disinfecting surfaces and infection control. *Colloids and Surfaces B: Biointerfaces* 178: 8–21.

Riordan, L., Smith, E.F., Mills, S. et al. (2019). Directly bonding antimicrobial peptide mimics to steel and the real world applications of these materials. *Materials Science and Engineering: C* 102: 299–304.

Schweizer, M. and Kolar, J.W. (2012). Design and implementation of a highly efficient three-level T-type converter for low-voltage applications. *IEEE Transactions on Power Electronics* 28 (2): 899–907.

Simmons, S.E., Carrion, R., Alfson, K.J. et al. (2021). Deactivation of SARS-CoV-2 with pulsed-xenon ultraviolet light: implications for environmental COVID-19 control. *Infection Control and Hospital Epidemiology* 42 (2): 127–130.

Smither, S.J., Eastaugh, L.S., Findlay, J.S. et al. (2020). Experimental aerosol survival of SARS-CoV-2 in artificial saliva and tissue culture media at medium and high humidity. *Emerging microbes & infections* 9 (1): 1415–1417.

Sportelli, M.C., Izzi, M., Kukushkina, E.A. et al. (2020). Can nanotechnology and materials science help the fight against SARS-CoV-2? *Nanomaterials* 10 (4): 802.

Tang, S., Mao, Y., Jones, R.M. et al. (2020). Aerosol transmission of SARS-CoV-2? Evidence, prevention and control. *Environment International* 144: 106039.

Thomson, S. (1955). The numbers of pathogenic bacilli in faeces in intestinal diseases. *Epidemiology and Infection* 53 (2): 217–224.

Usman, M., Farooq, M., and Anastopoulos, I. (2021). Exposure to SARS-CoV-2 in aerosolized wastewater: toilet flushing, wastewater treatment, and sprinkler irrigation. *Water* 13 (4): 436.

Van Doremalen, N., Bushmaker, T., Morris, D.H. et al. (2020). Aerosol and surface stability of SARS-CoV-2 as compared with SARS-CoV-1. *New England Journal of Medicine* 382 (16): 1564–1567.

Verani, M., Bigazzi, R., and Carducci, A. (2014). Viral contamination of aerosol and surfaces through toilet use in health care and other settings. *American Journal of Infection Control* 42 (7): 758–762.

Wang, J., Wang, L., Sun, N. et al. (2019). Viscoelastic solid-repellent coatings for extreme water saving and global sanitation. *Nature Sustainability* 2 (12): 1097–1105.

Wash, E. (2020). Boeing develops self-cleaning lavatory.

Yu I., Li Y, Wong TW et al. (2004). Evidence of airborne transmission of the severe acute respiratory syndrome virus. *New England Journal of Medicine* 350 (17): 1731–1739.

Zhao, J., Wang, X., Wang, H. et al. (2020). Occurrence and predictive factors of restenosis in coronary heart disease patients underwent sirolimus-eluting stent implantation. *Irish Journal of Medical Science (1971-)* 189 (3): 907–915.

Zhuang, X., Fang, D., and Ji, F. (2021). Beyond technology: a program for promoting urine-diverting dry toilets in rural areas to support sustainability. *Environmental Science: Water Research & Technology.* 7 (4): 789–796.

9

Industries and COVID-19

Pratik Kulkarni[1], Shyam Vasvani[2], Tejas D. Barot[1], Aayush Dey[1], and Deepak Rawtani[2]

[1] *School of Doctoral Studies and Research, National Forensic Sciences University (Ministry of Home Affairs, GOI), Gandhinagar, Gujarat, India*
[2] *School of Pharmacy, National Forensic Sciences University (Ministry of Home Affairs, GOI), Gandhinagar, Gujarat, India*

9.1 Introduction

There are six different coronaviruses (CoVs) identified in a human being (HCoVs) as of now: HCoV-HCoV-HKU1, HCoV-NL63, OC43.HCoV-229E, MERS-CoVs, and SARS-CoVs. The very first viruses appeared in the 1960s known as endemic HCoV-229E and HCoV-OC43, HCoV-NL63 in 2004, and HCoV-HKU1 in 2005 (Ye et al. 2020). The year 2002 recorded the first severe CoV disease epidemic in China, known as the novel serious acute respiratory syndrome CoV (SARS-CoV). The virus was assumed to have been spread to humans from bats or cats (Li et al. 2006) in 2012. The second novel CoV outbreak was reported in Saudi Arabia as the Middle East respiratory syndrome coronavirus (MERS-CoV) (Assiri et al. 2013), which was transmitted to humans from dromedary camels (Azhar et al. 2014). These outbreaks did not have an effect on the children extensively, due to the temporary, severe transmission route and nature of the epidemic of MERS. Compared to this, the latest SARS-CoV2 virus is believed to be spread through bats and pangolins and has created an unprecedented pandemic affecting all parts of the world. The virus was first spotted in Wuhan (China) and it possibly has an airborne route of transmission due to which its spread has been exponential (Campbell 2019).

More than 70 million confirmed cases and over 1.5 million deaths worldwide have resulted from the ongoing COVID-19 pandemic. Because of this, fears of a serious economic downturn and recession have been sparked. The workforce in all economic sectors and increased unemployment have been significantly diminished by self-isolation, social distancing, and travel restrictions. The demand for many goods and manufactured products has greatly reduced, and schools and colleges have also been shut down. Contrastingly, the need for medical supplies and food has increased substantially. Panic buying and stockpiling have increased the demand for foods and medicines (Ibeh et al. 2020).

As COVID-19 spreads globally, it has not remained a mere health problem now, but has also deeply impacted the world financial system and ecosystem in various methods. While its hurtful effect on the economy and society is apparent, the ecological area has demonstrated some guarantee as contamination has diminished essentially (Erokhin and Gao 2020). Because of exacting lockdown measures by the administrations all through the globe, the limited development of individuals, vehicles, and suspended modern exercises (He et al. 2020) have caused a critical decrease in air, water, and clamor contamination. For example, the degrees of ozone harming substance outflows, nitrogen dioxide (NO_2), black carbon (BC), and so forth and water contamination have radically diminished, giving indications of progress contrasted with the information of the most recent decade (Erokhin and Gao 2020; He et al. 2020; Simpson et al. 2014).

In Barcelona, Spain, a staggering 50% drop in the levels of air pollution levels has been recorded during the lockdown period. Notably, the emission levels of NO_2 and BC have shown a decline of 45–51% (Wehr 2011). Ozone (O_3) levels have also improved between 33 and 57% for the duration of the lockdown. In the same way, China has also witnessed a 25% decline in its carbon emission levels during the lockdown, which approximates around 1 million tons lesser than last year during the same period (Balsalobre-Lorente et al. 2020). Particulate matter (PM 2.5) levels in Malaysia fell by 58.4% during the lockdown (Huang et al. 2020) and water pollution in Venice, Italy showed signs of improvement as evidenced by more clear and transparent water canals of Venice prior to the lockdown period. In India, the surface water quality of Vembanad Lake increased significantly as suspended particulate matter (SPM) showed a 15.9% drop when related to the pre-lockdown period (Yunus et al. 2020). With such positive impacts, there have been some adverse consequences as well; for instance, a heavy amount of domestic and medical clutter has piled up and caused an absence of initiative to increase its subsequent recycling due to the fear of a surge in COVID-19 spread in the workers and to others connected with recycling activities (You et al. 2020).

As the positive and negative sides of the COVID-19 pandemic on the ecosystem are apparent, the opposite is also true, as the rate of COVID-19 transmission and mortality have been impacted by the environment or climate. Many studies cite a major correlation between COVID-19 transmissions, fatality, and climatic indicators like temperature, humidity, due point, rainfall, and wind speed (Elliott et al. 2020). Several studies have suggested the influence of temperature on the viral transmission rate, but have found diverse results as positive, negative, and insignificant impacts on its spread (Gilbert 2010). Air pollution is one of the most important indicators that govern the rate of COVID-19 spread and death (Comunian et al. 2020). For example, Northern Italy being the most polluted part of the country has relatively been affected by the virus more significantly with a higher incidence of infection-related casualties (Onder et al. 2020). While most research has concentrated on only one side or the other, a bidirectional study that explores the COVID-19 characteristics in much depth is needed to guide future research. Furthermore, a study on such a scale can help summarize the procedural development that can be applied in the perspective of other countries as well, apart from the ones already studied to investigate the connection between the environment and COVID-19 (Shakil et al. 2020) (Figure 9.1).

Figure 9.1 A schematic diagram listing out the industries impacted by the COVID-19 pandemic.

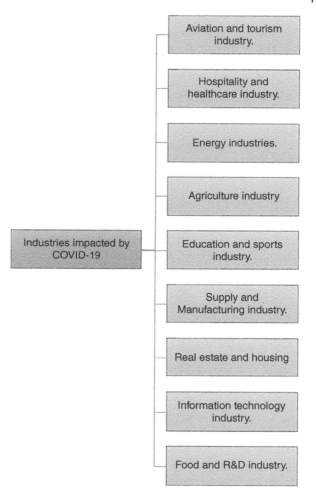

9.2 Renewable and Green Energy Industries

The current pandemic has presented several prospects for organic agri-food production and to promote and step up green modernization. When the pandemic subsides, it will call for sensible yet ambitious techno-economic recovery plans, for which necessary arrangements and planning must be carried out. Due to COVID-19, disruptive technologies may be developed that lead to improvements in agri-food, health, and the environment. Converging innovation hubs of a multiagency level hold the potential to accelerate the recovery of socio-economy during such situations (Colby 2020).

It is evident from the current situation that post-COVID-19, there will be a high demand for green innovative technologies and a specific focus on the sustenance of agri-food supply chains intensively. For example, Paludiculture, a technique for the development of new wet peatlands intensively sustains and blends agri-food and green innovation strategies, and methods like this may help post COVID-19 for a smooth transition to a better life (Colby 2020). As of now, the future looks promising for the development of novel sustainability as it helps multi-actor innovation hubs to recover and advance once the pandemic subsides, offering better funding, interactions, and companies. The nexus between the first "Green Contract" project, which funds 64 European startups, has been discussed in relation to cross-cutting innovations and the COVID-19 pandemic (Colby 2020). Future considerations will focus mainly on manufacturing and sustainable food manufacture, safety, digitization, climate action, and waste relief. Some recommendations have also been made, such as enabling community transition, enterprise training, and low-carbon employment (Moloney et al. 2010).

9.3   Agriculture Industry

The strength of the agricultural region has been tested by the COVID-19 pandemic. Due to the global decline in demand for hotels and restaurants, the cost of agricultural commodities has decreased considerably by 20% (Nicola et al. 2020). In almost all parts of the world, several strict measures have been imposed to curb the exponential spread of the virus. These measures include maintaining social distancing of at least 6 feet/1m, avoiding unwarranted travel, and a complete ban on congregations. In cases of contact with the suspected carriers, specific advice on self-isolation has to be followed in order to arrange the staff of inspectors and delivery agents available to ensure proper verification and shipping of the products. Such measures have had definite consequences for perishable goods such as meat, vegetables, and other poultry products. Furthermore, floor trading has also been shut down and has impacted the commodity exchange patterns, a recent example being The Chicago Mercantile Exchange (Baffes and Haniotis 2010). Also, panic buying further complicated the supply chain and led to shortages beyond supermarket shelves. The American Veterinary Medical Association (AVMA) have also expressed concern due to a lesser supply of animal pharmaceuticals (Nicola et al. 2020; Baffes and Haniotis 2010).

9.4   Petroleum and Oil Industry

During a recent meeting of the Organization of Petroleum Exporting Countries (OPEC) in Vienna on 6 March, Russia refused to cut its oil production, causing Saudi Arabia to retaliate by pumping more crude oil and giving buyers extraordinary discounts (Raphael 2000). As the de facto leader of OPEC, Saudi Arabia increased its oil supply by 25% in February, bringing its production volume to an unprecedented level. Due to this decision, there was the steepest one-day crash in oil prices in the last 30 years. On account of this, Brent Crude dropped its price per barrel by a staggering 24% on 23 March from $34/barrel to $25.70 (Hakes 2008). Despite some deceleration in the COVID-19 mortality rate and stabilization of oil costs, there is still indecision.

   As the pandemic has already dampened the demand for oil, the oil-price war is projected to have profound implications for the economic status globally. During ordinary times, the provision of cheap oil may be advantageous for the economies. On the contrary, the savings on petrol may become meaningless and could even lead to more spending once the pandemic situation subsides as social distancing has become mandatory and the working-class population has garnered fear regarding the security of employment. The harm caused to those relying on generating revenue from other sources and types of energy, such as shale gas (Binswanger-Mkhize and McCalla 2010), is also likely to overshadow any rise in customer activity. "Carbon Dividends" has been suggested by a prospective economic model from the Centre for Climate Finance and Investment of the Imperial College, citing the possibility of the same. This move has been supported as it gives an estimate to increase consumer spending while keeping the oil prices similar to that of February 2020. This, however, relies heavily on the turmoil between Saudi Arabia and Russia and should therefore not be regarded as sustainable in the long run.

9.5 Manufacturing Industry

The effect of the COVID-19 pandemic on manufacturing businesses was recently carried out in the United Kingdom through a brief survey by the British Plastics Federation (BPF). The results indicated a decline for the next two quarters as evident by the information given by over 80% of the respondents. More than 90% admitted concerns about the adverse impact of the pandemic on their business processes (Sibley et al. 2020). The main issues for businesses, caused by supply chain disruptions and self-isolation policies, were found to be issues relating to import and staffing deficiencies. A "work from home" option is not viable for several roles in a manufacturing firm. As the United Kingdom is also implementing similar measures like the rest of the world for curbing the virus transmission, this global overlap of supply chains is expected to elevate the anxieties to transcend borders. For the chemical industry, a 1.2% reduction in its global production is predicted to be the worst progress for the sector since the financial crisis in 2008 (Hutt 2020). Major chemical-manufacturing companies like BASF who were about to upscale their production capacities in China have faced a delay owing to COVID-19 and have predicted a slowdown in growth (Wild 2020).

9.6 Education

The COVID-19 pandemic has affected the education system at all levels, from preschool to tertiary education. Many countries like Germany, Italy, India, etc., have introduced various policies and regulations from a partial to complete closure of all the activities. Countries like the United Kingdom have followed a targeted closure approach for all, except the children of industrial workers (Mayilvaganan 2020). Additionally, nationwide closure of the educational facilities has been imposed in over 100 countries. As per the estimates provided by the UNESCO, approximately 900 billion learners have been altered due to COVID-19 and the subsequent closure of the educational institutions (Shah 2020). Such short-term disruptions have impacted many families globally as homeschooling has become a major burden for the parents affecting their productivity and also the social life of children and learning abilities. Owing to this, online platforms for teaching are rising as a substitute to live teaching, but their sudden rise is untested and unprecedented. Student activities and their assessments have also moved online with a lot of trial and error and increased uncertainty. Moreover, some assessments and final year exams in many universities have been cancelled. As a matter of fact, such measures are expected to have long-term implications for those affected and are likely to raise concerns about inequality. To tackle the issues related to this, many solutions have been suggested such as rebuilding necessary resources and their efficient use for reducing the losses faced (Burgess and Sievertsen 2020). Providing the most affected students and facilitating their needs remains a big question. For assessments, given their importance for learning, the schools and universities should consider postponing them rather than skipping them entirely. For fresh graduate students, special policies should be formed in order to ease their entry into the labor market to avoid unemployment (Burgess and Sievertsen 2020; Rana 2020).

9.7 Health Care Industry

In terms of risk factors, the health care industry has been largely impacted by the COVID-19 pandemic and has become challenging worldwide. Particularly, people working as health care workers are facing one of the greatest vulnerabilities currently. As most of them are unable to work remotely, they have an increased risk of getting infected as they deal with COVID-19 patients daily. In order to maintain their safety, it has become imperative to deploy viral testing at the earliest for asymptomatic and/or frontline health care workers (Sibley et al. 2020). Also, expensive health care facilities and the gaps in patient care delivery have been pointed out by shortages of safety equipment such as N95 face masks and smaller numbers of ICU beds and ventilators. Several uninsured individuals employed in such health care environments in the United States have risked predisposing themselves to the virus, which can place a financial burden on them in the event of illness. (Khan et al. 2020).

9.8 Pharmaceutical Industry

Dynamic changes in the health care system are likely to ensue, which may lead to huge amount of investments into disease preventing infrastructure and accelerating the health care delivery through digital transformation. Recent studies have highlighted some prominent changes in the health care policies and clinical management strategies as new evidence emerges (Burgess and Currie 2013). A large amount of active pharmaceutical ingredients (API) have been exported to the United States from Indi (18%), the EU (26%) and China (13%). Moreover, China is currently the biggest medical devices exporter compared to the United States, accounting for more than 39% than the US. Slowing down the production activities and limiting supplies would lead to revenue loss inadvertently (Kookana et al. 2014). AstraZeneca (United Kingdom), have indicated a huge loss in the revenue due to the COVID-19 situation (Datta 2020; EFPIA 2020).

On the other hand, opportunities have emerged for the companies for example, Johnson & Johnson, Vir Biotechnology, Novavax and NanoViricides to engage in vaccine with huge support from the government as well. Many scientists have started collaborating with such pharmaceutical companies in order to develop a robust and effective vaccine for combatting the viral transmission and providing immunity to the patients. Phase wise clinical trials are underway for many companies as of now like Pfizer, Moderna, University of Oxford, Gilead sciences, Zydus Cadila etc. (Datta 2020; EFPIA 2020).

9.9 Hospitality

The hospitality and travel industry has been hit hardest in terms of loss of income and unemployment, with hourly employees facing potentially stressful hardships and low wages. For example, Marriott International (comprising approximately >170 000 employees) is estimated to place >10 000 workers on furlough (Kunin 2012). Similarly, on March 5, Hilton Worldwide notified lenders of borrowing $1.75 billion under a revolving loan as a precautionary step in order to save money and maintain flexibility in the light of current uncertainty, which is evident in global markets.

In the United States, hotel industry revenue per space available fell by 11.6% on the week ending 7 March 2020, while in China, occupancy rates declined by 89% by the end of January 2020. Due to a dramatic decrease in demand, hotel businesses in the United States are seeking a $150bn amount as direct assistance for workers, along with a projected loss of $1.5bn since mid-February. MGM Resorts International, Las Vegas have also announced a temporary suspension in their casino operations effective from March 16, followed by hotel operations (Loi and Kim 2010). In Germany, a decrease of over 36% have been recorded in the hotel occupancy since 1 March 2020 (Goulden 2020). Also, Italian cities like Rome have been hugely affected due to the pandemic with a mere 6% occupancy rate. On the contrary, London has remained the most stable during the pandemic, showing an occupancy rate of approximately 47% (Fernandes 2020). In totality, the pandemic has led to distortions on an international level for the hospitality sector, and considerable slumps for the hotel markets (Gössling et al. 2020).

9.10 Tourism

Due to the COVID-19 situation, tourism has also been one of the hardest hit industries compared to the hospitality industry, leaving harmful effects on both supply and demand. According to the World Travel and Tourism Council, it is estimated that the pandemic will cost 50 million global travel jobs and that the tourism sector's risk is imminent (Fernandes 2020). In Europe, the European Tourism Manifesto alliance, which includes more than 50 European public and private tourism and travel organizations, has suggested the need for urgent action. These measures include a temporary state aid for both the sectors from national governments, as well as together with funds supplemented by the EU through the Corona Response Investment Initiative and fiscal relief schemes, providing fast, easy access to short- and medium-term loans to recover liquidity shortages (Cour-Thimann and Winkler 2012).This alliance has also led to the launch of a scheme termed as the European Unemployment Reinsurance Scheme (Pérez del Prado 2018).

In International tourism, Vietnam, during the first quarter of 2019 received more than a million Chinese visitors, which dropped to a shocking 644 000 in January 2020. Estimates suggest approximately a $5bn loss for Vietnam tourism given the COVID-19 pandemic extends into the second quarter of this year as well (Stern 2016). The Philippines has projected a 0.3–0.7% slowdown in its full-year GDP. In the United States, Canada, India, and many other countries, restrictions have been imposed to avoid all the nonessential travel, closure of borders, suspension of visa services etc., which may lead to a disruption of the economy. In the United Kingdom, along with many other countries as well, closure of parks and bans on recreational activities have been enforced in order to maintain social distancing and keep the spreading of the virus to the minimum (Stern 2016).

9.11   Air Travel

The travel industry is also dealing with many cancellations and declines in demands to sustain social distancing measures and restrict unnecessary travel in the light of strict governmental directions. Foreign nationals from China, Iran, India, and some EU countries are prohibited from entering worldwide, such as in the United States, as border closures are also on the increase (Schwartz 2016). This ban applies to all those who, within the 14-day period prior to their trip to the United States, have visited the above countries. The United Kingdom Foreign Office has advised its fellow nationals against all, if not only essential, international travel. In Europe, for all nonessential travel outside the EU, the EU Commission President has imposed a 30-day suspension. Similarly, travel suspensions have been implemented at a similar level in Asia and Africa (Shakil et al. 2020).

In the light of strict governmental guidelines, the travel industry is also dealing with many cancellations and declines in demands to preserve social distancing measures and reduce excessive travel. Border closures are also on the rise, with foreign nationals from China, Iran, India, and some EU countries being prohibited from entering globally, such as in the United States (Schwartz 2016) and in the industry (Guillén 2009). The United Kingdom airlines have also requested an immediate bailout emergency amounting to £7.5bn in order to avoid a widespread shutdown. In order to ensure the smooth functioning of Air France-KLM and Amsterdam's Schiphol airport, the Netherlands ministry has discussed the need to implement the essential strategies. On the contrary, the Government of Italy is projected to take full control of the ailing airline Alitalia (Shakil et al. 2020).

9.12   Real Estate and Housing Industry

The COVID-19 situation has caused a lot of uncertainty in the real estate industry. If we look at an individual level, the social distancing measures have decreased the number of house views, which remains a key part of the selling strategy and both the buyer and seller parties are reconsidering their plans due to which the sellers due to a natural fear are reassuring the health status of all the potential buyers in order to curb the viral spread of the infection to the properties and surroundings (Taylor 2019). This has led some brokers to offer a virtual tour of the house options via digital technologies like to minimize the risk of diseases, Skype and FaceTime. In the United States, brokers have begun to ask prospective customers to preregister for viewing in order to assess their preferences and the probability of purchase (Auerbach and Thachil 2019). Furthermore, thousands of workers globally have been dismissed or laid off on temporary or unpaid leave of absence. This has created an inevitable impact on the individuals, making it difficult to manage their lifestyles in terms of paying house rental, mortgages and various other household expenses. As an answer to such difficulties, the United Kingdom government as a part of the £350bn lifeline offered a three-month mortgage holiday for those having financial instabilities (Auerbach and Thachil 2019). The buyers and lenders have been advised by the governments to delay any negotiations during the lockdown in order to halt any transactions (DePamphilis 2019). The glooming threat of repeating the financial crisis back in 2008 is visible to many and has shaken the confidence of the real estate industry. Banks in the United Kingdom have started taking precautions such as approving the requirements of up to 40% deposits to high street lenders for new mortgages. The impact of COVID-19 on the housing market is still too early to speculate, as the infection has not had a substantial impact on it (Comas-Herrera et al. 2020).

9.13   Sports Industry

With the imposition of lockdown measures and social distancing rules, COVID-19 has created a substantial impact on most sporting schedules in 2020, some of the important examples being football, cricket, hockey, baseball, etc. Football's much anticipated Euro premier league is one prime example. Being one of the most popular sports events where thousands of fans flock to the stadium, it was postponed for 12 months. However, after careful consideration, it has been currently running successfully. Similarly, the Olympics being the grandest event for the player of several sports was previously scheduled to be hosted by Tokyo in summer without delay. However, the International Olympic Committee has postponed it to 2021, which was well supported by all the athletes and their respective nations (Schinke et al. 2020). In the same way, racing ventures like the Australian Formula One Grand Prix were also postponed until further notice. However, after approvals from the respective governments, they have started hosting the races with necessary precautions and 50% or even lesser occupancy for viewers. Apart from major sports many others like golf, athletics, tennis, rugby, basketball, boxing, cycling, ice skating, and snooker were cancelled, delayed, or postponed in order to curb the spread of the viral disease. Unavoidably, this is going to cause a significant financial burden on the teams and their respective managements, the gravity of which has yet to be determined (Nelson et al. 2020).

9.14   Information Technology, Media, Research and Development

With the number of COVID-19 cases increasing day by day, it has become a high time for more than 35 companies and institutions racing toward finding a cure for the infection in the form of an effective vaccine. Till now, several potential vaccine candidates have shown initial promises and further warrant detailed clinical trial studies in larger groups to obtain a conclusion. Clinical trial studies have been carried out on both animals and human patients with the disease and without it. For example, Moderna is a company, which has passed the Phase 3 stage of the trials and has started rolling out the first doses to the patients (Pang et al. 2020). The Coalition for Epidemic Preparedness Innovations (CEPI) has been actively involved with other government agencies in order to obtain funding for vaccine research and development for better coordination (Salami et al. 2020). CEPI has announced a partnership worth $4.4m in funds with the company Novavax and the University of Oxford to develop a viable and effective solution to COVID-19. The Gates Foundation run by Bill Gates, Wellcome, and Mastercard are some more examples of the companies that have committed an amount of $125m to find new treatments for the disease (Morningstar 2019).

Social distancing measures have been paramount in order to contain the spread of the virus. COVID-19 has left many hospitals in a state of turmoil as they have reached their maximum capacity due to which various countries have started using technological solutions for better patient care and at the same time, minimizing person-to-person transmission. In China, for example, various cities have developed 5G powered tele-response bots with wireless networks to enable health care staff to communicate better with patients, monitor their health, and provide them with necessary medical supplies. Special drones that could deliver drugs and work-from-home applications are also accepted as potential solutions to overcome any deficiencies. As service automation has always been a major objective for China, the COVID-19 pandemic has assisted to accomplish that objective (Allen et al. 2020).

Due to the respiratory complications caused due to the virus, the demand for respiratory ventilators has climbed sharply. At the current stage, it has become clear that the current supply does not fulfill the demands set forth by the United States, Europe, and other countries around the world. At a point of time, the United States had only 160 000 ventilators, which were 580 000 short of what was actually required for a pandemic of this intensity. Currently, the demand has been fulfilled. However, the shortage of expert staff to run them has become a problem for their maximum use (Jacobs 2020). In the United Kingdom, the prime minister requested major stalwart companies like Rolls Royce and Dyson to sidetrack their manufacturing power to produce medical supplies (Wunderlich and Martinez 2018). However, industry leaders argue that the manufacturing of ventilators in companies, which do not produce any kind of medical goods require specific equipment and strict regulations, which can make this request a lengthy process. Hence, collaborative efforts need to be made in such cases and in difficult times like this in order to fulfill the patient's needs and save their lives.

9.15 Food Sector

Due to the problem of panic-buying and stockpiling of food by most of the population, the food sector, which includes its proper distribution and retailing, has been put under immense strain. Such drastic incidences have led to increased concerns like food shortage of necessary products like milk, rice, and tinned vegetables. For example, panic buying has created a shocking increase in food worth £1bn in the UK homes. Seemingly, such high demand has impacted the online food delivery as well with companies struggling to keep up with excessive bookings and demands and delivering them either late or not at all. Food banks and food stockpiling have also been affected due to lesser donations. This is an alarming concern as running out of food increases the vulnerability of those who cannot afford to stockpile (Just Food 2020).

As a response to such concerns, governments and many NGOs have come forward to help distribute food packets and daily necessities to the poor and vulnerable. Facilities like food parcels, collect-and-go free meals, fruit juices, etc., have been distributed in many countries like the United Kingdom, India, the United States, etc. Examples of the vulnerable population include elderly individuals who lack any support network and school children specifically from low-income families (Just Food 2020).

To allow their stores to be replenished with the basic food products, governments in almost all countries have reduced restrictions on retail delivery hours. In addition, many organizations such as the British Retail Consortium (BRC) and the USFDA, regardless of the low inventory of certain food products and their availability in local stores, have reassured the public about the food shortage and continue to meet their demands (Manning 2018).

Moreover, despite the governmental reassurance, many stores have made radical changes by limiting per individual amount to buy a specific product in order to tackle shortages. This has provided over 30 000 new jobs to meet the high demands of shelve replenishment and to facilitate special shopping hours for elderly, vulnerable populations and NHS employees in particular. Some other noteworthy changes in the manufacturing industries are limiting the production of a range of products and rather focusing on those which are in dire need during the current situation. Independent supermarkets have also been impacted severely due to high demands for food products. These supermarkets and other local stores have started providing free delivery of food products to the customers in order to stop panic buying (IAAM 2020). They have also started restricting the number of customers entering the facility at a time in order to avoid crowding and hence maintain social distancing as well. Expanding the number of available suppliers from whom they buy their products have also been implemented to avoid food shortage.

While supermarkets saw an increase in demand for food products, cafes and restaurants were forced to close. This has increased the risk of permanently shutting down and many staff members have thus lost their jobs. The impact of COVID-19 has forced a UK fast-food chain called Leon to adopt a different business model, turning 65 of its outlets into shops that sell refrigerated ready-to-eat meals delivered in plastic pouches (IAAM 2020).

9.16 Conclusion

Times like these, with the emerging fears of a new recession and economic turmoil, call for resilient and strong leadership strategies in health care, government, industry, and wider society. It must be done with utmost caution to enforce immediate relief steps and change those which might slip through the cracks. Medium- and long-term preparation would be required to rebalance and re-enervate after the crisis. In order to make robust and supportive business models thrive, even more, socio-economic growth, including sector-wise plans and an ecosystem fueled by entrepreneurial efforts, is in dire need. As it is clear that the changing situation is continually reassessed and re-evaluated by governments and financial institutions, it must be ensured that the commitments are fulfilled to favor longevity and stay prepared for such setbacks in the coming future.

References

Allen, J., Burns, N., Garrett, L. et al. (2020). How the World will look after the coronavirus pandemic. *Foreign Policy* 20: 2020.

Assiri, A., Al-Tawfiq, J.A., Al-Rabeeah, A.A. et al. (2013). Epidemiological, demographic, and clinical characteristics of 47 cases of middle east respiratory syndrome coronavirus disease from Saudi Arabia: a descriptive study. *The Lancet Infectious Diseases* 13 (9): 752–761.

Auerbach, A.M. and Thachil, T. (2019). Cultivating clients: reputation, responsiveness, and ethnic indifference in India's slums. *American Journal of Political Science* 64: 471–487.

Azhar, E.I., El-Kafrawy, S.A., Farraj, S.A. et al. (2014). Evidence for camel-to-human transmission of MERS coronavirus. *New England Journal of Medicine* 370 (26): 2499–2505.

Baffes, J. and Haniotis, T. (2010). Placing the 2006/08 commodity price boom into perspective. World Bank Policy Research Working Paper-5371 (1 July 2010).

Balsalobre-Lorente, D., Driha, O.M., Bekun, F.V. et al. (2020). Consequences of COVID-19 on the social isolation of the Chinese economy: accounting for the role of reduction in carbon emissions. *Air Quality, Atmosphere and Health* 13: 1–13.

Binswanger-Mkhize, H. and McCalla, A.F. (2010). The changing context and prospects for agricultural and rural development in Africa. In: *Handbook of Agricultural Economics*, vol. 4 (ed. C.B. Barret and D.R. Just), 3571–3712. Elsevier.

Burgess, N. and Currie, G. (2013). The knowledge brokering role of the hybrid middle level manager: the case of healthcare. *British Journal of Management* 24: S132–S142.

Burgess, S. and Sievertsen, H.H. (2020). Schools, skills, and learning: the impact of COVID-19 on education. *VoxEu. org*, p.1.

Campbell, F. (2019). Developing methodologies and software for bayesian inference of transmission trees from epidemiological and genetic data. Phd thesis. Imperial College London.

Colby, A. (2020). *Subsistence Agriculture in the US: Reconnecting to Work, Nature and Community*. Routledge.

Comas-Herrera, A., Zalakaín, J., Litwin, C. et al. (2020). Mortality associated with COVID-19 outbreaks in care homes: early international evidence. LTCcovid. org, International Long-Term Care Policy Network. https://ltccovid.org/2022/02/22/international-data-on-deaths-attributed-to-covid-19-among-people-living-in-care-homes/ (accessed 22 February 2022).

Comunian, S., Dongo, D., Milani, C., and Palestini, P. (2020). Air pollution and covid-19: the role of particulate matter in the spread and increase of covid-19's morbidity and mortality. *International Journal of Environmental Research and Public Health* 17 (12): 4487.

Cour-Thimann, P. and Winkler, B. (2012). The ECB's non-standard monetary policy measures: the role of institutional factors and financial structure. *Oxford Review of Economic Policy* 28 (4): 765–803.

Datta, A. (2020). Is a Vaccine the Only Answer to the COVID-19 Pandemic? www.fit.thequint.com/coronavirus/is-a-vaccine-the-only-answer-to-the-covid-19-pandemic (accessed 13 December 2020).

DePamphilis, D. (2019). *Mergers, Acquisitions, and Other Restructuring Activities: An Integrated Approach to Process, Tools, Cases, and Solutions*. Academic Press.

Elliott, R.J., Schumacher, I., and Withagen, C. (2020). Suggestions for a Covid-19 post-pandemic research agenda in environmental economics. *Environmental and Resource Economics* 76: 1–27.

Erokhin, V. and Gao, T. (2020). Impacts of COVID-19 on trade and economic aspects of food security: evidence from 45 developing countries. *International Journal of Environmental Research and Public Health* 17 (16): 5775.

Fernandes, N. (2020). Economic effects of coronavirus outbreak (COVID-19) on the world economy. University of Navarra, IESE Business School, European Corporate Governance Institute (ECGI).

Gilbert, L. (2010). Altitudinal patterns of tick and host abundance: a potential role for climate change in regulating tick-borne diseases? *Oecologia* 162 (1): 217–225.

Gössling, S., Scott, D., and Hall, C.M. (2020). Pandemics, tourism and global change: a rapid assessment of COVID-19. *Journal of Sustainable Tourism* 1–20.

Goulden, J.C. (2020). *Korea: The Untold Story of the War*. Dover Publications.

Guillén, M.F. (2009). *The Global Economic & Financial Crisis: A Timeline, the Lauder Institute*, 1–91. University of Pennsylvania.

Hakes, J. (2008). *A Declaration of Energy Independence: How Freedom from Foreign Oil can Improve National Security, Our Economy, and the Environment*. Wiley.

He, G., Pan, Y., and Tanaka, T. (2020). The short-term impacts of COVID-19 lockdown on urban air pollution in China. *Nature Sustainability* 3: 1–7.

Huang, L., Liu, Z., Li, H. et al. (2020). The silver lining of COVID-19: estimation of short-term health impacts due to lockdown in the Yangtze River delta region, China. *GeoHealth* 4: e2020GH000272.

Hutt, R. (2020). The economic effects of COVID-19 around the world. World Economic Forum. Vol. 22. https://www.weforum.org/agenda/2020/02/coronavirus-economic-effects-global-economy-trade-travel/ (accessed 14 May 2020).

Ibeh, I.N., Enitan, S.S., Akele, R.Y. et al. (2020). Global impacts and Nigeria responsiveness to the COVID-19 pandemic. *International Journal of Healthcare and Medical Sciences* 6 (4): 27–45.

Jacobs, A. (2020). Now the U.S. has lots of ventilators, but too few specialists to operate them. https://www.nytimes.com/2020/11/22/health/Covid-ventilators-stockpile.html

Khan, N., Naushad, M., Akbar, A. et al. (2020). Critical review of COVID-2019 in Italy and impact on its economy. 3632007. SSRN.

Kookana, R.S., Williams, M., Boxall, A.B. et al. (2014). Potential ecological footprints of active pharmaceutical ingredients: an examination of risk factors in low-, middle-and high-income countries. *Philosophical Transactions of the Royal Society, B: Biological Sciences* 369 (1656): 20130586.

Kunin, M. (2012). *The New Feminist Agenda: Defining the Next Revolution for Women, Work, and Family*. Chelsea Green Publishing.

Li, W., Wong, S.K., Li, F. et al. (2006). Animal origins of the severe acute respiratory syndrome coronavirus: insight from ACE2-S-protein interactions. *Journal of Virology* 80 (9): 4211–4219.

Loi, K.I. and Kim, W.G. (2010). Macao's casino industry: reinventing Las Vegas in Asia. *Cornell Hospitality Quarterly* 51 (2): 268–283.

Manning, L. (2018). *Food and Drink-Good Manufacturing Practice: A Guide to its Responsible Management (GMP7)*. Wiley.

Mayilvaganan, M. (2020). COVID-19 Pandemic in the Indo-Pacific: How the Countries are Dealing Amidst Changing Geopolitics *(NIAS/CSS/ISSSP/U/RR/15/2020)*.

Moloney, S., Horne, R.E., and Fien, J. (2010). Transitioning to low carbon communities – from behaviour change to systemic change: lessons from Australia. *Energy Policy* 38 (12): 7614–7623.

Morningstar, C. (2019). The show must go on. Event 201: The 2019 Fictional Pandemic Exercise (World Economic Forum, Gates Foundation et al.).

Nelson, A. (2020). Here are all the major events that have been cancelled due to coronavirus. www.rugbyadvertiser.co.uk/read-this/here-are-all-major-events-have-been-cancelled-due-coronavirus-2448492 (accessed on 13 December 2020).

Nicola, M., Alsafi, Z., Sohrabi, C. et al. (2020). The socio-economic implications of the coronavirus pandemic (COVID-19): a review. *International Journal of Surgery (London, England)* 78: 185.

Onder, G., Rezza, G., and Brusaferro, S. (2020). Case-fatality rate and characteristics of patients dying in relation to COVID-19 in Italy. *JAMA* 323 (18): 1775–1776.

Pang, J., Wang, M.X., Ang, I.Y.H. et al. (2020). Potential rapid diagnostics, vaccine and therapeutics for 2019 novel coronavirus (2019–nCoV): a systematic review. *Journal of Clinical Medicine* 9 (3): 623.

Pérez del Prado, D. (2018). A European unemployment benefit scheme: looking for real alternatives. *Cross Border Benefits Alliance Europe Review* 33–55.

Rana, P. (2020). The impact of COVID-19 on the education sector. www.yourstory.com/mystory/impact-covid-19-education-sector (accessed 13 December 2020).

Raphael, B. (2000). *King Energy: The Rise and Fall of an Industrial Empire Gone Awry*. iUniverse.

Salami, K., Gsell, P.S., Olayinka, A. et al. (2020). Meeting report: WHO consultation on accelerating Lassa fever vaccine development in endemic countries, Dakar, 10–11 September 2019. *Vaccine* 18: 4135–4141.

Schinke, R., Papaioannou, A., Henriksen, K. et al. (2020). Sport psychology services to high performance athletes during COVID-19. *International Journal of Sport and Exercise Psychology* 18: 269–272.

Schwartz, J.D. (2016). *Water in Plain Sight: Hope for a Thirsty World*. St. Martin's Press.

Shah, S. (2020). Economy impact of covid-19-a case study of India. Doctoral dissertation. Caucasus International University.

Shakil, M.H., Munim, Z.H., Tasnia, M., and Sarowar, S. (2020). COVID-19 and the environment: a critical review and research agenda. *Science of the Total Environment* 745: 141022.

Sibley, C.G., Greaves, L.M., Satherley, N. et al. (2020). Effects of the COVID-19 pandemic and nationwide lockdown on trust, attitudes toward government, and well-being. *American Psychologist* 75.

Simpson, D., Arneth, A., Mills, G. et al. (2014). Ozone – the persistent menace: interactions with the N cycle and climate change. *Current Opinion in Environmental Sustainability* 9: 9–19.

Stern, R.J. (2016). Oil scarcity ideology in US foreign policy, 1908–97. *Security Studies* 25 (2): 214–257.

Taylor, S. (2019). *The Psychology of Pandemics: Preparing for the Next Global Outbreak of Infectious Disease*. Cambridge Scholars Publishing.

Wehr, K. (ed.) (2011). *Green Culture: An A-to-Z Guide*, vol. 11. Sage.

Wild, P.S. (2020). *Cooperation on Renewable Energy Transition: A Study of the Sino-German Energy Relationship*. University of Amsterdam.

Wunderlich, S.M. and Martinez, N.M. (2018). Conserving natural resources through food loss reduction: production and consumption stages of the food supply chain. *International Soil and Water Conservation Research 6* (4): 331–339.

European Federation of Pharmaceutical Industries and Associations (2020). European pharmaceutical industry response to COVID-19. www.efpia.eu/covid-19/member-updates/ (accessed 13 December 2020).

Advancements of materials to sustainable and green world (2020). Adaptations and lessons from COVID-19: a perspective on how some industries will be impacted. www.iaamonline. org/blog/adaptations-lessons-from-covid19-perspective-how-industries-will-be-impacted (accessed 13 December 2020).

Just Food (2020). COVID 19 impact on food industry. www.just-food.com/news/covid-19-food-industry-updates-monday-24-august-free-to-read_id143295.aspx (accessed on 13 December 2020).

Ye, Z.W., Yuan, S., Yuen, K.S. et al. (2020). Zoonotic origins of human coronaviruses. *International Journal of Biological Sciences 16* (10): 1686.

You, S., Sonne, C., and Ok, Y.S. (2020). COVID-19's unsustainable waste management. *Science* 368 (6498): 1438.

Yunus, A.P., Masago, Y., and Hijioka, Y. (2020). COVID-19 and surface water quality: Improved lake water quality during the lockdown. *Science of the Total Environment* 731: 139012.

10

Ramifications of Coronavirus on the Environment

Elisa Kalugendo[1], Manka Marycleopha[1], Piyush K. Rao[1], and Dharmesh Silajiya[2]

[1] *School of Doctoral Studies & Research (SDSR), National Forensic Sciences University (Ministry of Home affairs, GOI), Gandhinagar, Gujarat, India*
[2] *School of Forensic Sciences, National Forensic Sciences University (Ministry of Home affairs, GOI), Gandhinagar, Gujarat, India*

10.1   Introduction

After a cluster of patients with respiratory illness was reported in 2019, the Health Committee of Wuhan notified the WHO about the suspected variant of the coronavirus family of viruses (Vittori et al. 2020). The coronavirus pandemic, which is caused by SARS-CoV-2, is a highly infectious illness that has caused outbreaks in almost all the countries in the world. As of 2021, it has infected more than 156 million people. This led to the need for the use of protective materials such as face shield, PPE (personal protective equipment), and sanitizers. In order to prevent the transmission of the virus, it is obligatory for individuals to put on face masks/face shields in public areas and workplace and wash hands frequently with soap or use sanitizers, and all these products were used once and dumped, which led to high accumulation of wastes (GOV.UK 2021). Despite various measures taken by governments to improve the water and sanitation conditions in developing nations, about 2 billion people still have no access to clean water and sanitation. This also became a challenge since people instead of using water were using sanitizers, which have chemical substances to the environment. Quantifying the pollution level of carbon dioxide during road restrictions is a step toward maintaining the environment's health. This can be done by estimating the amount of COVID-19 in each area (Dong et al. 2021). The process of lockdown due to COVID-19 led to various industrial units and public transportation systems going offline due to non-operation, which led to the reduction of harmful pollutants that are responsible for thousands of deaths each year (Info 2021). The masks and PPE gloves and sanitizers are emerging pollutants that are contaminating the environment (Benson et al. 2021). Coronavirus disrupted the global economy, and lowered energy consumption and CO_2 release plus several environmental consequences. The outbreak forced many countries to impose quarantines. The environment has its advantages and disadvantages in this new period Figure 10.1.

The Environmental Impact of COVID-19, First Edition. Edited by Deepak Rawtani and Chaudhery Mustansar Hussain.
© 2024 John Wiley & Sons Ltd. Published 2024 by John Wiley & Sons Ltd.

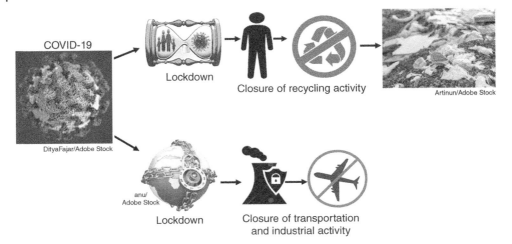

Figure 10.1 A summary of the ramification of coronavirus on the environment.

Thomas et al. (2021) provided information on government responses tracking design, which was provided by Oxford on the pandemic outbreak across different places, timing, and various perspectives. It also reported whether the limitations on internal travel applied to the full or part in a particular country. Consequences of coronavirus pandemic traveling restrictions, there has been a major decline in worldwide human mobility, particularly travel, resulting in the stoppage of anthropogenic activities (Lorreto et al. 2020). Number of attacks caused by deadly elasmobranchs (sharks) in French has increased during this coronavirus pandemic and has been taking place throughout the years 2020–2021, an event which has never been regularly seen in the region. Furthermore, the same events have been reported in Australia at large, whereby a number of people have been attached by these dangerous Sharks. It has been reported in India that Apes had attacked residents, though these animals have been friendly to human beings. Not surprisingly the change in behavior of these animals is due to the explosion of coronavirus pandemic, which has resulted in the change in lifestyles, and replicated aggressive and unpredicted behavior of different animals around the globe (Amada et al. 20201).

10.2 Footprints of Coronavirus Pandemic on the Surroundings (Mother Nature)

Coronavirus diseases have extensively affected the home of living and nonliving things (environment) in various ways, and it has affected both plants and animals so differently. Humans have been more prominently affected by COVID-19 than animals or other living things. Our environment, being the habitat for both living and nonliving things, has been observed to be affected both positively and negatively by COVID-19. Following are some of the footprints left by COVID-19 on our environment since its emergence in 2019.

10.3 Increase in Hospital Wastes

The coronavirus pandemic has increased the amount of hospital waste in China (Sarkodie and Owusu 2021). This waste has been deposited in the environment and causing the death of aquatic animals and also to the surface causing harm to the soil. In China, the expansion of waste treatment plants has led to the rise of medical waste. In Barcelona, the gloves and face masks used for health care have increased by 50% (Asumadu et al. 2021). Due to the implementation of the social distancing measures designed to prevent the COVID-19 spread, the use of plastic medical items such as sanitizers and face shields has increased. This causes the accumulation of plastic particles in marine environments like rivers, lakes, ponds, and litter in the cities, which led to the death of aquatic organisms (Cheval et al. 2020). This type of marine pollution is expected to increase in the future due to the lack of proper solutions to address it (De-la-torre and Aragaw 2020). Mismanagement of medical waste has been a growing concern worldwide. It can lead to infections, toxic effects, and air pollution (Mihai 2020). There are various types of medical waste that can be classified as nonhazardous waste, hazardous waste, and its derivatives Figure 10.2. Some of these include pathological waste and infectious waste, e.g. discarded blood and unwanted microbiological culture, and also chemical waste (WHO 2018). Due to the pandemic, various countries have reported an increase in medical waste. For instance, India has had to deal with an influx of medical waste from the use of safeguarding materials, such as gowns, gloves, and goggles. Due to the increasing number of COVID-19 patients, the volume of hospital medical waste has reached 240 metric tons. In Barcelona alone, the waste generated by individuals has increased by 350%, which resulted in around 1200 tons of waste (Calma 2020). Medical waste is generated by health care facilities. It includes all the materials that could come into contact with a person's body during a medical procedure or treatment; examples include drugs, COVID-19 testing kits, and so forth. Besides being toxic, it also has various derivatives such as cytotoxic waste like syringes and tubings, and pathological waste like body parts, carcasses, and body fluids. Medical waste can be handled by burning it in an incinerator or by irradiating it. This waste can also be reused. Reusing medical waste will maintain the cleanliness of the rivers, lakes, and oceans and this will rescue the aquatic life.

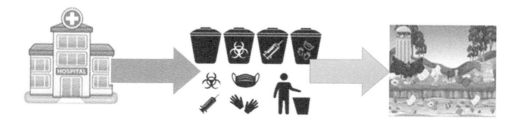

Figure 10.2 Releasing of the biomedical waste into the environment.

10.4   COVID-19 Declined Global Warming

Carbon dioxide release had fallen by negative 17% from the beginning year around the early months of the year 2020. This was quite different from that in the previous year; carbon dioxide emission might have been lowered due to traveling restrictions and the closing of manufacturing industries. The peculiar country observed that the decline of carbon emissions by negative 26 mean level were at their highest level (Gupta et al. 2020). Furthermore, there has been a decline in air pollution since the emergence of the COVID-19 pandemic (Howard and Huston 2019). This has contributed to the decline of global temperature by 50 °C over the course of the current pandemic. Due to traveling restrictions, lockdowns, shutting down of industries, and vehicles not frequently used, this has resulted in a decline in global temperature (Schwartz 2020).

This might have both positive and negative impacts on our planet. The global temperature may seem to have cooled down but soon it may result in catastrophic events like a change of seasons and climate in general, which may result in the outbreak of hunger, depopulation, the eruption of various diseases, hurricanes, floods, and unexpected volcanic eruption (Gribble et al. 2020).

World Scientific (WS) has highlighted that COVID-19 is not the first disease to be linked with climate change. A number of pandemics like malaria, HIV, influenza, and cholera were reported. It is because when any disease emerges in a population, most of the public sectors are not well prepared to encounter its effects after its emergence (Scientific 2021).

This is accompanied by a change in human behavior and results in a direct impact on the environment. Furthermore, the phenomenon has been well researched and explained well by international groups of scientists from the United Kingdom, Germany, and the United States. They published this article in the journal named Science of the Environment in January 2021. These scientists linked the COVID-19 pandemic with climate changes that have occurred in our surroundings (Adamescu et al. 2020).

Global temperatures have declined since the emergence of COVID-19 as observed from different studies by different authors. This has an implication for change of weather or can result in great seasonal variations, which can have big negative impacts on agricultural activities, which depend on the timing of different rainy seasons. This change of seasons can cause various natural disasters (Wuq Qiu 2018) and human catastrophes. This is why the organizations should prepare themselves to prevent these unforeseen effects like famine.

10.5   Poor Management of Waste

The rise in the use of plastic has environmental impacts such as poor decomposition and the release of toxic substances when they perish. The lifecycle of these chemicals has very negative effects on the environment (Dharmaraj et al. 2021). In addition, the discarded glove, sanitizer bottles and face masks on the sidewalks contribute to the pollution of the city (Asumadu et al. 2021). Due to the outbreak of COVID-19, the demand for protective equipment such as face shields and goggles has increased globally. Due to the rise of

COVID-19 cases globally, the demand for plastic-based protective equipment has increased. However, since the increasing number of these products are dumped in open areas, these contribute to environment pollution (Singh et al. 2020). The lifecycle of these products is very risky and has a high environmental cost. The increasing use of protective gears like PPE, gloves, goggles, and plastic items during hygiene measures can contribute to the transmission of COVID-19. This disease can be triggered by the discarded mask from people who regularly use them (Emily 2020). In Hong Kong, it is widely believed that plastic bottles and masks filled with nonbiodegradable materials end up in the ocean as they get discarded along beaches and nature trails. This leads to the depletion of marine habitats (Staff 2020). Not disposing of sanitizer bottles properly has a great impact on marine life and wildlife. The COVID-19 pandemic has also affected the recycling market. The price of virgin plastics has decreased due to the low oil price and the demand for recycled plastics. This has affected the profitability of the recycling industry. There have been reports of massive waste disposal in Thailand due to the amount of plastic food products that were brought to homes. In the UK, the waste disposal rate went up during the lockdown period (Word Economy Forum 2020). The pandemic has highlighted the need for households to separate their waste. In Milan, Italy, the strict lockdown led to a drop in the total waste manufacture, which included a decline in residual waste such as notepaper and cardboard waste. The decline in waste manufacturing can be attributed to various factors, such as the reduction in waste production and reprocessing. In addition, the implementation of certain restrictions on commercial and tourist activities in the city limits reduced waste generation by 25% in Barcelona (ACR+ 2021). There is a need for introducing recycled plastic, gloves, and mask in order to prevent environmental pollution. People should be advised and taught how to handle waste so as to keep the environment's well-being.

10.6 Reset of Nature

In the twenty-first century, nature has been treated differently due to the expansion of technology and the need for high development by human beings. Industries, vehicles, and the clearing of the land for agriculture or the building of infrastructure have impacted our planet so differently.

This has resulted in the accumulation of toxic gases into the atmosphere, destruction of the natural land, cutting down of trees, and so forth. Since the emergence of COVID-19, the world has observed the restoration of nature in various ways. Shutting down of industries and travelling restrictions have reduced the sending of bad gases into the atmosphere (Qiu 2018).

On the other hand, according to published papers, during the coronavirus pandemic, there is a common myth saying that our motherland has "taken time off" away from humankind. Instead, there were seizing, cutting down of trees, unauthorized extraction of minerals, and illegal hunting of animals, which have been taking place in many remote areas lying roughly on the globe. Some jobs were lost in the urban areas and made some individuals return to the rural areas, thus putting more strain on natural resources, and resulting in quick transmission of the coronavirus disease (Bates et al. 2021). Meanwhile, significant deforestation has been reported in Asia, Africa, and Latin America. Illegal mineral extractors plus cruisers are rushing back to their motherland and increasing the reparability of aboriginal individuals to get affected by rapidly emerging pandemic (Bashir et al. 2020).

All in all, from the studies and research published on the subject matter, it is obvious that the nature has at least rested for a while, though in the near future, it might have another serious implication. The government should put more effort into environmental restoration, this will help to show how living organisms connect with nature and interact with it. Traveling restrictions, for example, made most people use most of their free chance with their families and loved ones, especially in the cities (Greenwood-Hickman et al. 2020). We can learn from these changes that nature has been frequently subjected to the contact of human beings, but this has been th opposite during the time of the pandemic, whereby a higher human contact has been observed than the nature, for example, interactions, which are due to human activities intensively observed and more pronounced (Duffy et al. 2020). Reduced interactions of humans with mother nature can result in some bad impacts on the behavior of wild animals and changing their habitat as well as affecting the dynamics of human–nature interactions. During the pandemic, there was a spike in demand for various resources directed toward nature (environment) in European countries (as measured by humans' online extraction of data) (Sandra and Nick 2020).

10.7 Soil Contamination

The implementation of COVID-19 has affected various facets of the earth's environment. It has resulted in the reduction of air pollution, but it also led to various problems such as the improper disposal of waste (Rume and Islam 2020).

Without proper treatment, the release of toxic substances into the environment could cause severe effects like loss of fertility of the soil, and change of soil pH, which could affect agriculture. It is very important that waste disposal operators are well trained to properly dispose of the medical and industrial wastes that are generated (Nazir 2021).

In Iran, the Ministry of Industry and Trade has listed the importance of washing hands with soap and water. The properties of soaps can severely affect the water and soil in the long-term such as the presence of NaOH, which can cause soil adhesion. About two hundred people participated in the survey, and among them were those who increased the consumption of detergents. Due to the properties of soap, they can severely affect the water and soil quality in the long run. In addition, these chemicals can also cause cancer among soil and water users. The presence of detergents in water increases the soil permeability, which can allow microorganisms to enter the soil. It can also cause microbiological contamination. The entry of detergents into water sources will result in the development of harmful algae, foam production, and other environmental problems (Rad 2021).

Solid wastes are often dumped in open areas and on landfill sites. Not only are these conditions harmful to the environment but they can also contribute to the contamination of soil. Over 700 million people in Africa are estimated to use PPE such as face shields and gloves. This level of use poses a variety of environmental health hazards if done improperly

(Nzediegwu and Chang 2020). In order to avoid soil contamination, the waste materials should be well disposed of, and the wastewater should be well treated before disposing of to the environment.

10.8 Destruction of Arable Land

COVID-19 has claimed a greater number of people all over the world. This has resulted in insufficient places reserved for burials of dead bodies (Agencies, G. Staff 2021). Here a large part of the land has been used to bury dead bodies instead of intended activities like farming, pasturing, or any other profitable activity in the community. Other dead bodies were being dumped randomly on the ground and near the community housing. Hence, this has created a chaotic condition for both humans and animals due to the poor environment management during the COVID-19 pandemic (Gale 2021). We all know that agriculture is the backbone of any developed or developing country. The outbreak of hunger and different diseases may occur due to the lack of arable land for this precious and productive activity Figure 10.3.

Alternatively, the post-COVID period may observe increased soil fertility because dead bodies, when decomposed, result in the release of different minerals and various nutrients into the soils which may have a positive impact to farmers after COVID-19. Also, after a few years, the fossil fuel in the ground may be prompted due to the fact that these dead bodies will be compacted in the ground and contribute to the increase of fossils (O'Reilly 2021).

Most of the people in India are not buried when they die. Instead, they are cremated at very high temperatures. This has been an Indian ritual for so many years, but during COVID-19, this could not efficiently suffice for all the people who died during the pandemic. Instead, bodies of some of the dead were burned using firewood in open spaces, while the dead bodies of some were dumped randomly. Other people were forced to change their rituals of last rites and bury the dead bodies instead of cremating them (Spennemann 2021).

Due to multiple deaths within a short period of time, hospitals were overwhelmed with dead bodies, which resulted in the burying of the bodies randomly under the government supervision and sometimes relatives could not be allowed to witness the funerals of their loved ones. Due to a huge number of deaths, many last rite rituals were ignored, which resulted in random dumping of the corpses.

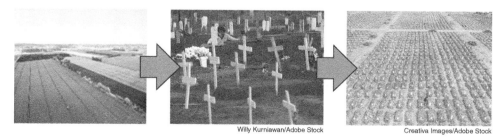

Willy Kurniawan/Adobe Stock   Creativa Images/Adobe Stock

Figure 10.3 The destruction of arable land during COVID-19.

10.9   Increased Poaching Activity

Poaching refers to the killing of wild animals for their meat or recreation. The trading of these animals has been considered one of the biggest threats to global biodiversity. It has been estimated that the demand for exotic pets and luxury goods has increased significantly (Mock et al. 2017).

The need for wild animals has increased due to illegal poaching. This causes the ecosystems to become imbalanced. Poaching is a global issue that can affect various species and regions. It can cause the disappearance of certain species, or it can affect the distributions of other species. It can also alter the structure and functioning of protected areas (Moore et al. 2021).

According to Matt Brown of the Nature Conservancy, African countries are going to experience a huge increase in wild meat poaching due to the economic crisis. This will cause demand for high-value products such as rhino horns and ivory to increase. For instance, the Environmental Protection Agency (US EPA) has stopped enforcing multiple environmental regulations (Mantur 2020). China has also temporarily suspended its environmental regulations (Quinete and Hauser-Davis 2021).

During the time of lockdown, many of the countries' woodlands were under pressure due to illegal hunting and smuggling. The reduced law enforcement led to a rise in illegal activities such as hunting and trapping, which are also disturbing the wildlife. Since the number of wildlife fatalities has increased in areas near human settlements, the effects of lockdowns have been negative for the local communities. However, the armed forces personnel lost their jobs and could be the main facilitators of poaching activities in their working area (Narayan Prasad Koju 2021). This will destroy the ecosystem and its inhabitants.

It will also cause the extinction of certain animals in the long run. During the coronavirus pandemic, the people who were protecting the wild animals went into quarantine. Due to the suspension of environmental regulations such as taking care of the wildlife and zoo, so many animals were killed.

10.10   COVID-19 Resulted in the Loss of a Great Number of People

COVID-19 allegedly killed approximately 2 million individuals all over the world. While the top global causes of fatality for 2020 have not yet been disclosed, COVID is one of the top five major causes of mortality in 2019. As of 6:19 p.m. CEST on 27 September 2021, WHO has received 200 000 000 reports on COVID-19, with approximately 4 000 000 000 individuals dying. Around 5 million shots of vaccinations have been jabbed as reported in September 2021 (Haddad 2021).

On 27 September 2021, John Elflein published that the coronavirus (COVID-19) outbreak had spread to six continents by this date and over 4.7 million people had perished as a result of infected with the respiratory virus. It is estimated that 131 000 people died in Italy.

Most of the people lost their lives due to COVID-19 through 27 September 2021. This was recorded from 206 countries when the study was done to compare deaths caused by coronavirus. Currently, there are more than 231.8 million individuals globally who have been affected by this dangerous pandemic, and more than 4.7 million deaths have been observed. Furthermore, the rates of testing for coronavirus are quite different from one nation to another. There was an emergence of disparities between the confirmed cases and deaths of coronaviruses when the two were put to comparison. The source appears to make no distinction between COVID-19's "Wuhan strain" (2019-nCOV), "the Kent mutation" (B.1.1.7), which was first shown in the UK by late 2020, and the 2021 Delta variation (B.1.617.2) from India (Agencies 2021).

Due to data on top, this led to the loss of workforce, whose professions are attached to the environment and conservations. Most environmental service workers were directly exposed to COVID-19 due to the nature of their work, which led to the negligence of cleanliness to the environment. Zookeepers, animal guards, and national park officers were highly affected by COVID-19 due to their interaction with the tourists, who came from the affected countries. Hence, this led to the loss of manpower and professionals toward environment conservation and management.

10.11   Negligence of Environmental Sanitation

Before the pandemic, the waste disposal industry was already facing many challenges. One of these was the lack of proper disposal of waste. Since the infections caused outdoor rodents to become more active, the indoor rat population had also increased (Sarkodie and Owusu 2021).

The high infection rate caused uncontrolled deaths in most of the developed countries like the United States of America, the United Kingdom, France, Spain, and Germany (Bar 2021). The high number of dead bodies led to the improper disposal of corpses. This caused the body to decompose and contaminate the environment and produce a bad smell. The precautionary measures taken by the authorities to overcome the spread of coronavirus caused an increase in the depletion of nonmedical products such as gloves, sanitizers, and PPE, which were deposited everywhere, and this led to poor hygiene.

The use of face shields, gowns, and goggles to decrease the transmission of COVID-19 has increased the global sales of these protective materials by US$166 billion since 2020 (UN 2020). This anticipated harsh social distancing measures to be imposed on waste pickers. They were no longer picking waste, which led to the poor management of waste Figure 10.4.

In 2019, Turkey banned over 8000 waste pickers due to COVID-19 containment measures. Although the government provided food aid and shelters for the workers, many of them were still able to work due to this ban. The improper disposal of waste and lack of sanitation in the environment are some of the elements that lead to the poor sanitation of communities. Not disposing of plastic bottles properly has been regarded as a common source of viral disease spread in developing countries. In many cases, the discarded bottles could be contaminated with the virus, and this led to high transmission of COVID-19.

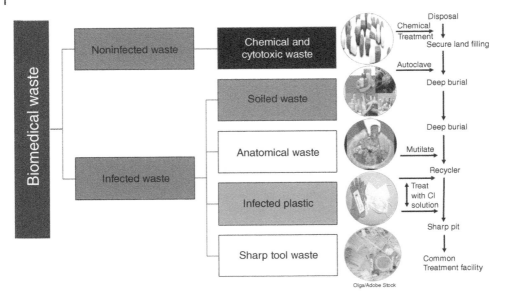

Olga/Adobe Stock

Figure 10.4 The types of biomedical waste.

10.12 Decrease of Municipal Wastewater Particles

Australia was one of the nations where coronavirus was firstly reported in raw sewage. Societies are apprehensive because if coronaviruses are able to escape medicants in municipal wastewater points, it will take a lot of energy and time to eliminate them from the environment. Methods like chlorination, UV irradiation, and ozonation are all potential therapies for coronavirus in water. However, in water with few dispersed or suspended salts, all of these treatment techniques are successful (Ghernaout and Ghernaout 2020).

As a consequence, if the virus will be difficult to be detected and removed from the wastewater, there is a probability that it may be taken back to the surroundings. Moreover, if the microbe creates its way and stays in cross-contact with human beings, it can result in the resistance of chlorination or ozonation, and the virus will flourish. If cryptosporidium, adenovirus, or giardia are prevalent, coronavirus is also likely to be detected in effluent water or wastewater in general. The authors of this study examined an abrupt decline in sewage collection point inflow and outflow for studying any differences in carbon–oxygen demand (COD) and total suspension of solids (Aydın et al. 2021).

There was an observation or study of differences in sewage treatment points in Australia on the efficiency of effluent and influent in different places. The daily flow rates of the two plants are remarkably similar. During the coronavirus pandemic, there were no flow rate alterations. At the time of shutdown, COD effluent of some Australian wastewater treatment points increased.

Because the sewage collection points for inflows and outflows remained unchanged, this is safe to assume that any coronavirus-contaminated water was effectively treated by the wastewater treatment system. There was an analysis of wastes from hospitals in the same area, and it was observed that the number of wastes increased in April 2020 and in May 2020, the generation of wastes had gone back to the normal level. Due to the predicament of COVID scenarios handled only by hospitals during the pandemic, there was no increase in waste creation (Lokhandwala and Gautam 2020).

Wastewater/sewage system has been observed to have some of the dissolved particles from different backgrounds including pharmaceuticals waste from industries and hospitals. During the COVID-19 pandemic, there has been a noticeable decline in water-dissolved particles due to the shutting down of industries or some hospitals could not manufacture too much of the waste products, and otherwise, it may be evident that there was complete and satisfying wastewater treatment during the pandemic.

10.13 Future Implications

Treatment and reuse of wastewater: This can help minimize water pollution. Also, it can reduce a load of water withdrawn from the non-production processes. Waste recycling and reuse are the processes of disposing of waste in order to reduce environmental pollution. Both industrial and municipal wastes should be reused and recycled. This can be done by using a circular economy or by following the guidelines of the WHO (Rahman et al. 2020).

Ecotourism and ecological restoration are two interrelated concepts that should be pursued in order to conserve the environment. For environmental restoration, certain tourist spots should be temporarily closed to prevent pollution and promote sustainable development (Rume and Islam 2020). COVID-19 is the cause of the pandemic that has affected the world. There was a discount in energy, coal, and power demand. Outdoor pollutant concentrations withinside the surroundings had been reduced with the aid of using authority's lockdown orders; nevertheless, interior pollutants range expanded because of expanded in-domestic activity.

For starters, the COVID-19 pandemic decreased water intake because of lower electricity power generation. Water intake withinside the business region declined while it climbed withinside the residential region. The incorrect disposal of plastic merchandise wreaked havoc on the environment. These items fall apart into microplastics, which might be dangerous to land and water environments. The emission of microplastics is a very risky environmental issue. The disposal of unwanted and spoiled vaccination doses also has an environmental impact. Yet, the majority of the COVID-19 outcomes in the environment were handled here; however, researchers must continue to investigate the effects of this type of epidemic condition.

As a result, combining public databases from trials research and advanced technical analysis modeling can be used to forecast the types of disasters, which can occur in the surroundings. As a result, further studies should focus on the improvement of social life through giving potential opinions or indirectly affecting the environment and the global economy. It also teaches us how to address the threats posed by climate change and human activities.

The toxic chemicals found in water pollution can harm aquatic life and worsen air quality. Without proper environmental management, this issue could lead to the disappearance of certain species in the ecosystem and may cause mutation. Suppose the soil contamination is not corrected in the future. In that case, it will eventually lead to the eruption of hunger, which will cause the soil to lose its fertility and the death of microorganisms. It is time for all of us to put in place strong techniques and enforce the law, which can be sustained for a long time in our environment. By reacting to the coronavirus disease, the global response has been well acknowledged, and united efforts have been made to safeguard the well-being of humans.

References

ACR+ (2021). Municipal waste management and COVID-19.

Agencies, G. Staff (2021). India's Covid crisis: Delhi crematoriums forced to build makeshift pyres. 7. https://www.theguardian.com/world/2021/apr/28/india-covid-funeral-pyres-delhi-crematoriums-spacehttps://www.acrplus.org/en/municipal-waste-management-covid-19#data_catalonia (accessed 13 June 2022).

Asumadu, S., Phebe, S., and Owusu, A. (2021). Impact of COVID - 19 pandemic on waste management. *Environment, Development and Sustainability* 23 (5): 7951–7960. https://doi.org/10.1007/s10668-020-00956-y.

Aydın, S., Nakiyingi, B.A., Esmen, C. et al. (2021). Environmental impact of coronavirus (COVID-19) from Turkish perceptive. *Environment, Development and Sustainability* 23 (5): 7573–7580. https://doi.org/10.1007/s10668-020-00933-5.

Bar, H. (2021). COVID - 19 lockdown: animal life, ecosystem and atmospheric environment. *Environment, Development and Sustainability* 23 (6): 8161–8178. https://doi.org/10.1007/s10668-020-01002-7.

Bashir, M.F., Ma, B., and Shahzad, L. (2020). A brief review of socio-economic and environmental impact of Covid-19. *Air Quality, Atmosphere and Health* 13 (12): 1403–1409. https://doi.org/10.1007/s11869-020-00894-8.

Bates, A.E., Primack, R.B., and Duarte, C.M. (2021). Global COVID-19 lockdown highlights humans as both threats and custodians of the environment. *Biological Conservation* 109175. https://doi.org/10.1016/j.biocon.2021.109175.

Benson, N. U., Bassey, D. E., & Palanisami, T. (2021). COVID pollution: impact of COVID-19 pandemic on global plastic waste footprint. *Heliyon*, 7(2), e06343. https://doi.org/10.1016/j.heliyon.2021.e06343

Calma, J. (2020). The COVID-19 pandemic is generating tons of medical waste. https://www.theverge.com/2020/3/26/21194647/the-covid-19-pandemic-is-generating (accessed 13 June 2022).

Cheval, S., Adamescu, C.M., Georgiadis, T. et al. (2020). Observed and potential impacts of the covid-19 pandemic on the environment. *International Journal of Environmental Research and Public Health* 17 (11): 1–25. https://doi.org/10.3390/ijerph17114140.

De-la-torre, G.E. and Aragaw, T.A. (2020). What we need to know about PPE associated with the COVID-19 pandemic in the marine environment. *Marine Pollution Bulletin* 111879. https://doi.org/10.1016/j.marpolbul.2020.111879.

Dharmaraj, S., Ashokkumar, V., and Hariharan, S. (2021). Chemosphere the COVID-19 pandemic face mask waste: a blooming threat to the marine environment. *Chemosphere* 272: 129601. https://doi.org/10.1016/j.chemosphere.2021.129601.

Duffy, C. R., Hart, J. M., Modest, A. M., Hacker, M. R., Golen, T., Li, Y., Zera, C., Shainker, S. A., Mehrotra, P., Zash, R., & Wylie, B. J. (2020). Lymphopenia and severe acute respiratory syndrome coronavirus 2 (SARS-CoV-2) infection among hospitalized obstetric patients. *Obstetrics and Gynecology*, 136(2), 229–231. https://doi.org/10.1097/AOG.0000000000003984

Gale, A.A.-D. (2021). *Protecting the Environment During Armed Conflict*. IHL and Islamic law https://blogs.icrc.org/law-and-policy/2021/06/03/protectintons-of-medical-waste.

Ghernaout, D., & Ghernaout, B. (2020). Controlling COVID-19 Pandemic through Wastewater Monitoring. *OALib*, 07(05), 1–20. https://doi.org/10.4236/oalib.1106411

GOV.UK (2021). Face coverings: when to wear one, exemptions, and how to make your own.

Greenwood-hickman, M.A., Dahlquist, J., Cooper, J. et al. (2020). Kaiser Permanente Washington Health Research Institute, Seattle, Washington, United States, 2. Kaiser Permanente Washington, Seattle, Washington, United States. 4(July), 2020.

Gribble, K., Marinelli, K.A., Tomori, C., and Gross, M.S. (2020). Implications of the COVID-19 pandemic response for breastfeeding, maternal caregiving capacity and infant mental health. *Journal of Human Lactation* 36 (4): 591–603. https://doi.org/10.1177/0890334420949514.

Gupta, N., Tomar, A., and Kumar, V. (2020). The effect of COVID-19 lockdown on the air environment in India. *Global Journal of Environmental Science and Management* 6: 31–40. https://doi.org/10.22034/GJESM.2019.06.SI.04.

Haddad, M. (2021). Infographic: How has the world changed since COVID-19? *Aljazeera* https://www.aljazeera.com/news/2021/3/22/how-has-the-world-changed-since-covid-19.

Howard, C. and Huston, P. (2019). The health effects of climate change: know the risks and become part of the solutions. *Canada Communicable Disease Report* 45 (5): 114–118. https://doi.org/10.14745/ccdr.v45i05a01.

Info, S. (2021). The effect of COVID-19 lockdown on the air environment in India. *Global Journal of Environmental Science and Management* 6: 31–40. https://doi.org/10.22034/GJESM.2019.06.SI.04.

Koju, N.P. (2021). COVID-19 lockdown frees wildlife to roam but increases poaching threats in Nepal. *Ecology and Evolution 11*: 17. https://doi.org/https://doi.org/10.1002/ece3.7778.

Lai, T. H. T., Tang, E. W. H., Chau, S. K. Y., Fung, K. S. C., & Li, K. K. W. (2020). Stepping up infection control measures in ophthalmology during the novel coronavirus outbreak: an experience from Hong Kong. *Graefe's Archive for Clinical and Experimental Ophthalmology*, 258(5), 1049–1055. https://doi.org/10.1007/s00417-020-04641-8

Lokhandwala, S. and Gautam, P. (2020). Indirect impact of COVID-19 on environment: a brief study in Indian context. *Environmental Research* 188: 109807. https://doi.org/10.1016/j.envres.2020.109807.

Mantur, N.G. (2020). Impact of Covid-19 on environment. *Mukt Shabd Journal* IX (Vi): 1545–1552.

Mendenhall, E. (2020). The COVID-19 syndemic is not global: context matters. The Lancet, 396(10264), 1731.

Mihai, F.C. (2020). Assessment of COVID-19 waste flows during the emergency state in romania and related public health and environmental concerns. *International Journal of Environmental Research and Public Health* 17 (15): 1–18. https://doi.org/10.3390/ijerph17155439.

Charles N. Mock, Rachel Nugent, Olive Kobusingye, Kirk R. Smith (2017). Disease control priorities, third edition (volume 7): injury prevention and environmental health.

Disease Control Priorities, Third Edition (Volume 7): Injury Prevention and Environmental Health, (Volume 7), 7–8. Washington, DC: World Bank. https://doi.org/10.1596/978-1-4648-0522-6

Moore, J.F., Uzabaho, E., Musana, A. et al. (2021). What is the effect of poaching activity on wildlife species? *Ecological Applications* 1–12. https://doi.org/10.1002/eap.2397.

Nazir, A. (2021). Management of Tannery Solid Waste (TSW) through pyrolysis and characteristics of its derived biochar. https://web.a.ebscohost.com/abstract?direct=true&profile=ehost&scope=site&authtype=crawler&jrnl=12301485&AN=146335171&h=uzXMsxyU5mTZbGQ5IrM1CecRIyqe%2F8qJsr%2BteaZMSQ03vR8MSROs4rQtHV9ldzAAFw6x3gKCEFmhbqj0x0cQKA%3D%3D&crl=c&resultNs=AdminWebAuth&resultLoca.

Nzediegwu, C. and Chang, S.X. (2020). Improper solid waste management increases potential for COVID-19 spread in developing countries. *Resources, Conservation and Recycling 161*: 104947. https://doi.org/10.1016/j.resconrec.2020.104947.

O'Reilly, L. (2021). New Delhi forced to build makeshift funeral pyres as India coronavirus death toll climbs.

Qiu, W. (2018). The impacts on health, society and economy of SARS and H7N9 outbreaks in China: a case comparison study. *Journal of Environmental and Public Health* 2018: 7.

Quinete, N. and Hauser-davis, R.A. (2021). Drinking water pollutants may affect the immune system : concerns regarding COVID-19 health effects. *Environmental Science and Pollution Research* 28 (1): 1235–1246.

Rad, A.K. (2021). Marine science: research & development the impacts of the Covid-19 crisis on water and soil safety and health with emphasis on Iran situation. *Journal of Marine Science: Research & Development* 11 (3): 8.

Rahman, M.M., Bodrud-Doza, M., Griffiths, M.D., and Mamun, M.A. (2020). Biomedical waste amid COVID-19: perspectives from Bangladesh. *The Lancet Global Health* 8 (10): e1262. https://doi.org/10.1016/S2214-109X(20)30349-1.

Rume, T. and Islam, S.M.D. (2020). Heliyon environmental effects of COVID-19 pandemic and potential strategies of sustainability. *Heliyon 6*: e04965. https://doi.org/10.1016/j.heliyon.2020.e04965.

Sarkodie, S.A. and Owusu, P.A. (2021). Impact of COVID-19 pandemic on waste management. *Environment, Development and Sustainability* 23 (5): 7951–7960. https://doi.org/10.1007/s10668-020-00956-y.

Schwartz, D.A. (2020). An analysis of 38 pregnant women with covid-19, their newborn infants, and Mafrtenal-Fetal Transmission of SARS-CoV-2 (p. 7). https://meridian.allenpress.com/aplm/article/144/7/799/441923/An-Analysis-of-38-Pregnant-Women-With-COVID-19 (accessed 30 September 2021).

Scientific, W. (2021). *The Impacts and Implications of the COVID-19 Pandemic on the Global Response to Climate Change* (p. 2). https://www.worldscientific.com/doi/10.1142/S234574812150007X

Singh, V., Singh, S., Biswal, A. et al. (2020). Diurnal and temporal changes in air pollution during COVID-19 strict lockdown over different regions of India. *Environmental Pollution* 266: 115368. https://doi.org/10.1016/j.envpol.2020.115368.

Spennemann, D.H.R. (2021). Covid-19 on the ground: managing the heriatge sites of pnademic. *Heritage* 4 (3): 23.

Staff, R. (2020). Discarded coronavirus masks clutter Hong Kong's beaches, trails. https://www.reuters.com/article/us-health-coronavirus-hongkong-environme-idUSKBN20Z0PP (accessed 30 September 2021).

UN (2020). Use of masks for UN personnel in non-healthcare settings in areas of Covid-19 community transmission. https://www.un.org/sites/un2.un.org/files/ddcoronavirus_ppeforwardfacingstaff.pdf (accessed 12 October 2021).

Vittori, A., Lerman, J., Cascella, M. et al. (2020) 'COVID-19 pandemic acute respiratory distress syndrome survivors: pain after the storm?', *Anesthesia and Analgesia*, pp. 117–119. doi: https://doi.org/10.1213/ANE.0000000000004914.

WHO (2018). Health-care waste. https://www.who.int/news-room/fact-sheets/detail/health-care-waste. p. 5 (accessed 29 October 2021).

WHO (2021). Respondingto.COVID-19. https://www.gavi.org/covid19?gclid=CjwKCAjwkvWKBhB4EiwA-GHjFnYtlE9w0BZxPOypcYxyMyVgmbqZRU20y_NXAlxjOgjDR_tKTnctRxoCPiYQ (accessed 20 October 2021).

Word economy forum (2020). Protector or polluter? The impact of COVID-19 on the movement to end plastic waste. https://www.weforum.org/agenda/2020/05/plastic-pollution-waste-pandemic-covid19-coronavirus-recycling-sustainability/.3.

11

Management of Risks Associated with COVID-19

Shrutika Singla, Shruthi Subhash, and Amarnath Mishra

Amity Institute of Forensic Sciences, Amity University, Noida, Uttar Pradesh, India

11.1 Introduction

A new strain of coronavirus has become a risk to all the continents as it is spreading at a very high rate. It is named after SARS-CoV ddue to its analogy with that phylogenetically and in its genomic composition by ICTV. SARS-CoV-2 induced commencement of pneumonia in Wuhan, Hubei Province, China in December 2019. China was having a large burden on its economic condition due to COVID-19 but the cases were also increasing gradually in the countries like Europe and the United States of America. According to the WHO, the whole globe is at high risk due to the SARS-CoV-2 outbreak (Chen et al. 2020; WHO 2019).

From the beginning, coronavirus is known to infect humans, birds, and various animals. The classification of coronavirus is given next (Contini et al. 2020):

Virus classification:

Order	Nidovirales
Family	Coronaviridae
Subfamily	Coronavirinae
Genus	*Betacoronavirus*
Sub-genus	*Sarbecovirus*

SARS-CoV-2 belongs to beta-coronavirus groups of viruses, which have a **positive single-stranded RNA** of size **26–32 kilobases** and are surrounded by an envelope (Lu et al. 2020). There is a high possibility of error in the genetic material due to its enormous size, which results in rapid mutation. Due to mutation arising in the genetic material of the virus, there are high chances that these viruses will get new properties to infect new cells and cause several symptoms having flu-like characteristics and respiratory diseases.

Subfamily is segregated into four genera, ***Alpha***, ***Beta***, ***Gamma***, and ***Delta***. *Alpha* and *Beta* genera of coronavirus are claimed to be derived from the gene pool of bat, which is known to infect animals and humans, whereas *Gamma* and *Delta* genera of coronavirus are claimed to be derived from the gene pool of aves and pigs, which is known to infect birds and rarely mammals including rodents and bats (Drexler et al. 2013).

11.2 Types

Coronaviruses are zoonotic coronaviruses, most of which are known to infect animals and birds. There are many strains, which are known to infect humans also.

Other viruses are also known that spread in animals and birds and infect humans due to transmission from animals. Earlier, a pneumonia outbreak was persuaded in Guangdong, China in 2002 by the Severe Acute Respiratory Syndrome-Coronavirus. After this, a new coronavirus appeared in Jeddah, Saudi Arabia in 2012, which was MERS-CoV. This virus enters the human body and causes respiratory and gastrointestinal diseases (Lau et al. 2005).

The common symptoms include common cold, pneumonia, fever, cough, sore throat, and severe Acute Respiratory Distress Syndrome (ARDS). Studies show that these viruses have originated from the bat as their genome is similar to the genome of the virus detected in the bat and then transmission of the virus occurs via different means.

It has been reported that *Nycteris* and *Pipistrellus* bats are the reservoirs of MERS-CoV. Many bat samples were taken from Saudi Arabia and there was an association between the part of the genome derived from the Taphozous bat and humans (Woo et al. 2012).

There are many intermediate hosts known for transmitting viruses. To identify the reservoir of MERS-CoV, many samples were taken from camels from different countries. Similarities between camels and MERS-CoV were established and those camels were used for the preparation of vaccines against MERS-CoV (Muller et al. 2014). Bats, snakes, and pangolins were identified as the transitional host of COVID-19.

The transmission rate of coronavirus is very high in comparison to other coronaviruses, yet the mortality rate is the lowest, the main reason for high spreading being that the infected individual remains asymptomatic for many days. The period of infection of SARS-CoV-2 varies between 2 and 14 days. That's why people who are positive for the virus are being quarantined for 14–15 days to make sure whether they are infected or not (Meyer et al. 2014).

Certain affinity and distinctions among SARS-CoV, MERS-CoV, and COVID-19 or SARS-CoV-2 are briefed next.

As shown in Table 11.1, the possible natural reservoirs of all the coronaviruses are believed to be bats as their genome is similar to the coronavirus identified in bats. There are many possible intermediate hosts like camels, palm civets, pangolins, etc., for the virus and there may be more which have not been identified yet. SARS-CoV and SARS-CoV-2 bind to the ACE-2 receptor and MERS-CoV binds to the DPP-4 receptor. The mortality rate of MERS-CoV is the highest, which is 34.4% and SARS-CoV-2 is the lowest, which is 2.9% (Reusken et al. 2014; Muhairi et al. 2016).

Table 11.1 Certain features of different coronavirus.

	SARS-CoV	MERS-CoV	SARS-CoV-2
Year of detection	November 2002	June 2012	December 2019
Place of detection	Guangdong, China	Jeddah, Saudi Arabia	Wuhan, China
Natural reservoir	Bat	Bat	Bat
Intermediate host	Palm Civets	Camels	Bats, Snakes, Pangolin (not confirmed yet)
Receptor to which virus binds	Angiotensin Converting Enzyme (ACE-2) Receptor	Dipeptidyl Peptidase 4 (DPP4 or CD26) Receptor	ACE-2 Receptor
Confirmed cases	8422	2494	4 525 497 (till 17 May 2020)
Mortality rate	9.19%	34.4%	2.9%

11.3 Origin

An increase in pneumonia cases took place in Guangdong Province, China in 2002 by SARS-CoV, which is claimed to be originated from the bat (Guan et al. 2003). This virus then spreads rapidly to other countries including Hong Kong. This virus caused infection in the lower respiratory system. And then another outbreak occurred by MERS-CoV in Jeddah, Saudi Arabia, 2012, which is claimed to be originated from dromedary camels and transmitted from bats only (Ahn et al. 2020). This also caused lower respiratory tract infections (Peiris et al. 2004).

How coronavirus originated has not been established yet but reports said that SARS-CoV-2 might be disseminated through the help of bats, snakes, or pangolins (Zimmermann and Curtis 2020).

From these studies (in Table 11.2), it is shown that the RaTG13 region of RNA-dependent RNA polymerase and genetic content of COVID-19 are very close, about 96.2–98.7%. Then come the genomes of bat coronavirus, Bat-SL-CoVZC45 and Bat-SL-CoVZXC21, which are approx. 88% close. The genome of SARS-CoV-2 is about 80% in resemblance to the SARS-CoV and 50% analogous to the MERS-CoV (Liu et al. 2020).

From the phylogenetic studies, it is shown that there is a close relation between SARS-CoV-2 and coronavirus identified in bats. That's why it is believed that the origin of this virus are also bats but this has not been proved yet. A study of phylogeny says that this virus is in close resemblance with the virus found in **Rhinolophus** (horseshoe bat) and have 98.7% similarity with the RdRp gene of the bat coronavirus strain BtCoV/4991 and 87.9% similar nucleotide sequence with the bat coronavirus strains bat-SL-CoVZC45 and bat-SL-CoVZXC21 (Meo et al. 2020).

Many studies showed that coronavirus detected in pangolins is in resemblance to SARS-CoV-2. This proves that pangolins are intermediate reservoirs of SARS-CoV-2. This also shows that the Wuhan seafood market is not the only one responsible for the spreading of the virus and there may be another source of SARS-CoV-2, which has to be established yet (Lai et al. 2020; Guo et al. 2020).

Table 11.2 Genetic association of SARS-CoV-2 with other bat coronaviruses.

Studied by	\multicolumn{5}{c}{The similarity with the genome of SARS-CoV-2 (%)}				
	RaTG13 region of RdRp Gene	Bat-SL-CoVZC45	Bat-SL-CoVZXC21	SARS-CoV	MERS-CoV
Lu (Drexler et al. 2013)	—	87.99	87.23	79.0	50.0
Wu (Wu et al. 2020a)	—	Closer	Closer	—	Distant
Paraskevis (Paraskevis et al. 2020)	96.3	—	—	—	—
Chen (Chan et al. 2020a)	98.7	87.9	87.9	79.7	—
Chan (Chan et al. 2020b)	—	89.0	89.0	82.0	—
Chan (Chan et al. 2020b)	—	89.0	—	—	—
Wu (Wu et al. 2020b)	—	89.1	—	—	—
Zhou (Zhou et al. 2020)	96.2	88.1	88.0	79.5	—

11.4 Structure

Coronaviruses are single-stranded, positive-sensed and enveloped viruses with a large genome (Su et al. 2020). It has a capping at 5′ end and poly-A-tail at 3′ end as given in Figure 11.1. The genome of SARS-CoV-2 has many **Open Reading Frames** (ORFs). The first open reading frame (ORF1a and ORF1b) has about two-thirds of the genome and translates two polyproteins, namely pp1a and pp1ab, which encode non-structural proteins, which consist of the RdRp enzyme (Chan et al. 2020a; Ge et al. 2020).

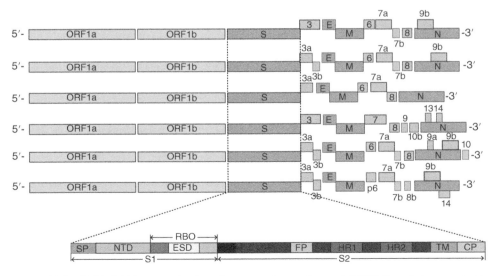

Figure 11.1 SARS-CoV-2 – organization of genome. *Source:* Ge et al. (2020). Permission granted by Dr. Xiao.

Figure 11.2 Structure of SARS-CoV-2.

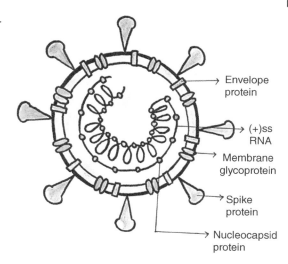

Rest one-third part of the genome codes for four essential structural proteins, which are (i) Spike Glycoprotein [S], (ii) Envelope Protein [E], (iii) Matrix Protein [M], and (iv) Nucleocapsid Protein [N] and some accessory proteins (shown in Figure 11.2).

Coronavirus got its name due to its structure, which is crown-like. It has many protrusions on its surface due to the presence of Spike protein on its, which gives it a structure like that of a crown (Figure 11.2).

S protein is a protrusion from the surface of the virus and helps in the transfer of genetic material of viruses into the host cell by binding with the ACE2 receptor. S1 and S2 are subunits of S protein, S1 sticks to the receptor, and S2 gets stuck with the cell membrane. **M protein** takes the responsibility for the transference of nutrients across the membrane and it also helps in the formation of a new virus and its spreading. **N** and **E proteins** and other accessory proteins get involved in the working of the host innate immune response (Shanmugaraj et al. 2020).

11.5 Risk Associated with COVID-19

The abrupt outspread of COVID-19 has afflicted all spaces of day-to-day existence, including clinical consideration. Significant mediations to slow sickness spread have been physical distancing, hand and respiratory cleanliness, and remaining at home however much as could be expected (Li et al. 2020). Conveying care for patients with malignant growth during this emergency is testing given the contending dangers of death from disease versus demise or genuine difficulties from SARS-CoV-2, and possible higher lethality of COVID-19 in immune-compromised hosts. Clinicians should adjust the dangers of postponing disease medicines as compared to the dangers for SARS-CoV-2 openness and the likely expanded weakness to unfriendly results from SARS-CoV-2 contamination, amidst exploring interruption in care related to restricted medical care assets. While a majority of the people are staying indoors and trying to cope with the situation, few people are facing mental health issues and are prone to develop certain antisocial behavior (Yang et al. 2020).

A report from China explains a surge in the levels of stress, anxiety, and insomnia amongst health care workers. Potential risk factors such as economic loss, the prolonged period of staying quarantined, losing closed ones, fear of unemployment, and the impact of social and mass media tend to deviate one's mind to commit self-harms and violent activities. Reports of suicide because of extreme fear and anxiety have been reported in India.

11.5.1 Risk at Hospitals or Point-of-Care Centers

Notable laborers who are the first-line fighters of this crisis are likely to develop psychological distress due to work overload (Bo et al. 2020). Fear of contracting this disease has led to a significant increase in fear, anxiety, and subsyndromal to syndromal levels of depression amongst many individuals. Citizens are also expected to face monotony, irritability, and disappointment during quarantine. A review of previous works regarding behavioral aftermath on survivors revealed an immense level of perplexity amongst the populace (Ebrahim et al. 2020). During the first wave of the pandemic, overstretched medical care frameworks left wellbeing laborers in hard-hit nations battling with long working hours, exhaustion, and outrageous mental pressure. Quickly disappearing supplies, public lockdowns, and a feeding frenzy on the open market for individual defensive hardware (PPE) prompted deficiencies. Medical services laborers frequently needed to really focus on patients with suspected or affirmed coronavirus contamination without appropriate preparation or satisfactory PPE. This added to an expanded danger to medical care laborers during the underlying period of the pandemic.

Most nations battled with a deficient testing limit in the first few months of the pandemic, which hampered the early location of arising outbreaks and implementation of contamination control measures. Expanding experience currently proposes that every suspected medical care-related disease should trigger a heap of quick contamination control measures, including broad evaluation for extensive screening for respiratory condition COVID 2 (SARS-CoV-2), isolating of all patients on the influenced ward, physical distancing among the workforce, and use of PPE during all contact with patients on the influenced ward, to forestall bigger outbreaks. Frontline health care workers play an extremely important role in treating patients testing positive for COVID-19, having a greater danger of the occurrence of stress due to workloads, insomnia, and depression. According to one of the studies, the frequency of occurrence of stress among the medical staff was found to be 27.33% and the PSTD was 42.92% among 230 respondents. Another study comprising 1563 health care professionals described that 50.7% of respondents experienced discouraging manifestations, 44.7% of them had nervousness and an estimated 36.1% suffered from changes in sleep patterns and habits. Insufficient resources and the absence of specific treatments for COVID-19 added to the challenges of managing severely ill patients. Medical care laborers needed to really focus on colleagues who were sick, offer solace to dying patients who were confined from their friends and family, and educate and console patients' relatives distantly (Goyal et al. 2020). Some medical services' laborers were troubled with genuinely and morally fraught choices about resource rationing and retaining revival or ICU affirmation. They shared the pain of patients without COVID-19, who had their medical procedures or other fundamental therapies dropped or deferred. The weight of COVID-19 on wellbeing frameworks and medical services laborers was considerable in low-income and middle-income countries (LMICs), where troublesome day-by-day emergency choices must be made with regard to grave deficiencies of essential equipment. LMICs saw an internal drain on human resources as medical care laborers were pulled from clinical practice to join COVID-19 boards and teams. In the generally extended spaces of sedation and concentrated consideration, a high clinician burnout rate may have added to more regrettable results for patients with COVID-19. An expansion in non-COVID-related medical issues and deaths (e.g. those made by disruptions in vaccinations or evaluating programs for other infections), including individual wellbeing challenges for medical services laborers (e.g. deterioration of diabetes control), further stressed inadequately resourced wellbeing frameworks.

LMICs experienced high rates of health care-associated COVID-19, due to a shortage of PPE, increased workload, inadequate training and infection control practices, and pandemic fatigue. Guilt and stigma associated with COVID-19 were common. Cases of health care workers abandoning their posts or refusing to attend to patients suspected of having COVID-19 were not uncommon. Health-care workers have been subjected to denigration from various sources during the pandemic, including political leaders and hospital administrators. In some LMICs, such as Uganda, health professionals were targeted by the public because of their roles on scientific advisory committees, and their policy decisions were met with mistrust and hostility.

11.5.2   Risk at Airport and Other Transport Mediums

Air travel amidst the COVID-19 pandemic is demanding for travelers, airlines, airports, health officials, and governments. Flights are diminished by 43% in comparison to 2019. Sanitation measures, mask use, and isolation techniques are adequate, while temperature screening has been indicated to be inconsistent. Albeit the hazard of in-flight spreading is viewed as particularly less, estimated at one case per 27 million travelers, proved in-flight cases have been reported. Travelers are effortless victims of contagious diseases. Tourists experience an inconceivable degree of grimness, anxiety, and viability to epidemic and pandemic outbreaks when traveling globally. Anticipated risk is explored as an added factor that alters consequent travel intentions, information searches, the parting of information, and visiting decision-making. Travelers look for information to lessen the extent of risk correlated with their travel. Risk consciousness is noticed as the precursor of risk information-seeking conduct. Mass communication equips the crowd with symbolic data about risk.

11.5.3   Environmental Risk Due to COVID-19

The unforeseen COVID-19 has disseminated around the globe and has afflicted 213 countries with more than 10 million people. Many cities and countries have opted for isolation measures confining people to their homes and exceedingly diminishing social and commercial activities. The lockdown measures are affecting the environment due to the shutdown of industries, factories, construction, schools and offices and reduced vehicular activity.

The pandemic has halted both ground and air travel. Vehicular activity significantly contributes to greenhouse gas (GHG) emissions. The ramping down of industries and transport has reduced the release of GHG's and effluents, lessening the environmental pollution.

The European Space Agencies' Copernicus Sentinel 5P satellite has mapped changes in air pollution. Nitrous oxide (NO_2) is an important air pollutant produced due to human activities. Unlike other gases, NO_2 has a short life span and satellite images reveal a reduction in NO_2 levels, especially in urban and industrial areas. COVID-19 restrictions have given residents of highly polluted cities an experience of clean air and blue sky. Air Quality Index across cities has improved. However, this improved air quality is not sustainable as it is the indirect impact of the virus on the environment.

11.6 Risk Management and Mitigation

COVID-19 has been a major illness these years. There are many risks due to COVID-19, which need to be taken care of. Many steps are being taken for managing the risk of COVID-19 spread. Not only at the personal level but also at domestic and global levels, steps have been taken to prevent COVID-19. One of the major steps taken up by the government is avoidance of human-to-human transmission. Various other ways to stop the spreading of COVID-19 have been explained under this subtopic.

11.6.1 Gathering Information from Different Sources

SARS-CoV-2 onset had been dominant defiance to everyone. All the countries are working against COVID-19 to prevent its propagation. In Taiwan, TCDC (Taiwan Centers for Disease Control) were maintaining real-time screening to monitor the spreading of COVID-19 in other countries to warn citizens of Taiwan (Jian et al. 2021). Regular journals, news, broadcasting channels, the Internet and social media were seen to gather relevant information. Protocols released by WHO and ECDC were followed in response to the COVID-19 outbreak (ECDC 2019).

Taiwan was maintaining daily risk management on the basis of a few factors including daily transmission generation, exported cases, status of infection, and number of confirmed cases (Bogoch et al. 2020).

In India, there were websites developed to check the regular updates regarding the spread of coronavirus. Even an app, namely "Arogya Setu" was developed to check the vulnerability of coronavirus at surrounding places within a 5-km radius. These websites and apps helped people stay away from places which are highly infected.

11.6.2 Preventing National and International Traveling

The Central Epidemic Command Center (CECC) was keeping a check on travelers from different countries. Travelers from low COVID-19 risk countries with no past travel history were allowed to enter any country with the condition of being quarantined for 14 days (Taiwan CDC 2019).

People traveling to different countries are divided into two zones – Green and Red. People from the Red zone mean they are from high-risk COVID-19 countries and they are strictly told to be quarantined or not travel. People from green zones were from low-risk COVID-19 countries. They were also kept in the quarantine period in hotels (Whitelaw et al. 2020).

All these precautions were followed in many countries including the United States, New Zealand, India, Korea, etc.

11.6.3   Vaccination

After a few months of the spreading of the virus, our scientists started working to make a cure for this disease and soon they were out with vaccines against the coronavirus (Rab et al. 2020).

Vaccines can be classified as virus- or protein-based. Suspended/inactivated or dead or live-attenuated viruses are incorporated in virus-based vaccines. Against these viruses, our body will produce antibodies. During the course of life, if such a virus enters our body, then our body knows how to eliminate such a virus from the body (van Riel and de Wit 2020).

Many countries have worked on vaccines against the coronavirus. "Sputnik-V" is the first vaccine approved by Russia. India had been working on the cure of coronavirus and released many vaccines, two among which have been taken up by most of Indian citizens, namely "covishield and covaxin" (Lurie et al. 2020).

Not only virus- or protein-based, but DNA-based vaccines also have been developed to prevent this disease (Coban et al. 2013). DNA-based vaccines activate humoral as well as cell-mediated response. The DNA antigen containing virus DNA as an antigen is injected to start the transcription of the viral gene using the host cell, which activates antigen- presenting cells (APCs). The genes get transcripted into protein, which then binds to MHC (major histocompatibility complex), which then exposes the antigen to CD4 and CD8 receptors, which then start working against the antigen (Li et al. 2012).

mRNA-based vaccines were also developed. It consists of mRNA having more stability and efficiency (Zhang et al. 2019). It directly encodes for protein antigen. The first mRNA vaccine is the mRNA-1273 vaccine developed to treat COVID-19. mRNA covered with lipid nanoparticles has been used for injecting purposes (Chakraborty and Parvez 2020).

11.6.4   Self-Isolation and Quarantine

People suffering from coronavirus were instructed to live in a 14-day quarantine to avert the escalation of the virus. They were given all the facilities they needed to live. People are quarantined so that they do not spread the virus to uninfected ones. Earlier, special quarantine wards were made to keep people, for example, in hospitals, hotels and schools, but later they were told to go for self-isolation in their homes by keeping themselves away from other family members, especially senior citizens and kids.

11.6.5   Clinical Management

Artificial intelligence has played a major role in diagnosing and developing methods to prevent coronavirus. In China, CT images were used to differentiate between infection in lungs due to coronavirus and other lung diseases, which helped in treating the disease at the earliest (Liu 2020).

11.6.6   Masks and PPE Kits Use

One of the major steps taken up by all the countries is the use of a mask to curtail the human-to-human transmission of the virus. If the mouth of a person remains covered and they stand some distance away from each other, then there are lower chances of getting infected with the coronavirus. The use of a mask is efficient only when used with proper hygiene of hands such as using sanitizer frequently.

Medical practitioners and other people are suggested to wear PPE kits while treating infected patients. Children were advised to use face shields along with masks. Double masking was started when the spreading of coronavirus was at its peak. This prevention method is majorly accepted all over the globe and still going on (Wang et al. 2020).

11.7 Conclusion and Future Perspectives

Contagion caused by these viruses is a colossal health hazard. They lead to fatality and possess conflicting socioeconomic effects that are continually aggravated. Therefore, possible alternatives to treatment and approaches need to be developed. Firstly, India is following crucial measures to inhibit viral transmission as much as possible. Secondly, the Ministry of AYUSH and ICMR administered needful guidelines to use accustomed and precautionary treatment approaches to boost immunity against COVID-19. This guidance could help lessen the grimness of the viral infection in comparatively old patients and raise the life expectancy. India has proficiency in specially designed therapeutically/pharmaceutical industries with manufacturing skills and the government has entrenched fast-tracking analysis and investigative research to flourish accelerated diagnostic test kits and vaccines at low cost. India is seeking to augment its research facilities and deviate from examining the mass population, as endorsed by medical experts in India and international countries.

References

Ahn, D.G., Shin, H.J., Kim, M.H. et al. (2020). Current status of epidemiology diagnosis, therapeutics, and vaccines for novel coronavirus disease 2019 (COVID-19). *J Microbiol Biotechnol* 30 (3): 313–324.

Bo, H.X., Li, W., Yang, Y. et al. (2020). Posttraumatic stress symptoms and attitude towards crisis mental health services among clinically stable patients with COVID-19 in China. *Psychology of medicine* 27: 1–2.

Bogoch, I.I., Watts, A., Thomas-Bachli, A. et al. (2020). Pneumonia of unknown aetiology in Wuhan, China: potential for international spread via commercial air travel. *J Travel Med* 27: 2.

Chakraborty, R. and Parvez, S. (2020). COVID-19: an overview of the current pharmacological interventions, vaccines, and clinical trials. *Biochemical pharmacology.* 180: 114184.

Chan, J.F., Kok, K.H., Zhu, Z. et al. (2020a). Genomic haracterization of the 2019 novel human-pathogenic coronavirus isolated from a patient with atypical pneumonia after visiting Wuhan. *Emerg Microbes Infec* 9: 221–236.

Chan, J.F., Yuan, S., Kok, K.H. et al. (2020b). A familial cluster of pneumonia associated with the 2019 novel coronavirus indicating person- to- person transmission: a study of a family cluster. *Lancet* 395: 514–523.

Chen, L., Liu, W., Zhang, Q. et al. (2020). RNA based mNGS approach identifies a novel human coronavirus from two individual pneumonia cases in 2019 Wuhan outbreak. *Emerg Microb Infect* 9: 313–319.

Coban, C., Kobiyama, K., Jounai, N. et al. (2013). DNA vaccines: a simple DNA sensing matter? *Hum Vaccin Immunother* 9: 2216–2221.

Contini, C., Nuzzo, M.D., Barp, N. et al. (2020). The novel zoonotic COVID-19 pandemic: an expected global health concern. *J Infect Dev Ctries* 14 (3): 254–264.

Drexler, J.F., Corman, V.M., and Drosten, C. (2013). Ecology, evolution and classification of bat coronavirus in the aftermath of SARS, Germany. *Antiviral Research* 101: 45–56.

Ebrahim, S.H., Ahmed, Q.A., Gozzer, E. et al. (2020). Covid-19 and community mitigation strategies in a pandemic. *BMJ* 17: 368.

European Centre for Disease Prevention and Control (ECDC) (2019). *Operational Tool on Rapid Risk Assessment Methodology*. Stockholm: ECDC.

Ge, H., Wang, X., Yuan, X. et al. (2020). The epidemiology and clinical information about COVID-19. *Eur J Clin Microbiol Infect Dis* 39 (6): 1011–1019.

Goyal, K., Chauhan, P., Chhikara, K. et al. (2020). Fear of COVID 2019: first suicidal casein India! *Asian Journal of Psychiatry* 49: 101989.89.

Guan, Y., Zheng, B.J., He, Y.Q. et al. (2003). Isolation and characterization of virus related to the SARS coronavirus from animals in Southern China. *Science* 302 (5643): 276–278.

Guo, Y.R., Cao, Q.D., Hong, Z.S. et al. (2020). The origin, transmission and clinical therapies on coronavirus disease 2019 (COVID-19) outbreak- an update on the status. *Military Medical Research* 7: 11.

Jian, S.W., Kao, C.T., Chang, Y.C. et al. (2021). Risk assessment for COVID-19 pandemic in Taiwan. *International Journal of Infectious Disease* 104: 746–751.

Lai, C.C., Shih, T.P., Ko, W.C. et al. (2020). Severe acute respiratory syndrome coronavirus 2 (SARS-CoV- 2) and coronavirus disease-2019 (COVID-19): the epidemic and the challenges (2020). *International Journal of Antimicrobial Agents* 7: 4.

Lau, S.K.P., Woo, P.C.Y., Li, K.S.M. et al. (2005). Severe acute respiratory syndrome coronavirus- like virus in Chinese horseshoe bat. *PNAS* 102 (39): 14040–14045.

Li, L., Saade, F., and Petrovsky, N. (2012). The future of human DNA vaccines. *Journal of biotechnology* 162: 171–182.

Li, Z., Ge, J., Yang, M. et al. (2020). Vicarious traumatization in the general public, members, and non-members of medical teams aiding in COVID-19 control. *Brain Behav Immun* 88: 916–919.

Liu, J. (2020). Deployment of IT in China's fight against the Covid-19 pandemic. April 2 2020.

Liu, Y.H., Lai, C.C., Wang, C.Y. et al. (2020). Asymptomatic carrier state, acute respiratory disease, and pneumonia due to severe acute respiratory syndrome coronavirus 2 (SARS-CoV-2): facts and myths. *Journal of Microbiology, Immunology and Infection* 53 (3): 404–412.

Lu, R., Zhao, X., Li, J. et al. (2020). Genomic characterisation and epidemiology of 2019 novel coronavirus; implications for virus origins and receptor binding. *Lancet* 395: 565–574.

Lurie, N., Saville, M., Hatchett, R., and Halton, J. (2020). Developing Covid-19 vaccines at pandemic speed. *The New England journal of medicine* 382: 1969–1973.

Meo, S.A., Khlaiwi, T.A., Usmani, A.M. et al. (2020). Biological and epidemiological trends in the prevalence and mortality due to outbreaks of novel coronavirus COVID-19. *Journal of King Saud University-Science* 32 (4): 2495–2499.

Meyer, B., Muller, M.A., Corman, V.M. et al. (2014). Antibodies against MERS coronavirus in dromedaries, United Arab Emirates, 2003 and 2013. *Emerging Infectious Disease* 20 (4): 552–559.

Muhairi, S.A., Hosani, F.A., Eltahir, Y.M. et al. (2016). Epidemiological investigation of middle east respiratory syndrome coronavirus in dromedary camel farms linked with human infection in Abu Dhabi Emirates, United Arab Emirates. *Virus Genes* 52: 848–854.

Muller, M.A., Corman, V.M., Jores, J. et al. (2014). MERS coronavirus neutralizing antibodies in Camels, Eastern Africa, 1983-1997. *Emerging infectious Diseases* 20 (12): 2093–2095.

Paraskevis, D., Kostaki, E.G., Magiorkinis, G. et al. (2020). Full-genome evolutionary analysis of the novel coronavirus (2019- nCoV) rejects the hypothesis of emergence as a result of a recent recombination event. *Infect Genet Evol* 79: 104212.

Peiris, J.S.M., Guan, Y., and Yuen, K.Y. (2004). Severe acute respiratory syndrome. *Nature Medicine Supplement* 10 (12): S88–S97.

Rab, S., Afjal, Javaid, M. et al. (2020). An update on the global vaccine development for coronavirus. *Diabetes & metabolic syndrome* 14: 2053–2055.

Reusken, C.B.E.M., Messadi, L., Feyisa, A. et al. (2014). Geographic distribution of MERS coronavirus among dromedary camels, Africa. *Emerging Infectious Disease* 20 (8): 1370–1374.

van Riel, D. and de Wit, E. (2020). Next-generation vaccine platforms for COVID-19. *Nature materials* 19: 810–812.

Shanmugaraj, B., Siriwattananon, K., Wangkanont, K., and Phoolcharoen, W. (2020). Perspective on monoclonal antibody therapy as potential therapeutic intervention for Coronavirus disease- 19 (COVID-19). *Asian Pac I Allergy Immunol* 38: 10–18.

Su, S., Wong, G., Shi, W. et al. (2020). Epidemiology, genetic recombination, and pathogenesis of coronavirus. *Trends in Microbiology* 24 (6): 490–502.

Taiwan Centers for Disease Control (Taiwan CDC) (2019). COVID-19 (2019-nCoV). Press release.

Wang, J., Pan, L., Tang, S. et al. (2020). Mask use during COVID-19: a risk adjusted strategy. *Environmental Pollution* 266 (Pt 1): 115099.

Whitelaw, S., Mamos, M.A., Topol, E., and Spall, H.G.C.V. (2020). Application of digital technology in COVID-19 pandemic planning and response. *Lancet Digital Health* 2 (8): e435–e440.

Woo, P.C.Y., Lau, S.K.P., Li, K.S.M. et al. (2012). Genetic relatedness of the novel Human group C betacoronavirus to *Tylonycteris* bat coronavirus HKU4 and *Pipistrellus* bat coronavirus HKU5. *Emerging Microbes and Infection* 1: e35.

World Health Organization (2019). Coronavirus Disease 2019 (COVID-19) Situation Report-118; 17 May 2020.

Wu, A., Peng, Y., Huang, B. et al. (2020a). Genome Composition and Divergence of the novel coronavirus (2019- nCoV) originating in China. *Cell Host Microbe* 27 (3): 325–328.

Wu, F., Zhao, S., Yu, B. et al. (2020b). A new coronavirus associated with human respiratory disease in China. *Nature* 579: 265–269.

Yang, Y., Li, W., Zhang, Q. et al. (2020). Mental health services for older adults in China during the COVID-19 outbreak. *The Lancet Psychiatry* 7 (4): 19.

Zhang, C., Maruggi, G., Shan, H., and Li, J. (2019). Advances in mRNA vaccines for infectious diseases. *Frontiers in immunology* 10: 594.

Zhou, P., Yang, X.L., Wang, X.G. et al. (2020). A pneumonia outbreak associated with a new coronavirus of probable bat origin. *Nature* 579: 270–273.

Zimmermann, P. and Curtis, N. (2020). Coronavirus infection in children including COVID-19: an overview of the epidemiology, clinical features, diagnosis, treatment and prevention options in children. *Pediatr Infect Dis J* 39: 355–368.

12

Case Studies: COVID-19 and the Environment

Aayush Dey[1], Pratik Kulkarni[1], Piyush K. Rao[1], Nitasha Khatri[2], and Deepak Rawtani[3]

[1] School of Doctoral Studies and Research, National Forensic Sciences University (Ministry of Home Affairs, GOI), Gandhinagar, Gujarat, India
[2] Department of Forest and Environment, Gujarat Environment Management Institute (GEMI), Gandhinagar, Gujarat, India
[3] School of Pharmacy, National Forensic Sciences University (Ministry of Home Affairs, GOI), Gandhinagar, Gujarat, India

12.1   Introduction

It is a well-established fact that particulate matter in the ambient air surroundings is a prominent source of fatal diseases. Amid the COVID-19 epidemic and forced lockdowns across the globe, the levels of particulate matter in the air have dropped drastically (Wang and Su 2020). COVID-19 and different particulate matter in the ambience have a conceivable relationship, which can be comprehended further via this chapter. Severe implications such as economic crashes and hefty losses in private small-scale businesses have been observed on a global scale due to COVID-19. Major geographical regions such as China, Southeast Asia, European countries such as Italy, and South American countries such as Brazil, Spain, and Turkey have faced major setbacks due to the onset of COVID-19. This chapter would emphasize primarily the rate of spread of COVID-19 primarily due to particulate matter and temperature within the aforementioned regions. Preliminary assessments of the pandemic have been carried out using different models, for instance, a 3-staged model such as e-ISHR has been utilized in the Wuhan province of China to predict the number of confirmed SARS-CoV-2 cases (Li et al. 2020b). In another study conducted in China, the spatial extent and the magnitude of variations in air pollution concentrations were measured by cross-referring different sets of data from satellites, ground-tethered devices, and different models (Marlier et al. 2020). Southeast Asian regions amidst the lockdown period have observed declinations in the levels of aerosols and pollutants. Urban settlements in this region have reported declinations in the levels of tropospheric NO_2, i.e. around 27–34% (Kanniah et al. 2020). Studies regarding aerosol optical depth (AOD) levels in south-southeast Asia, the USA, and Europe regions have also been reported in this chapter in order to impart a different perspective to its readers (Acharya et al. 2021).

This chapter will also accentuate the major preliminary assessments in other major geographical regions as well.

12.2 COVID-19 and Its Impact on the Environment – A Case Study of China

The absolute effect of the pandemic caused by the novel coronavirus on the environment has been studied extensively. Several other case studies and the analysis provided in such reports have revealed several positive implications that include aspects, such as augmentation in statistics regarding the air quality in China and a significant drop in the global carbon emission levels. However, it remains to be seen whether this impact will stay in the long run. The rise in the levels of gases causing the greenhouse effect and energy exploitation is expected once China resumes the large-scale industrial activities and lifts the lockdown. The pandemic caused by the novel coronavirus has caused a significant reduction in nitrogen dioxide (NO_2) concentration as well. According to a report, the curb in environmental pollutant levels was noticed first in severely affected Chinese cities as they imposed strict restrictions and lockdown protocols (Dey et al. 2022). Following China's decision, more regions started applying similar restrictions resulting which the air quality improved significantly throughout the country. It has been evident that the lockdown measures have curbed the environmental pollution levels, but a steady declination has also been observed in the economic growth as well. Hence, it would be justifiable to relate economic growth or declination rates to the environmental pollution levels. The Wuhan province of China, where the novel coronavirus emerged, saw a declination in the economic growth as well as the environmental levels first and later the same was observed throughout the country (Lian et al. 2020; Ruiz Estrada et al. 2020). Hence, this indicates that declination in the economic curve and imposing restrictions on vehicular movements can cause a direct change in the country's energy consumption and prevent environmental pollution (Phadke and Rawtani 2022). The study also stated that following strict quarantine measures can protect everyone from getting infected and also lead to a positive effect on the environment. This study has become a tool that enriches the theoretical research on economic and environmental pollution during such extreme events like the COVID-19 pandemic (Purohit et al. 2022; Rao and Rawtani 2022). A systematic analysis has to be performed for developing a relationship between the economic growth and environmental pollution during such outbreaks, as they can provide a reference for other countries to assess the impact of the situation on many other factors including the imminent impact on the environment (Rawtani et al. 2022).

This particular assessment has emerged as a tool that augments the academic research on environmental pollution during such extreme events like the COVID-19 pandemic. A systematic analysis has to be performed for developing an association amid the economic boom and environmental pollution during such outbreaks, as they can act as a referral for different nations to evaluate the impact of the situation on many other factors including the imminent impact on the environment (Kaushik and Rawtani 2022).

12.3   Environmental Impact of Particulate Matter in Italy Due to COVID-19

In another study, the impact of PM2.5 and PM10 particulate matter surface levels were assessed to evaluate the impact due to COVID-19 in Milan, Italy. Its degree of accelerated diffusion and COVID-19 lethality in the city were also studied (Lovarelli et al. 2020). Data regarding particulate matter (PM) in two distinctive size portions i.e., PM 2.5 and PM 10 and climatic factors that include average temperature, humidity, air velocity, atmospheric pressure, and planetary boundary layer height were procured within a time span of four months, i.e. 1 January to 30 April 2020, and these data were examined in accordance to COVID-19 transmission (Fattorini and Regoli 2020). Aerosol from an infected individual is considered the primary mode of transmission. Despite this fact, the aforementioned factors have been emphasized regarding the transmission of COVID-19, and it has been found that these factors directly corelate with the transmission of COVID-19 (Parikh and Rawtani 2022). It concurred that in Milan, ambient temperature showed a direct correlation to COVID-19 transmission rates and the relationship between the COVID-19 transmission and humidity is inversed (Mohite et al. 2022).

A negative relationship between the prevalence of COVID-19 and different environmental aspects such as airspeed, humidity, etc., were observed in this study. Unlike other aspects such as temperature, a positive association was observed. The association between COVID-19 prevalence and the aforementioned environmental aspects proved that dry air can act as a potential medium for the transmission of the novel coronavirus, whereas ambient temperature and warm season are somewhat effective in stopping the COVID-19 transmission. On the contrary, particulate matter can combine with viruses or bacterial cells, which would definitely impact human health and immunity (Setti et al. 2020). Fomite or aerosols infected with the SARS-CoV-2 penetrate the alveoli, causing the lung function to cease at a steady rate, and further causing pneumonia. There is an urgent requirement to devise novel strategies for controlling the SARS-CoV-2 spread, and this could be achieved by understanding the dynamics of transmission of the virus via air. This study also emphasized the importance of cleaner air and its role in better health and immunity of humans in the context of the ongoing pandemic (Zoran et al. 2020).

12.4   Impact Upon the Atmospheric Environment of the Southeast Asia Region

Malaysia and adjacent Southeast Asian countries following the steps of the superpower China, imposed nationwide lockdowns in order to mitigate the spread of the COVID-19 virus. The lockdown measures imposed by the Southeast Asian countries observed a positive impact on the environment (Kanniah et al. 2020). The impact on air pollution has been positive due to the reduction in the use of fossil fuels, but the same positive impact cannot be seen upon the economy as the lockdown measures imposed by the governments have forced small scale industries and businesses to shut down (Wong et al. 2021). In this particular study, the fluctuations in the level of AOD were observed by accumulating data from the Himawari-8 satellite. The changes in the levels of NO_2 were quantified through Aura-OMI. Several stations across Malaysia carried out measurements for ground-based pollution for obtaining quantifiable changes in aerosol and air pollutant levels due to the overall closure of working in industries during the pandemic (Fauzi and Paiman 2021). During the lockdown, AOD levels in the sea and the contamination discharge over the oceanic waters have decreased significantly. Tropospheric NO_2 has also shown a significant decrease (27–30%), especially in areas not affected by seasonal biomass burning. Concentrations of $PM_{2.5}$, PM_{10}, SO_2, NO_2, and CO in Malaysia have shown a decrease of 23–32%, 26–31%, 9–20%, 63–64%, and 25–31%, respectively, in the urban areas (Latif et al. 2021). Compared to a similar period in 2018–2019, this decrease has been quite evident this year owing to the lockdown. Industrial, suburban, and rural areas across the country have shown notable reductions in the levels of particulate matter since the initiation of the lockdown. Further research is needed to quantify the reductions in harmful air pollutant levels via health-related research and studying the changes in air quality and climate change (Suhaimi et al. 2020).

Assessment of the fluctuations in the primary air contaminants or pollutants over Southeast Asia was carried out via spatiotemporal studies and data accumulated from such studies were utilized to evaluate the impact of the lockdown (Yang et al. 2020). Information regarding the amalgamation of aerosols, i.e. (AOD, $PM_{2.5}$, PM_{10}) and air pollutants such as (SO_2, NO_2, CO, and O_3) were accumulated via the help of the Himawari-8 satellite (Zang et al. 2021). The ground stations in Malaysia and Aura-OMI were also involved in collection of data. According to the data collected, values for AOD were found to be substantially reduced over the Southeast Asian regions in countries like Singapore, Brunei, the Philippines, and Malaysia (Nguyen et al. 2019). Data regarding aerosol composition were also recorded over the industrial regions in Malaysia, which exhibited around 40–70% reduction in AOD values. On the contrary, the northern part of the SEA peninsula of Malaysia exhibited an elevated level of AOD although the lockdown was enforced. Forest fires and the burning of agricultural wastes contributed to the elevated levels of AOD. The level of air pollutants, such as NO_2 was also seen to be extensive in such areas, i.e. approximately $(4 \times 10^{-15}\,\text{moles/cm}^2 – 5 \times 10^{-15}\,\text{moles/cm}^2)$. Cities like Ho Chi Minh and Yangon exhibited a drop in the NO_2 levels, i.e. approximately (27–34%) (Kanniah et al. 2020; Takahashi et al. 2020). Measures such as restrictions in transport and movement across countries and reduction in industrial and business operations contributed to the reduction in NO_2 levels in the aforementioned countries. Enforcement of aggressive lockdown measures was adopted by countries such as Malaysia, Singapore, and Brunei, with the assistance of the armed forces. Some of the lockdown measures included rules such as restriction of religious activities and gathering of people in a group or a crowd, prohibiting any forms of travel, transportation, etc. Other countries such as Indonesia and Thailand including the Philippines and Myanmar enacted rather liberal measures of lockdown (Aung et al. 2021). In Malaysia, strict measures enforced on 18 March exhibited a significant decline in particulate matter levels, i.e. approximately, 28–39% and 26–31% for PM_{10} and 20–42% and 23–32% for $PM_{2.5}$. These statistics conferred for industrial and urban areas. For the NO_2 level, a greater decline was obtained (33–46% and 64%) in the industrial sites and the urban centres, respectively. Reductions for SO_2 and CO were lower than the other pollutants, and

O_3 reduction did not show any significant changes compared to the past readings. These results from the research designate the impact of restraint measures and the regional lockdown during such times as affected by regional air pollution showing elevated heights of aerosol and pollutant content due to nontraffic factors, for example, industrial operations. The effect of the pandemic on the air quality index is necessary and rather challenging. It becomes more challenging just before the onset of the monsoon season, i.e. during March–April. Other factors that contribute to the increase in the aerosol and pollutant levels include agricultural and forest fires as mentioned prior in this section. A rather detailed assessment by the meteorology department is required to quantify the increasing aerosol and pollutant content.

12.5 Impact of COVID-19 Lockdown on PM_{10}, SO_2, and NO_2 Concentrations in Salé City, Morocco

The ruling government of Morocco professed national emergency due to COVID-19 on 2 March, 2020. Since then, for curbing the transmission of COVID-19, rigorous protocols have been devised that constituted nationwide lockdown and restrictions on transport and traveling, restricting human movement and barring all public and group mediated activities (Otmani et al. 2020). The current research deals with the evaluation of changes in some air pollutant levels namely PM_{10}, NO_2, and SO_2 in Salé city, which lies in the Northwestern region of Morocco. These evaluations were carried out during the lockdown period. Constant quantification of particulate matter and the air pollutants were carried out prior to and within the lockdown phase (He et al. 2020). The results exhibited a sharp decline in their levels as emanations from vehicles and industrial processes were condensed to a greater extent. There were 96, 49, and 75% in the NO_2, SO_2, and PM_{10} levels. PM_{10} level reduction was lesser than the NO_2 level reduction (He et al. 2020). Using the HYSPLIT model, the advantages of PM_{10} level deductions were explained by a 3-D air mass backward trajectory (Maneesh and El Alaoui 2020). Additionally, remarkable dissimilarities were noted in the air mass back trajectories and the meteorology during these two periods.

12.6 Correlation of Pandemic-Induced Lockdown and Stone Quarrying and Crushing – An Indian Perspective

The decrease in the levels of PM_{10}, SO_2, and NO_2 concentrations can be mainly credited to the rigorous lockdown procedures restraining industrial activities and human mobility in the ongoing pandemic scenario that has caused a momentous drop in vehicle exhaust emanations and industrial procedures (Tobías et al. 2020). These decreases are projected to go on further during the lockdown period. The COVID-19 pandemic persuaded lockdown effects on the environment over stone quarrying and crushing areas. One of the major threats to the environment, ecosystem and human health is stone quarrying and crushing that releases a large amount of stone dust (Janati Idrissi et al. 2020). Despite creating an economic crisis during the emergency lockdown in India, it has facilitated an improvement in the environmental quality in all aspects (Lancet 2020). A qualitative benefit has already been proven by the global scale study for air quality; however, its impact on the regional level is yet to be investigated. Dwarka river basin in the eastern peninsula of India (middle catchment) is a well-established part popularly known for stone quarrying and crushing activities, due to which the region remains highly polluted (Pal and Mandal 2021). Another study published by (Pal and Mandal 2019) explores the effect of lockdown on the environmental particulate matter like PM_{10} emission, river water quality, land surface temperature (LST), and noise using image and field-derived data before and during the lockdown period. Results in the selected stone-crushing clusters show a marked decrease in the maximum particulate matter concentration from 189–278 µg/m^3 prior to the lockdown phase to approximately 50–60 µg/m^3 after just 18 days during the lockdown. LST has also decreased by 3–5 °C, and the noise level dropped to 65 dBA from 85 dBA during the lockdown in parts where stone crushing is dominant. Also, the quality of river water has improved due to the stoppage of the dust released into the water (Mandal and Pal 2020). A quantitative parameter to evaluate the water quality termed as total dissolved solids (TDS) level has reduced almost two times that of its safety level. During this unprecedented crisis of COVID-19, nations on a global scale have enforced apt strategies for curbing pollution levels in the environment such as nationwide-lockdown (Lokhandwala and Gautam 2020). These strategies have been proved to be a successful attempt to manage pollution sources. Also due to these enforced measures an improvement in the environment and the ecosystem has been observed.

12.7 Temperature vs. COVID-19 Transmission – Brazil

Rio de Janeiro, São Paulo, Brasília, Fortaleza, and Manaus were among the five major Brazilian cities that were selected to enumerate the impact of meteorological conditions on the spread of COVID-19 (Auler et al. 2020). As of 13 April, 2020, these cities were worst affected by the novel coronavirus or SARS-CoV-2 infection. The variables that were shortlisted in this research constituted collective cases, new infection cases, and transmission speeds. Contradicting reports regarding transmission speeds of SARS-CoV-2 in colder countries, the transmission of SARS-CoV-2 in Brazilian cities was supported due to higher mean temperatures and relative humidity (Qi et al. 2020). The need for intersectoral strategies and approaches in the aforementioned cities was indicated by the SARS-CoV-2 transmission speeds. Appropriate strategies against the spread of COVID-19 must be enforced in order to prevent the collapse of the health system. This particular research is novel as it evaluates the impact of meteorological aspects on the novel coronavirus transmission in tropical climate ambience. The transmission of COVID-19 in Brazil was favored due to higher ambient temperatures, i.e. 27.5 °C and relative humidity that measured to be around 80% (Coelho et al. 2020). However, this study is only based on preliminary findings and has some limitations, indicating a need for a more extended study period to provide a broad perspective of the meteorological conditions and their effects upon the COVID-19 transmission.

Other researchers, especially those specialized in studying epidemics and meteorology, are further advised to conduct further studies on how different climatic conditions are responsible for the transmission of COVID-19 in a tropical setting. However, factors such as living and health conditions of the population apart from meteorological conditions are examples of some complex aspects that are also responsible for spreading the virus. These factors highlight individual and collective coverage, such as economic, political, social, and cultural conditions. Due to the complex nature of the analysis and lack of the updated data, only some factors were emphasized. However, the results described here are aimed to provide an understanding of the role of tropical climate conditions in the transmission of the disease. In the future, the research must be focused on the issue of the basic sanitation in these Brazilian cities, as evidenced by the survival of the virus in untreated wastewater. Wind speed, presence of pollutants in the atmosphere, and socio-economy of the population are some other factors which must be considered in future studies (Auler et al. 2020).

12.8 Correlation of COVID-19 and Air Quality in Spain

Similar to studies in other countries, the improvement of air quality in Madrid, Spain due to the COVID-19 pandemic has been attributed to the imposition of lockdown, which has reduced the traffic and caused a substantial decrease in air pollution levels (Martorell-Marugán et al. 2021). In Madrid and Barcelona, a 75% decrease in traffic was observed, which led to a reduced NO_2 concentration (62 and 50%) in Spain's two largest cities – Madrid and Barcelona (Baldasano 2020). The promising results show the limits that can be achieved post low emission zones (LEZs) and the total contamination, which can be eliminated (55%) in the case of these two cities. This value indicates the need to put together collective efforts in order to ensure a clean and healthy atmosphere in both cities in terms of NO_2 (Baldasano 2020).

12.8.1 Conclusive Statements

The concentration levels dropped lower than the standards set by the EU and WHO, i.e. $40\,\mu g/m^3$ after a fortnight in the month of March. The concentration values of NO_2 during the latter half of March were recorded to be lower when compared to the standards set by the EU and WHO, i.e. ($40\,\mu g/m^3$). In the past recent years, the NO_2 concentrations in the environment were recurrently found to be exceeding in urban traffic stations. After a few decades, although there are several implications to COVID-19 health-wise, the skies appear to be more transparent and the surrounding air is cleaner. Apart from 62 and 50% reduction in the NO_2 levels in Madrid and Barcelona, the maximum hourly peak values have also reduced significantly, with ratios between 1.2 and 1.7. During the pandemic, the meteorological conditions in March 2020 played a significant role. Motor vehicles with the internal combustion system and increased traffic are one of the most important sources of air pollution in cities and are well-known to be a terrible dilemma (Air 2020). With this pandemic and its positive effect on the environment, it has become a major idea among the population regarding the feats that are yet to be achieved regarding refining the air in urban areas (Muhammad et al. 2020; Ogen 2020).

12.9 Weather Impacts COVID-19 Transmission – A Case Study of Turkey

This study conducted across nine cities in Turkey correlates different dynamics of weather and COVID-19. The primary dynamics of weather that were considered for this study included ambient/surrounding temperature (°C), relative humidity (%), dew point, and wind speed (mph). As per literature, the incubation period of the SARS-CoV-2 virus varies from 1 to 14 days. Therefore, following 1st, 3rd, 7th, and 14th days, the effects of each parameter are examined. Additionally, the population has been included as an active evaluation parameter. Spearman's correlation coefficients have been used to conduct the analysis. The highest correlations were observed on day 14 for population, wind speed, and day for temperature (Şahin 2020).

This particular study that was carried out in the major cities of Turkey was different from previously conducted studies of COVID-19 as it primarily focuses on specific days of the preliminary COVID-19 infection, i.e. days 1, 3, 7, and 14. The dynamics that were previously mentioned in this section were directly correlated to these specifically mentioned days (Li et al. 2020a). Another factor, i.e. the population density was also considered for this study. The population density was directly correlated to the prevalence of COVID-19 in the environment. It was observed that the population density was directly related to the prevalence of COVID-19 as higher population density resulted in higher positive infection cases. Wind speed alike the population density as a parameter for checking the COVID-19 prevalence exhibited a similar phenomenon in which higher wind speeds resulted in greater cases of COVID-19 infections (Chen et al. 2020). The accuracy of the results can be improved with the availability of weather data from Sakarya and Zonguldak (Şahin 2020), where the case density of the COVID-19 infection may be considered high. Moreover, city-wise case updates could help broaden the results. Also, keeping track of people moving to and fro in the city and those under quarantine could help in increasing the accuracy of the study. These points may be considered for future analysis and data from different cities in different countries may help generalize the overall results.

12.10 COVID-19 vs. Ambient Temperature – A Perspective of Canada

In the January–May period of the year 2020, more than 77 000 individuals with positive COVID-19 infections were selected to conduct a study in order to correlate the surrounding temperature of Canada and the prevalence of the novel coronavirus. Cases from four different provinces of Canada, i.e. Ontario, Alberta, British Columbia, and Quebec were selected (To et al. 2021). A positive correlation was found in the study after considering other environmental factors such as wind speed and precipitation. However, there was no statistical significance (14.2 per 100 000 people; 95% CI: −0.60–29.0). Likewise, no statistical significance between the R_0, i.e. the basic reproduction number of the novel coronavirus and the surrounding temperature. The findings do not support the hypothesis of higher temperatures reducing the viral transmission rate and warn the public to stay vigilant and keep practicing precautionary measures such as wearing facial masks, hand washing, and social distancing despite the warming climates (Berry et al. 2020).

In a study, a total of 49 regions across four provinces of Canada were selected that accounted for almost 99.6% of the total affirmed COVID-19-affected individuals. This data accounts for the time period starting from 25 January to 18 May, 2020. Higher latitudes showed a decrease in the mean temperature and total precipitation. Areas around the urban centers showed the highest number of overall collective cases and increased collective prevalence rates. The results from the study did not show any statistical significance after altering the rainfall, wind velocity, and province between temperature and R-value ($p = 0.74$). Various regression models, tuned for wind velocity, rainfall, and province, an increase in ambient temperature amplified the figure for confirmed COVID-19 cases. However, this equation established between ambient temperature and the amplification in the figures for confirmed COVID-19 cases was deemed to be insignificant (To et al. 2021).

Among all the studies that have been conducted to study the transmission of COVID-19, this research is the first that utilizes quotidian meteorological data. Meteorological data from four different provinces were gathered and utilized to study the coalition between ambient temperature and COVID-19. Other examples of researches, for instance (Pawar et al. 2020; Sarwar et al. 2021), also utilized meteorological data to study the influence of environmental factors in the transmission of COVID-19. Several studies based on evaluating the coalition between the novel coronavirus and ambient temperature have shown an inverse relationship, and the results obtained from this study are in accordance with those. For example, a study in Wuhan and a Canadian study comprising 144 geopolitical areas found no association (Jüni et al. 2020). Likewise, a study based on the data obtained from 21 countries and French administrative regions showed an inverse association at high temperatures but doubted its association at lower and seasonal temperatures. From these results, it is likely that Canada experienced these lower seasonal temperature changes rather than at high temperatures that were needed to affect COVID-19 cases, as seen in the study published by (Demongeot et al. 2020). Besides, studies in Iran on various climate variables, the spatiotemporal analysis of Spain and a preprint study in Nigeria during the early wave of COVID-19 did not find any association between temperature and COVID-19 (Lu et al. 2020). Despite the fact that this study showed a statistically nonsignificant association between COVID-19 cases and temperature, the positive regression coefficient indicated that COVID-19 revealed that with increasing temperature, the infection rate also increases (Bashir et al. 2020). During the study period, severe spikes in COVID-19 cases were observed in April and May, meat processing plants in Alberta, and several long-term care homes in Ontario and Quebec reported outbreaks (Abdeen et al. 2021). These might have formed a skewed association away from the null independent of increasing temperatures in the provinces studied. Canada has a robust heterogeneous climate, and a considerable variation in its temperature and a comparison of results between the provinces studied allowed better identification of the association between COVID-19 cases and temperature (Jüni et al. 2020). Moreover, an analysis based on the health region level and accurate representation of area-wide climate patterns were possible. Despite this advantage, the limitation of using health regions as a geographical unit could not be further disaggregated like in cities, which can be studied at a more granular level. Factors like testing rates, local public health policies, and urbanization drives exert a confounding effect on the ecological nature of this study (To et al. 2021).

In summary, this study disregarded the hypothesis of high temperature, reducing the viral transmission rate due to a lack of strong evidence. Hence, as the studies show very fewer signs of curtailing the current pandemic, it advises everyone to stay vigilant and continue practicing safety measures such as wearing face masks, washing hands frequently, and maintaining social distancing despite the warming of climates. These findings also shed some light on preparing future potential strategies for resurging COVID-19. In the coming times, future studies will be able to encompass more data on climate and COVID-19 cases as they are substantially increasing globally in the summer months. Therefore, meteorological factors must be studied in detail to elucidate the relationship between COVID-19 and the climate in a better way (To et al. 2021).

12.11 Conclusion

In conclusion, this chapter provides comprehensive detail on the effect of the COVID-19 pandemic on the environment in regards to change in the climate and several other factors. Casewise study has been discussed throughout by giving examples from various parts of the world. As the current situation indicates a need for a long-term and extensive study, collective efforts must be implemented in order to form better policies and strategies to curb the spread of the virus. From all the studies outlined here, it has become clear that air pollution plays a crucial role in the formation of chronic diseases and other complications, which has resulted in a pandemic situation. This should be taken as a warning, and the governing bodies must act accordingly and favour sustainable approaches more along with keeping the economy stable by finding novel solutions and preventing pandemics like COVID-19 from occurring again and increasing the preparedness in the future during such situations.

References

Abdeen, A., Kharvari, F., O'Brien, W., and Gunay, B. (2021). The impact of the COVID-19 on households' hourly electricity consumption in Canada. *Energy Build.* 250: 111280. https://doi.org/10.1016/j.enbuild.2021.111280.

Acharya, P., Barik, G., Gayen, B.K. et al. (2021). Revisiting the levels of aerosol optical depth in south-southeast Asia, Europe and USA amid the COVID-19 pandemic using satellite observations. *Environ. Res.* 193: 110514. https://doi.org/10.1016/j.envres.2020.110514.

Air, I.Q. (2020). COVID-19 air quality report.

Auler, A.C., Cássaro, F.A.M., da Silva, V.O., and Pires, L.F. (2020). Evidence that high temperatures and intermediate relative humidity might favor the spread of COVID-19 in tropical climate: a case study for the most affected Brazilian cities. *Sci. Total Environ.* 729: 139090. https://doi.org/10.1016/j.scitotenv.2020.139090.

Aung, M.N., Stein, C., Chen, W.T. et al. (2021). Community responses to COVID-19 pandemic first wave containment measures: a multinational study. *J. Infect. Dev. Ctries.* 15: 1107–1116. https://doi.org/10.3855/jidc.15254.

Baldasano, J.M. (2020). COVID-19 lockdown effects on air quality by NO_2 in the cities of Barcelona and Madrid (Spain). *Sci. Total Environ.* 741: 140353. https://doi.org/10.1016/j.scitotenv.2020.140353.

Bashir, M.F., Ma, B.J., Bilal et al. (2020). Correlation between environmental pollution indicators and COVID-19 pandemic: a brief study in Californian context. *Environ. Res.* 187: 109652. https://doi.org/10.1016/j.envres.2020.109652.

Berry, I., Soucy, J.-P.R., Tuite, A., and Fisman, D. (2020). Open access epidemiologic data and an interactive dashboard to monitor the COVID-19 outbreak in Canada. *Can. Med. Assoc. J.* 192: E420–E420. https://doi.org/10.1503/cmaj.75262.

Chen, B., Liang, H., Yuan, X. et al. (2020). Roles of meteorological conditions in COVID-19 transmission on a worldwide scale. *medRxiv* https://doi.org/10.1101/2020.03.16.20037168.

Coelho, M.T.P., Rodrigues, J.F.M., Medina, A.M. et al. (2020). Exponential phase of Covid19 expansion is driven by airport connections. *medRxiv* https://doi.org/10.1101/2020.04.02.20050773.

Demongeot, J., Flet-Berliac, Y., and Seligmann, H. (2020). Temperature decreases spread parameters of the new Covid-19 case dynamics. *Biology* https://doi.org/10.3390/biology9050094.

Dey, A., Rao, P.K., and Rawtani, D. (2022). Chapter 11 – risk management of COVID-19. In: *COVID-19 in the Environment* (ed. D. Rawtani, C.M. Hussain and N.B.T. Khatri), 217–230. Elsevier https://doi.org/10.1016/B978-0-323-90272-4.00018-X.

Fattorini, D. and Regoli, F. (2020). Role of the chronic air pollution levels in the Covid-19 outbreak risk in Italy. *Environ. Pollut.* 264: 114732. https://doi.org/10.1016/j.envpol.2020.114732.

Fauzi, M.A. and Paiman, N. (2021). COVID-19 pandemic in southeast Asia: intervention and mitigation efforts. *Asian Educ. Dev. Stud.* 10: 176–184. https://doi.org/10.1108/AEDS-04-2020-0064/FULL/PDF.

He, G., Pan, Y., and Tanaka, T. (2020). COVID-19, city lockdowns, and air pollution: evidence from China. *medRxiv* https://doi.org/10.1101/2020.03.29.20046649.

Janati Idrissi, A., Lamkaddem, A., Benouajjit, A. et al. (2020). Sleep quality and mental health in the context of COVID-19 pandemic and lockdown in Morocco. *Sleep Med.* 74: 248–253. https://doi.org/10.1016/j.sleep.2020.07.045.

Jüni, P., Rothenbühler, M., Bobos, P. et al. (2020). Impact of climate and public health interventions on the COVID-19 pandemic: a prospective cohort study. *Can. Med. Assoc. J.* 192: E566–E573. https://doi.org/10.1503/cmaj.200920.

Kanniah, K.D., Kamarul Zaman, N.A.F., Kaskaoutis, D.G., and Latif, M.T. (2020). COVID-19's impact on the atmospheric environment in the southeast Asia region. *Sci. Total Environ.* 736: 139658. https://doi.org/10.1016/j.scitotenv.2020.139658.

Kaushik, K. and Rawtani, D. (2022). Chapter 5 – sensor-based techniques for detection of COVID-19. In: *COVID-19 in the Environment* (ed. D. Rawtani, C.M. Hussain and N.B.T. Khatri), 95–114. Elsevier https://doi.org/10.1016/B978-0-323-90272-4.00012-9.

Lancet, T. (2020). India under COVID-19 lockdown. *Lancet* 395: 1315. https://doi.org/10.1016/S0140-6736(20)30938-7.

Latif, M.T., Dominick, D., Hawari, N.S.S.L. et al. (2021). The concentration of major air pollutants during the movement control order due to the COVID-19 pandemic in the Klang Valley, Malaysia. *Sustain. Cities Soc.* 66: 102660. https://doi.org/10.1016/j.scs.2020.102660.

Li, Q., Guan, X., Wu, P. et al. (2020a). Early transmission dynamics in Wuhan, China, of novel coronavirus-infected pneumonia. *N. Engl. J. Med.* 382: 1199–1207. https://doi.org/10.1056/NEJMoa2001316.

Li, S., Song, K., Yang, B. et al. (2020b). Preliminary assessment of the COVID-19 outbreak using 3-staged model e-ISHR. *J. Shanghai Jiaotong Univ. Sci* 25: 157–164. https://doi.org/10.1007/s12204-020-2169-0.

Lian, X., Huang, J., Huang, R. et al. (2020). Impact of city lockdown on the air quality of COVID-19-hit of Wuhan city. *Sci. Total Environ.* 742: 140556. https://doi.org/10.1016/j.scitotenv.2020.140556.

Lokhandwala, S. and Gautam, P. (2020). Indirect impact of COVID-19 on environment: a brief study in Indian context. *Environ. Res.* 188: 109807. https://doi.org/10.1016/j.envres.2020.109807.

Lovarelli, D., Conti, C., Finzi, A. et al. (2020). Describing the trend of ammonia, particulate matter and nitrogen oxides: the role of livestock activities in northern Italy during Covid-19 quarantine. *Environ. Res.* 191: 110048. https://doi.org/10.1016/j.envres.2020.110048.

Lu, R., Zhao, X., Li, J. et al. (2020). Genomic characterisation and epidemiology of 2019 novel coronavirus: implications for virus origins and receptor binding. *Lancet* 395: 565–574. https://doi.org/10.1016/S0140-6736(20)30251-8.

Mandal, I. and Pal, S. (2020). COVID-19 pandemic persuaded lockdown effects on environment over stone quarrying and crushing areas. *Sci. Total Environ.* 732: 139281. https://doi.org/10.1016/j.scitotenv.2020.139281.

Maneesh, P. and El Alaoui, A. (2020). How countries of south mitigate COVID-19: models of Morocco and Kerala, India. *SSRN Electron. J.* https://doi.org/10.2139/SSRN.3567898.

Marlier, M.E., Xing, J., Zhu, Y., and Wang, S. (2020). Impacts of COVID-19 response actions on air quality in China. *Environ. Res. Commun.* 2: 075003. https://doi.org/10.1088/2515-7620/ABA425.

Martorell-Marugán, J., Villatoro-García, J.A., García-Moreno, A. et al. (2021). DatAC: a visual analytics platform to explore climate and air quality indicators associated with the COVID-19 pandemic in Spain. *Sci. Total Environ.* 750: 141424. https://doi.org/10.1016/j.scitotenv.2020.141424.

Mohite, V., Vyas, K., Phadke, G., and Rawtani, D. (2022). Chapter 7 – Challenges and future aspects of COVID-19 monitoring and detection. In: *COVID-19 in the Environment* (ed. D. Rawtani, C.M. Hussain and N.B.T. Khatri), 131–150. Elsevier https://doi.org/10.1016/B978-0-323-90272-4.00013-0.

Muhammad, S., Long, X., and Salman, M. (2020). COVID-19 pandemic and environmental pollution: a blessing in disguise? *Sci. Total Environ.* 728: 138820. https://doi.org/10.1016/j.scitotenv.2020.138820.

Nguyen, T.T.N., Pham, H.V., Lasko, K. et al. (2019). Spatiotemporal analysis of ground and satellite-based aerosol for air quality assessment in the southeast Asia region. *Environ. Pollut.* 255: 113106. https://doi.org/10.1016/j.envpol.2019.113106.

Ogen, Y. (2020). Assessing nitrogen dioxide (NO_2) levels as a contributing factor to coronavirus (COVID-19) fatality. *Sci. Total Environ.* 726: 138605. https://doi.org/10.1016/j.scitotenv.2020.138605.

Otmani, A., Benchrif, A., Tahri, M. et al. (2020). Impact of Covid-19 lockdown on PM_{10}, SO_2 and NO_2 concentrations in Salé City (Morocco). *Sci. Total Environ.* 735: 139541. https://doi.org/10.1016/j.scitotenv.2020.139541.

Pal, S. and Mandal, I. (2019). Impact of aggregate quarrying and crushing on socio-ecological components of Chottanagpur plateau fringe area of India. *Environ. Earth Sci.* 78: 661. https://doi.org/10.1007/s12665-019-8678-1.

Pal, S. and Mandal, I. (2021). Impacts of stone mining and crushing on environmental health in Dwarka river basin. *Geocarto Int.* 36: 392–420. https://doi.org/10.1080/10106049.2019.1597390.

Parikh, G. and Rawtani, D. (2022). Chapter 10 – environmental impact of COVID-19. In: *COVID-19 in the Environment* (ed. D. Rawtani, C.M. Hussain and N.B.T. Khatri), 203–216. Elsevier https://doi.org/10.1016/B978-0-323-90272-4.00001-4.

Pawar, S., Stanam, A., Chaudhari, M., and Rayudu, D. (2020). Effects of temperature on COVID-19 transmission. *medRxiv* https://doi.org/10.1101/2020.03.29.20044461.

Phadke, G. and Rawtani, D. (2022). Chapter 13 – impact of waste generated due to COVID-19. In: *COVID-19 in the Environment* (ed. D. Rawtani, C.M. Hussain and N.B.T. Khatri), 251–276. Elsevier https://doi.org/10.1016/B978-0-323-90272-4.00005-1.

Purohit, S., Rao, P.K., and Rawtani, D. (2022). Chapter 4 – sampling and analytical techniques for COVID-19. In: *COVID-19 in the Environment* (ed. D. Rawtani, C.M. Hussain and N.B.T. Khatri), 75–94. Elsevier https://doi.org/10.1016/B978-0-323-90272-4.00008-7.

Qi, H., Xiao, S., Shi, R. et al. (2020). COVID-19 transmission in Mainland China is associated with temperature and humidity: a time-series analysis. *Sci. Total Environ.* 728: 138778. https://doi.org/10.1016/j.scitotenv.2020.138778.

Rao, P.K. and Rawtani, D. (2022). Chapter 6 – modern digital techniques for monitoring and analysis. In: *COVID-19 in the Environment* (ed. D. Rawtani, C.M. Hussain and N.B.T. Khatri), 115–130. Elsevier https://doi.org/10.1016/B978-0-323-90272-4.00015-4.

Rawtani, D., Hussain, C.M., and Khatri, N. (2022). Part 1 – transmission of COVID-19 in environment. In: *COVID-19 in the Environment* (ed. D. Rawtani, C.M. Hussain and N.B.T. Khatri), 1–2. Elsevier https://doi.org/10.1016/B978-0-323-90272-4.00070-1.

Ruiz Estrada, M.A., Park, D., and Lee, M. (2020). The evaluation of the final impact of wuhan COVID-19 on trade, tourism, transport, and electricity consumption of China. *SSRN Electron. J.* 1–13: https://doi.org/10.2139/ssrn.3551093.

Şahin, M. (2020). Impact of weather on COVID-19 pandemic in Turkey. *Sci. Total Environ.* 728: 138810. https://doi.org/10.1016/j.scitotenv.2020.138810.

Sarwar, S., Shahzad, K., Fareed, Z., and Shahzad, U. (2021). A study on the effects of meteorological and climatic factors on the COVID-19 spread in Canada during 2020. *J. Environ. Health Sci. Eng.* 19: 1513–1521. https://doi.org/10.1007/s40201-021-00707-9.

Setti, L., Passarini, F., De Gennaro, G. et al. (2020). SARS-Cov-2RNA found on particulate matter of Bergamo in Northern Italy: first evidence. *Environ. Res.* 188: 109754. https://doi.org/10.1016/j.envres.2020.109754.

Suhaimi, N.F., Jalaludin, J., and Latif, M.T. (2020). Demystifying a possible relationship between COVID-19, air quality and meteorological factors: evidence from Kuala Lumpur, Malaysia. *Aerosol Air Qual. Res.* 20: 1520–1529. https://doi.org/10.4209/AAQR.2020.05.0218.

Takahashi, M., Feng, Z., Mikhailova, T.A. et al. (2020). Air pollution monitoring and tree and forest decline in east Asia: a review. *Sci. Total Environ.* 742: 140288. https://doi.org/10.1016/j.scitotenv.2020.140288.

To, T., Zhang, K., Maguire, B. et al. (2021). Correlation of ambient temperature and COVID-19 incidence in Canada. *Sci. Total Environ.* 750: 141484. https://doi.org/10.1016/j.scitotenv.2020.141484.

Tobías, A., Carnerero, C., Reche, C. et al. (2020). Changes in air quality during the lockdown in Barcelona (Spain) one month into the SARS-CoV-2 epidemic. *Sci. Total Environ.* 726: 138540. https://doi.org/10.1016/j.scitotenv.2020.138540.

Wang, Q. and Su, M. (2020). A preliminary assessment of the impact of COVID-19 on environment – a case study of China. *Sci. Total Environ.* 728: 138915. https://doi.org/10.1016/j.scitotenv.2020.138915.

Wong, J.J.M., Abbas, Q., Chuah, S.L. et al. (2021). Comparative analysis of pediatric COVID-19 infection in southeast Asia, south Asia, Japan, and China. *Am. J. Trop. Med. Hyg.* 105: 413–420. https://doi.org/10.4269/ajtmh.21-0299.

Yang, C., Sha, D., Liu, Q. et al. (2020). Taking the pulse of COVID-19: a spatiotemporal perspective. *Int. J. Digit. Earth* 13: 1186–1211. https://doi.org/10.1080/17538947.2020.1809723.

Zang, Z., Li, D., Guo, Y. et al. (2021). Superior $PM_{2.5}$ estimation by integrating aerosol fine mode data from the Himawari-8 satellite in deep and classical machine learning models. *Remote Sens.* https://doi.org/10.3390/rs13142779.

Zoran, M.A., Savastru, R.S., Savastru, D.M., and Tautan, M.N. (2020). Assessing the relationship between surface levels of $PM_{2.5}$ and PM_{10} particulate matter impact on COVID-19 in Milan, Italy. *Sci. Total Environ.* 738: 139825. https://doi.org/10.1016/j.scitotenv.2020.139825.

13

Effect of Waste Generated Due to COVID-19

Saeida Saadat[1], Piyush K. Rao[1], Nitasha Khatri[2], and Deepak Rawtani[3]

[1] *School of Doctoral Studies & Research, National Forensic Sciences University, (Ministry of Home Affairs, GOI), Gandhinagar, Gujarat, India*
[2] *Gujarat Environment Management Institute (GEMI), Gandhinagar, Gujarat, India*
[3] *School of Pharmacy, National Forensic Sciences University (Ministry of Home affairs, GOI), Gandhinagar, Gujarat, India*

13.1 Introduction

The novel coronavirus first arose from a meat market in Wuhan, China in the last month of the year 2019 and, therefore, was named COVID-19 (Corman et al. 2020; Espejo et al. 2020a; Wölfel et al. 2020). The genomic analysis of COVID-19 showed its association with severe acute respiratory syndrome (SARS) viruses, which could originate from bats (Das and Das 2020; Rume and Islam 2020). This virus became a worldwide pandemic very quickly, infecting more than 10 million people around the globe within six months (Somani et al. 2020). To reduce the pandemic curve, governments in different parts of the world applied many preventive actions (Christoforidis et al. 2020), for instance, limitations on social contact, applying social distancing guidelines, restrictions on travel and limitations on the transformation of goods and, most importantly, partial and complete lockdown. These restrictions not only reduced economic activities but also affected the environment in both negative and positive ways (Patrício et al. 2021). Due to the lockdown during the COVID-19 pandemic, different kinds of both domestic and biomedical wastes have been massively generated, which had affected the environment and created environmental problems worldwide (Shettya et al. 2020). For testing and treatment of COVID-19, a vast number of healthcare centers and hospitals have been established worldwide. These hospital/ healthcare centers along with the already existing hospitals have used a lot of healthcare tools and materials which created a lot of biomedical waste during this pandemic (Hellewell et al. 2020). As the fear of infection did not allow us to segregate and process the waste all the generated waste has gone to the environment and polluted both the landfill and water bodies (Allison et al. 2020). Also, there are several reasons which contributed to the high production of domestic wastes including high demand in online mood purchase, storing foods due to the lockdown panic without awareness of their shelf life, and using personal safety equipment (Kucharski et al. 2020; Wang et al. 2020b). For instance, to reduce the transmission of COVID-19, everyone has been using facemasks to keep themselves and their family members safe from the COVID-19 virus. Therefore, billions of facemasks which are made of plastic-based material have been used as a precautionary tool around the globe. However, there are different kinds of facemasks available in the market that are made of different materials (Liu and Zhang 2020). Among them, surgical masks are confirmed to be effective for the prevention of this virus. Surgical masks which are also known as N95 are categorized into two types FFP1 and EN149EU. These facemasks have the capability to filter the air particles at almost 95% and therefore are the most suitable one to be used against COVID-19 (Nghiem et al. 2020; Sangkham 2020). Surgical masks are made of different layers of a special type of fabric (nonwoven fabric) and a layer of cellulose. Nonwoven fabric is synthesized from polypropylene plastic which is non-biodegradable in nature (Mas-Comaa et al. 2020; Mccloskey and Heymann 2020). These facemasks are disposable as they get contaminated hence contribute to generating medical waste during this pandemic. Facemasks alone could be a good example which increased medical waste production during this pandemic which can be a serious environmental concern as plastic management is already extremely poor (Asumadu et al. 2020b; Kucharski et al. 2020). The mortality rate of this virus, which is somehow high, could also affect the environmental activists due to the usage of plastics and its poor management. For example, in the UK more than 128 000 tons of plastic waste is predicted to be generated during one year of which the majority is surgical facemask. Therefore, scientists are putting lots of effort to accelerate their search for solutions for plastic waste management around the world (Okoro et al. 2020). In this article, the impacts of the current global pandemic COVID-19 on waste generation, their management and future technical approaches for the generated waste post-pandemic world have been discussed.

13.2 Impact of COVID-19 on Waste Production

Due to COVID-19 outbreak governments all over the world implemented lockdown rules to avoid the spread of this contagious disease (Gaffney et al. 2020). To take precautionary actions, individuals were advised to use safety appliances such as facemasks (two types of facemasks N95 and FFP2 are confirmed to avoid COVID-19 transmission), gloves and use hand sanitizers multiple times daily. These items created a massive amount of waste globally (Chinazzi et al. 2020). Besides this, health care employees apart from masks and gloves have been instructed to use special glasses, aprons, boots, and special types of single-use shoes which also contributed to the waste generation around the world. Water bottles, single-use food containers, as well as other plastic-based materials like plastic bags, have also been majorly used during this pandemic time (Wang et al. 2020a). These human health precautionary actions caused an extremely high peak in waste generation affecting the environment, which has become a global environmental concern. This pandemic and its environmental impacts happened while the waste amount and its management were already a global problem (Rothan and Byrareddy 2020). While the COVID-19 pandemic created a lot of waste of both health care waste as well as domestic waste, environmental dealers are overwhelmed with this phenomenon as they are not able to deal with this problem satisfactorily (Parashar and Hait 2021). For instance, in Wuhan, China, prior to the COVID-19 pandemic, around 49 tons of waste were being generated daily, while during the COVID-19 pandemic, this amount raised to around 240 tons per day, which shows an enormous difference. The major amount of this waste is health care waste, while prior to the COVID-19 pandemic, the medical waste generation was 40 tons per day (Haque et al. 2020). Similarly, in the Hubei city in China, a 60% increase in waste generation has been reported during the COVID-19 outbreak. Literature reports that in the Southeast Asian countries, the COVID-19 pandemic caused additional 1000 tons of waste to the usually generated waste per day. For instance, in Manila, Philippines, health care waste generation is 280 tons per day, and in Jakarta, the medical waste generation is reported to be 212 tons daily. The studies have predicted that each infected individual can produce nearly 3.40 kg of hazardous health care waste (Ramteke and Sahu 2020).

13.3   Classification of Waste Generated Due to the COVID-19 Pandemic

The COVID-19 outbreak has affected all aspects of global citizens, especially the global economy (Boone 2020; Carlsson-szlezak et al. 2020). Almost all economic activities have been reduced or stopped, which led to reduction in the stock market (Fernandes 2020). All over the world, transportation systems have been shut down due to the lockdown rules and traveling has become extremely limited, which includes only emergency cases (Interim and Assessment 2020; Zhou et al. 2020). Also, to avoid spreading COVID-19, lockdown rules were applied that included closing schools, universities, hotels, restaurants, bars, gyms, and similar other public places resulting in the reduction of local business and traveling to a huge extent (Nilashi et al. 2020). Due to the lockdown, people are no longer able to attend entertaining areas such as beaches, bars, hotels, parks, and ski centers, which resulted in the reduction of waste production in public places (Arora et al. 2020). However, as people are asked to stay in quarantine and take extra care of cleanliness and hygiene (Paital et al. 2020), the waste generation of both domestic and biomedical has increased. Also, for the diagnosis of COVID-19 and in the case of positive cases, the treatment practices have created a lot of biomedical waste (Ramteke and Sahu 2020). Both the generated wastes have affected the environment in a very unexpected way as the processing and management of the wastes have also been stopped during this pandemic (Villani et al. 2020). In the following section, we will discuss the domestic and biomedical waste generated due to COVID-19 and their consequences on the environment. The classification of waste generated during lockdown due to the COVID-19 pandemic is shown in Figure 13.1.

13.3.1   Domestic Waste

There is a significant increase in the production of domestic waste due to the massive production of waste and closure of recycling industries and unsatisfactory waste management during the COVID-19 pandemic. One of the most widely generated domestic waste during the COVID-19 pandemic is considered to be food delivery containers (Yao et al. 2020). As restaurants remained closed during this pandemic time, the only option was ordering food

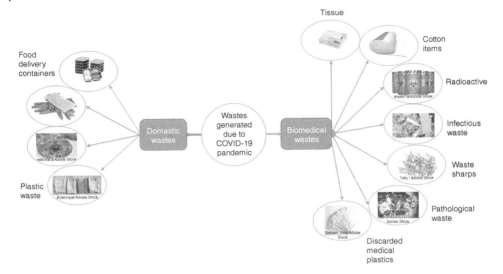

Figure 13.1 Classification of waste generated due to the COVID-19 pandemic.

from outside, which created a huge amount of waste and as the recycling system is also stopped due to infectious issues, these wastes are dumped in landfills, which directly affect the environment (Bogoch et al. 2020). As reported by the recent research in China, the quantity of domestic waste generation raised four times more compared to the pre-COVID-19 period. Also, a physical blockade for maintaining social distance and controlling people's traffic from restricted cities could add to the waste generated during this pandemic time (Asumadu et al. 2020a). These barriers are made up of methacrylate, which is a nonbiodegradable material and causes environmental pollution. Due to COVID-19, when there were predictions about starting a total lockdown, people started purchasing and storing food items without thinking about their storage life. The lockdown panic did not allow people to study the shelf life of the products that they are purchasing, which resulted in wasting a lot of food which directly affected the economy and environment (Xu et al. 2020). Food production majorly happens in the rural areas and very less in cities. COVID-19 has impacted the cities and towns more than the rural areas due to the high rate of population. Therefore, food production has been affected due to the lack of raw materials for farming activities, even though labor workers were available (Lipsitch et al. 2020). In addition, to prevent the spread of the virus, employees in the food supply system stopped their work in the cities and towns, which also affected the food supplement. Also, the food transportation system was disturbed or even stopped in the virus hotspot areas due to the blockage of borders (Lau et al. 2020). The processed food industry has been in a huge loss due to the lockdown regulations and social distancing practices. These issues hindered the food supply system, which led to the wastage of the available food product resources in the farms. There are reports that food products have been buried or dumped in landfills due to the broken food supply system (Sharma et al. 2020).

13.3.2 Biomedical Waste

As defined by the World Health Organization (WHO), the waste produced by health care organizations during health care-related activities is called biomedical/health care waste (BMW). The health care activities consist of precautionary, diagnostic, healing, and calming treatments in the field of medicine (Patrício et al. 2021). The waste generated while such activities at home by patients themselves or their family members are also considered BMW. The BMW contains a vast number of wastes, which are divided into the following categories including radioactive wastes, medical wastes, pathological wastes, infectious and sharps (Chinazzi et al. 2020). A huge amount of these wastes, about 85%, are nonhazardous wastes, while infectious waste is the second-largest group of this waste and is reported to be 10% in volume and the least amount of this waste is radioactive and chemical wastes (5%). Besides the transmission of diseases, while dealing with MBW, this waste could lead to negative environmental impacts such as soil and water contamination, degrading the useful microorganisms in septic systems, and physical harm by sharps (Agamuthu and Barasarathi 2020; Sharma et al. 2020). As novel coronavirus is highly contagious, millions of people got infected around the world, which paved the way for establishing millions of testing centers. Those testing centers have been using a lot of disposable materials usually made of plastic materials, which pollute the environment. Besides the testing centers, individuals are also advised to take precautionary actions, which include using facemasks and gloves, and using handwashes and sanitizers, which usually come in plastic containers and these materials contribute to waste generation worldwide (Espejo et al. 2020a). Pandemics like SARS-CoV and Ebola taught us to consider that there is a crucial need for the establishment of a serious waste management procedure for the processing and controlling of health care waste in a safe manner to reduce the risk of infection. Literature has reported that most of the infections have happened via accidental contact with waste by staff and health care workers at the moment of waste generation (Peng et al. 2020). In first-world countries such as the United States, this risk is low as all the hospitals are following the roles and guidelines and prevent infectious while dealing with BMW. But, in developing countries, the shortage of essential infrastructure such as wastebaskets and sealed bags results in discarding infected BMW together with other solid wastes. Sometimes, reselling of discarded sharps and other discarded items as reusables on black markets could contribute to the creation of diseases. There is a high probability of such incidents happening in developing countries due to the negligence of rules and guidelines (Daryabeigi et al. 2020; Kashyap et al. 2020). Another concern toward the usage of health care tools is the lack of onsite treatment equipment in medical centers, which leads to massive health care waste generation. A vast number of these tools need to be autoclaved or kept in a microwave, which makes it complicated and negligible. However, incineration or chemical treatment for disinfecting might also be a suitable method for most of these wastes (Hassan et al. 2020). The additional expenses and lack of education are the two major causes of failure toward skipping the pollution standard regulations. COVID-19 pandemic caused a crisis for BMW management, as this pandemic generated a massive amount of BMW worldwide. For instance, utilizing single-use facemasks and gloves alone added a huge amount of waste to the previously available waste (Ather et al. 2020). In addition, the establishment of temporary health centers, isolation camps, and COVID-19 test centers created an enormous amount of waste that could be considered an unexpected challenge in the waste management systems (Kalina and Tilley 2020). As COVID-19 is highly contagious, sorting BMW has been a severe problem due to the lack of trained staff. This, in turn, leads to the massive dumping of infectious waste into streams, landfills, etc., in many developing countries, which could be a big health concern for residents. Also, the high vitality rate of COVID-19 on different surfaces for an extended period is a warning for us to sort the BMW from the other solid wastes (Meo et al. 2020; Sharma et al. 2020). To avoid infection, most hospitals and health care centers no longer recycle glassware medical tools. They too can be considered part of the generated BMW during this pandemic. Wastewater from the hospitals and health care centers is often polluted with drugs in extremely high concentrations. For instance, hydroxychloroquine as well as chloroquine have been used for the treatment of COVID-19 patients. These medications such as pollutants in the water could be hazardous to aquatic organisms. There is a major concern about the presence of these pollutants in freshwater ecosystems as it is well known that the treatment of the wastewater system is not satisfactorily done in most countries around the globe (Anand et al. 2020; Celis et al. 2021; Ploeg 2020).

13.4 Reduction in Waste Recycling

Reduction in recycling is one of the most important environmental issues during the COVID-19 pandemic worldwide. Recycling is considered the most significant method to fight pollution, reduce the consumption of energy, and preserve natural energy resources globally (Zambrano-monserrate et al. 2020).

The main body of recycling waste comes from waste collection trucks and landfills. Due to lockdown ever since the COVID-19 pandemic started, recycling processes are being paused or significantly reduced because of contamination issues. In different parts of the world, governments put strict rules on hygiene and cleanliness strategies to prevent the spreading of this virus and, therefore, waste picker and manager's activities have been stopped. For instance, due to the total lockdown in the United Kingdom, about 45% of recycling activities and in the United States, about 30% of the same activities have been reduced (Somani et al. 2020). Similarly, in a majority of European countries, waste processing and recycling have been paused. Among the European countries, Italy can be an example where the residents were guided not to sort their waste due to the infection problems. Also, the plastic bag bans were cancelled due to the COVID-19 pandemic as they are single-use materials (Zambrano-monserrate et al. 2020).

13.5 Environmental Impacts of COVID-19

The COVID-19 pandemic has changed the world in a short period of time. Millions of people got infected by this virus and thousands have lost their lives, the ones who survived are not living the life as usual (Caballero-domínguez et al. 2020; Velavan and Meyer 2020). All over the world, people are staying in their homes due to the lockdown regulations to prevent the spreading of the virus and slow down the mortality rate (Valenzuela et al. 2020). Despite all the negative impacts of this pandemic such as increasing waste generation, a huge rise in plastic usage, and a sudden surge in BMW production, the lockdown rules brought some positive changes to the environment. One of the changes could be the air quality in some big cities in various countries (Mehran et al. 2021). Studies reported that the NO_2 and CO_2 levels in the air have decreased. Similarly, the improvement in water bodies has also been noticed, for example, the Ganga River in India (Kotnala et al. 2020; Nilashi et al. 2020). A study reported that during the COVID-19 pandemic, the air quality in China got better, which has a positive impact on carbon emissions worldwide. The level of energy consumption has also been reduced during this pandemic. With lower coal consumption, the levels of carbon dioxide and carbon monoxide have also decreased in the air (Wang and Su 2020).

Existing studies report that there is an estimation of about a 17% decrease in carbon dioxide emission. Also, a decrease in consumption of coal to about 50%, and oil to around 25% has been predicted, which directly affects climate change. Before the COVID-19 outbreak, glaciers were melting due to greenhouse gases (greenhouse gases create global warming), which could raise sea levels. Lockdown due to the COVID-19 outbreak has paused the economic activities, which has resulted in stopping global warming temporarily (Espejo et al. 2020b). There is a direct link between economic activities and air pollution level. Existing literature presents pollution surges with the growth of the economic activities, and the level of pollution decreases during the reduction of economic activities. COVID-19 stopped economic activities around the world and, therefore, the level of pollution has also dropped worldwide (Singh et al. 2020; Wang and Su 2020). In many countries around the globe, air pollution levels have fallen significantly. For in New York city of the United States, the air pollution level reduced by about 50% during the lockdown as compared to that in the pre-COVID-19 period. Also, there is a 25% air pollution reduction shown in China during the lockdown compared to normal time. The above-mentioned good air quality might directly be linked to the reduction in the use of coal and other fossil fuels. In Brazil, there is a significant reduction in the CO level (around 65%) during the COVID-19 pandemic (Celis et al. 2021). Another effect of lockdown due to COVID-19 is a significant decrease in the water pollutants level in different water bodies. For example, Venice of Italy have gotten much cleaner water canals while COVID-19 epidemic due to the lack of tourists compared to normal time. Now you can get amazed by watching fish swimming in clean and clear water in the canals instead of motorboats and water pollutants in these canals (Doremalen et al. 2020). However, it has been reported that rather than the positive environmental impacts of COVID-19, the negative impacts of this pandemic are more noticeable on the environment. The massive amount of domestic and health care waste generation, closure of the processing and recycling industries are all evidence of the negative impacts of this pandemic on the environment. In many countries in Asia, the presence of a huge number of facemasks and other safety equipment such as gloves have been seen on beaches and water bodies in the sea, these plastic-based materials could be dangerous to aquatic organisms. There is evidence that microplastics can even enter human bodies either through breathing or eating, which obviously have harmful effects on our health and well-being (Doremalen et al. 2020; Allen et al. 2020; Adyel 2020). Different environmental impacts of COVID-19 are shown in Figure 13.2.

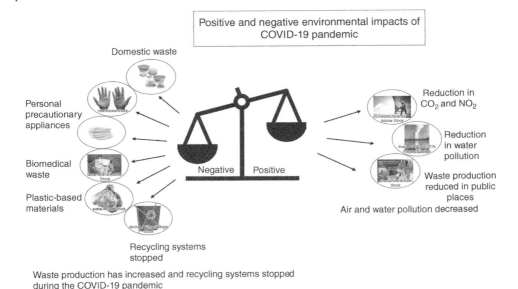

Waste production has increased and recycling systems stopped during the COVID-19 pandemic

Figure 13.2 Different environmental impacts of COVID-19.

13.6 Management of the Generated Waste Due to the COVID-19 Pandemic

As mentioned earlier, there is a surge in the production of the biomedical wastes by several health care activities conducted by medical laboratories, research institutions, hospitals, and similar other organizations, which are performing health-related activities during this pandemic (Nghiem et al. 2020). Also, during this pandemic, the consumption of plastic-based materials has increased, which is linked to environmental contamination. To prevent the spread of COVID-19, the usage of safety equipment such as facemasks and gloves, which are plastic-based materials are creating a vast number of pollutants to the environment around the world (Bogoch et al. 2020). The huge consumption of these materials has made waste management exceedingly difficult around the world. In the health care system, used plastic tools are contaminated by pathogenic microorganisms, which need special management as infectant disposals. Even prior to the COVID-19 outbreak, the management of plastic-based discards was a huge environmental concern due to their potential in contaminating the land and ocean (Fan et al. 2021; Klemeš et al. 2020).

The global protocols in disposal process and management are not able to regulate appropriately the present plastic discards, while with the beginning of the COVID-19 outbreak and its related waste discards doubled the problem around the world (Rothan and Byrareddy 2020). As mentioned earlier, medical waste from various health care organizations is overly complicated due to contamination issues. Inadequate process and management of these wastes can become serious transformants of secondary illnesses as health workers including cleaners, waste pickers, and patients are dealing with these materials. In medical waste management, it is mandatory to use a standard team for measurement and all the areas must get cross-checked (Anderson et al. 2020). The best monitoring method for medical waste management is to reduce the volume of contaminated waste as much as possible. The easiest approach to medical waste management is not to mix the contaminated and noncontaminated wastes and to process the contaminated wastes under special treatment and the uncontaminated ones must be treated in the same way as the domestic wastes (Ranjan et al. 2020). This method can be applied by training health care workers and employees as well as the formation of uniform medical waste flows and different colored trash bins (Nilashi et al. 2020). With the sudden burden of waste generated due to COVID-19, we can learn useful lessons from waste management in Wuhan, China, as they used effective strategies for this purpose, which can be a useful lesson for some other developing countries where still the virus is spreading and lots of wastes are getting produced due to this reason (Wang et al. 2020a). In Wuhan, medical wastes are being discarded in a sanitary landfill or burnt. Although, in a lot of developing countries, medical waste is being discarded in the open landfill where the movements of animals like cows, dogs, and other animals have been observed. A limited number of countries have applied innovative technology to treat medical waste through sterilization or chemical-based disinfectants, but these strategies are not applicable in most developing countries (Raja et al. 2021). From the COVID-19 pandemic, we got the experience that personal and public hygiene are extremely helpful in preventing infection risk and controlling the spreading of this virus. And for BMW processing and management, there are many methods including incineration, steam and gas sterilization, chemical treatment of the wastes, microwave as well as thermal methods. However, BMW management has not been extraordinarily successful around the world and still there are a lot of concerns about the same globally (Luan and Ching 2020; Sharma et al. 2020).

13.7 Technical Approaches to Waste Management for the Post-COVID-19 World

At present time, the few available waste management solutions are not adequate for waste management as COVID-19 caused a huge amount of waste worldwide. Therefore, there is a serious requirement for the establishment of novel technical solutions for solving this problem in a proper way (Rume and Islam 2020). With the already available problems due to the pre-COVID-19-existing waste, the generated waste due to this pandemic make us think of the establishment of innovative solutions to this challenge, which include both segregation of the BMW from other solid waste due to infectious issues and treatment of the wastes (Zhou et al. 2020). To enhance the applicability of available technologies, novel developments must be designed as a complementary part for supporting the waste management system to deal with the generated waste due to the COVID-19 pandemic. There are some scientific techniques through which we can inactivate viruses on the BMW and other wastes (Bogoch et al. 2020; Xu et al. 2020). One of the most significant methods is sterilization of the BMW of health care centers and hospitals. There are two types of sterilization including steam sterilization and gas sterilization according to the availability of the equipment and the type of the waste. Any of the above-mentioned sterilization techniques could be applied to stop the spreading of the COVID-19 virus through BMW

(Narayan et al. 2020). The second most significant method for disinfecting the medical wastes is energy-based methods such as radiowave and microwave. However, these techniques could not be applicable in most of the hospitals and health care centers in developing countries due to the lack of these equipment (Parashar and Hait 2021). The third method could be incineration (burning of infectious wastes), although this is not a suitable method as it creates air pollution, which, in turn, contributes to environmental problems. The last method is chemically disinfecting of the infectious waste. In this method, certain chemical-based materials are applied to the BMW to inactivate the microorganisms present in the waste. This method seems appropriate but still, the lack of chemicals and negligence of non-trained health care workers might make this method complicated (Li et al. 2020; Mas-Comaa et al. 2020). A major concern toward the usage of chemical disinfectants on nonbiodegradable waste is its harm to the environment, as these wastes will be dumped in the landfill and if animals like dogs and cows touch them, it might affect their health. Overall, the WHO claims that incineration at hot temperatures is the most appropriate method for disinfecting infectious waste (Raja et al. 2021; WHO 2020).

In case of the unavailability of the above-mentioned techniques, deep burial is the last option to deal with infectious wastes. In addition, the transformation of the infectious BMW from the generation site to the treatment place should be done with extra care as there is a considerable risk of infection during the collection, transformation, and discarding of the wastes (WHO 2005). One of the most important guidelines for waste pickers would be hygiene and sanitation while dealing with infectious wastes; personal safety tools such as facemasks and gloves would slow down the risk of infection (Di et al. 2020). In addition, the establishment of automatic smart systems for separation of the infectious wastes would significantly minimize the risk of infection and grant the safety of health care employees and particularly waste collectors. Automatic systems for waste separation not only reduce the risk of infection but also increase the speed of the work and recycling, which might even improve the quality of recycled materials (Chidepatil et al. 2020). During the COVID-19 pandemic and even after it, nonbiodegradable waste production will remain high because of hygienic issues. To process and control the COVID-19 period and post-COVID-19-generated waste, upgrading of the waste management systems must be done. To achieve this goal, recycling the recyclable plastic-based waste, which makes up most of the BMW would be an effective action to be taken care of. Post pandemic, it is expected that the production of infectious BMW comes down to the optimum usual levels due to the restarting of the recycling systems. Also, the incineration rate is predicted to reduce by restarting the recycling industry (Mascio et al. 2020). However, as mentioned earlier, the incineration and other similar waste management methods, which have negative environmental impacts, should be replaced with clean and safe energy-based novel systems to handle the environmental pollution crisis (Wang et al. 2020b). This important goal could only be obtained when the governments and the other parties who deal with environmental issues focus their attention on the innovative recycling systems through which all the landfill waste dumps turn into recycled and reusable materials. Through this method, the need for new produce production would also reduce and fewer resources would be utilized (Kumar et al. 2021; Zhang et al. 2020). Literature reports that feedstock recycling of those wastes, which contain 50% plastic and 50% other materials, has produced 50% less carbon dioxide compared to incineration in which the production of carbon dioxide is the same as the mechanical recycling of this waste. Therefore, the feedstock recycling of mixed plastic materials could be considered a safer and cleaner option for the environment (Raja et al. 2021). And at last, controlling the amount of waste generation could contribute to processing and controlling COVID-19-related wastes during and after this pandemic. However, reducing the BMW generation seems exceedingly difficult due to hygienic concerns at this pandemic time, but still reducing the waste quantity should be the top priority as much as possible. It is obvious that the production of health care waste is at its highest peak and reduction of this waste is not possible at the moment but to contribute to the waste management system, we can reduce the amount of plastic we use in our daily life (Klemeš et al. 2020). A research report suggests that post-COVID-19 pandemic, there is a need for an adjustment in the solid waste management system, which could be done by the aforementioned strategies which include: (i) Enhancing the recycling systems with special attention to recycling of the food delivery containers; (ii) Training waste-processing staff in order to consider safety issues while collecting, sorting, and transferring of the waste materials; and (iii) Serious observation of the BMW production and its treatment for estimation of expansion of the system in case if it was needed (Custodio et al. 2021).

13.8 Conclusion

For many decades, waste management and especially nonbiodegradable ones and their recycling have been one of the main environmental problems around the world. COVID-19 pandemic has doubled this problem, as an enormous amount of both domestic and biomedical/health care wastes are being produced due to total or partial lockdown regulations in all the countries worldwide. To stop the spread of the virus, people have been advised to stay home and, therefore, the online purchase of both food delivery and other goods has been highly practiced throughout this pandemic. In the online mood of services, the usage of plastic-based materials is extremely high, as every package must be well packaged for maintenance of the transformation and customer satisfaction, which could result in the generation of a lot of domestic wastes, which are mostly nonbiodegradable in nature. Also, precautionary equipment including facemasks, gloves, and hand sanitizers also contributed to waste production during this pandemic time. In addition, the testing centers for COVID-19, and in case of positive cases, the treatment has produced a lot of health care wastes and those too are majorly plastic-based materials, which could have dangerous impacts on the environment. As the risk of infection is extremely high, the biomedical waste as well as the domestic waste have not been processed, segregated, or recycled during the COVID-19 pandemic time and hence they are dumped in the landfill or thrown in the ocean, which harms the aquatic animals in case if they eat them mistakenly or disturb their free movement in the water. Or even they can be a source of infection if any animal like dogs and cows, which have connections with humans, comes in contact with these wastes. To deal with these wastes, there are several scientific methods suggested by scientists such as sterilization of the BMW, energy-based techniques consisting of radiowave and microwave, incineration, and chemical disinfecting. And the last option could be a deep burial, which is advised as the last option in case of the impossibility of the other mentioned techniques.

References

Adyel, T.M. (2020). Accumulation of plastic waste during COVID-19. *Science* 369 (6509): 1314–1315.

Agamuthu, P. and Barasarathi, J. (2020). Clinical waste management under COVID-19 scenario in Malaysia. *Waste Management & Research* 39 (1_suppl): 18–26. https://doi.org/10.1177/0734242X20959701.

Allen, S., Allen, D., Moss, K. et al. (2020). Examination of the ocean as a source for atmospheric microplastics. *PloS One* 15 (5): e0232746.

Allison, A. L., Ambrose-Dempster, E.T., Aparsi, D., et al. (2020). The environmental dangers of employing single-use face masks as part of a COVID-19 exit strategy.

Anand, K.S., & Sharma, B. Mahajan, R. K., Panesar, S., & Dubey, P. (2020). Coronavirus disease (covid-19) and public health issues in developing countries-focus on biomedical waste management. *Archives of Community Medicine and Public Health*, 6(2), 246–249.

Anderson, R.M., Heesterbeek, H., Klinkenberg, D., and Hollingsworth, T.D. (2020). How will country-based mitigation measures influence the course of the COVID-19 epidemic? *The Lancet* 395 (10228): 931–934.

Arora, S., Bhaukhandi, K.D., and Mishra, P.K. (2020). Coronavirus lockdown helped the environment to bounce back. *Science of the Total Environment* 140573. https://doi.org/10.1016/j.scitotenv.2020.140573.

Asumadu, S., Phebe, S., and Owusu, A. (2020a). COVID-19 and globalization. *Environment, Development and Sustainability*, 0123456789. https://doi.org/10.1007/s10668-020-00801-2.

Asumadu, S., Phebe, S., and Owusu, A. (2020b). Impact of COVID - 19 pandemic on waste management. *Environment, Development and Sustainability* https://doi.org/10.1007/s10668-020-00956-y.

Ather, A., Dds, B.D.S., Bds, B.P. et al. (2020). Coronavirus Disease 19 (COVID-19): implications for clinical dental care. *Journal of Endodontics* 19: 1–12. https://doi.org/10.1016/j.joen.2020.03.008.

Bogoch, I.I., Watts, A., Thomas-bachli, A. et al. (2020). Pneumonia of unknown aetiology in Wuhan, China : potential for international spread via commercial air travel. *Journal of Travel Medicine* 27 (2): taaa008. https://doi.org/10.1093/jtm/taaa008.

Boone, L. (2020). Coronavirus : the world economy at risk. March.

Caballero-domínguez, C.C., Jiménez-villamizar, M.P., Campo-arias, A., and Caballero-dom, C.C. (2020). Suicide risk during the lockdown due to coronavirus disease (COVID-19) in Colombia in Colombia. *Death Studies* 0: 1–6. https://doi.org/10.1080/07481187.2020.1784312.

Carlsson-szlezak, P., Reeves, M., and Swartz, P. (2020). What coronavirus could mean for the global economy what coronavirus could mean for the global economy. *Harvard Business Review* 3 (10): 1–10.

Celis, J.E., Espejo, W., Paredes-osses, E. et al. (2021). Plastic residues produced with con fi rmatory testing for COVID-19: classi fi cation, quanti fi cation, fate, and impacts on human health. *Science of the Total Environment* 760: https://doi.org/10.1016/j.scitotenv.2020.144167.

Chidepatil, A., Bindra, P., Kulkarni, D., and Qazi, M. (2020). From trash to cash : how blockchain and multi-sensor-driven artificial intelligence can transform circular economy of plastic waste? 2018: 1–16. https://doi.org/10.3390/admsci10020023.

Chinazzi, M., Davis, J.T., Ajelli, M. et al. (2020). The effect of travel restrictions on the spread of the 2019 novel coronavirus (COVID-19) outbreak. 368 (6489): 395–400.

Christoforidis, A., Kavoura, E., Nemtsa, A. et al. (2020). Coronavirus lockdown effect on type 1 diabetes management on children wearing insulin pump equipped with continuous glucose monitoring system. *Diabetes Research and Clinical Practice* 108307. https://doi.org/10.1016/j.diabres.2020.108307.

Corman, V. M., Landt, O., Kaiser, M., Molenkamp, R., Meijer, A., Chu, D. K. W., Bleicker, T., Schneider, J., Schmidt, M. L., Mulders, D. G. J. C., Haagmans, B. L., Veer, B. Van Der, Den, S. Van, Wijsman, L., Goderski, G., Ellis, J., Zambon, M., Peiris, M., Goossens, H., ... Drosten, C. (2020). Detection of 2019 novel coronavirus (2019-nCoV) by. *Eurosurveillance*, 25(3), 1–8. https://doi.org/10.2807/1560-7917.ES.2020.25.3.2000045

Custodio, R., Yuri, L., and Nakada, K. (2021). Science of the total environment COVID-19 pandemic : solid waste and environmental impacts in Brazil. *Science of the Total Environment* 755: 142471. https://doi.org/10.1016/j.scitotenv.2020.142471.

Daryabeigi, A., Azar, Z., and Heir, V. (2020). Environmental impacts of new Coronavirus outbreak in Iran with an emphasis on waste management sector. *Journal of Material Cycles and Waste Management* https://doi.org/10.1007/s10163-020-01123-1.

Das, S. and Das, S. (2020). The COVID - 19 pandemic : biological evolution, treatment options and consequences. *Innovative Infrastructure Solutions* 1–12. https://doi.org/10.1007/s41062-020-00325-8.

Di Mascio, D., Khalil, A., Saccone, G. et al. (2020). Outcome of coronavirus spectrum infections (SARS, MERS, COVID 1 -19) during pregnancy: a systematic review and meta-analysis. *American Journal of Obstetrics & Gynecology MFM* 100107. https://doi.org/10.1016/j.ajogmf.2020.100107.

Di, F., Beccaloni, E., Bonadonna, L. et al. (2020). Science of the total environment minimization of spreading of SARS-CoV-2 via household waste produced by subjects affected by COVID-19 or in quarantine. *Science of the Total Environment* 743: 140803. https://doi.org/10.1016/j.scitotenv.2020.140803.

van Doremalen, N., Morris, D.H., and Holbrook, M.G. (2020). Aerosol and surface stability of SARS-CoV-2 as Compared with SARS-CoV-1. *The New England Journal of Medicine* 728: https://doi.org/10.1016/j.scitotenv.2020.138870.

Espejo, A.P., Akgun, Y., Mana, A.F. et al. (2020a). Review of current advances in serologic testing for covid. *American Journal of Clinical Pathology* 154 (3): 293–304. https://doi.org/10.1093/AJCP/AQAA112.

Espejo, W., Celis, J.E., Chiang, G., and Bahamonde, P. (2020b). Environment and COVID-19: Pollutants, impacts, dissemination, management and recommendations for facing future epidemic threats. *Science of the Total Environment* 747: 141314. https://doi.org/10.1016/j.scitotenv.2020.141314.

Fernandes, N. (2020). Economic effects of coronavirus outbreak (COVID-19) on the world economy Nuno Fernandes Full Professor of Finance IESE Business School Spain. 0–32.

Gaffney, A.W., Woolhandler, S., and Himmelstein, D.U. (2020). Correspondence US law enforcement lockdown is not egalitarian: the costs fall. *The Lancet* 396 (10243): 21–22. https://doi.org/10.1016/S0140-6736(20)31422-7.

Haque, S., Uddin, S., Sayem, S., and Mohib, K.M. (2020). Coronavirus disease 2019 (COVID-19) induced waste scenario: a short overview. *Journal of Environmental Chemical Engineering* 9 (1): 104660. https://doi.org/10.1016/j.jece.2020.104660.

Hassan, M., Haque, Z., Tasnia, M., and Sarowar, S. (2020). Science of the total environment COVID-19 and the environment: a critical review and research agenda. *Science of the Total Environment* 745: 141022. https://doi.org/10.1016/j.scitotenv.2020.141022.

Hellewell, J., Abbott, S., Gimma, A. et al. (2020). Feasibility of controlling COVID-19 outbreaks by isolation of cases and contacts. *The Lancet Global Health* 8 (4): e488–e496. https://doi.org/10.1016/S2214-109X(20)30074-7.

Interim, O. and Assessment, E. (2020). Coronavirus: The world economy at risk 2.

Kalina, M. and Tilley, E. (2020). "This is our next problem": cleaning up from the COVID-19 response. *Waste Management* 108: 202–205. https://doi.org/10.1016/j.wasman.2020.05.006.

Kashyap, S., Ramaprasad, A., and Sastry, N. B. (2020). Waste quarantine to reduce COVID-19 infection spread. The international journal of health planning and management, 35(5), 1277.

Klemeš, J., Van Fan, Y., Tan, R.R., and Jiang, P. (2020). Minimising the present and future plastic waste, energy and environmental footprints related to COVID-19. *Renewable and Sustainable Energy Reviews* 127: 109883. https://doi.org/10.1016/j.rser.2020.109883.

Kotnala, G., Mandal, T.K., Sharma, S.K., and Kotnala, R.K. (2020). Emergence of blue sky over Delhi due to coronavirus disease (COVID - 19) lockdown implications. *Aerosol Science and Engineering* 4 (3): 228–238. https://doi.org/10.1007/s41810-020-00062-6.

Kucharski, A.J., Russell, T.W., Diamond, C. et al. (2020). Early dynamics of transmission and control of COVID-19 : a mathematical modelling study. *The Lancet Infectious Diseases* 20 (5): 553–558. https://doi.org/10.1016/S1473-3099(20)30144-4.

Kumar, V., Ramkumar, M., Baba, V., and Agarwal, A. (2021). Selection of the best healthcare waste disposal techniques during and post COVID-19 pandemic era. *Journal of Cleaner Production* 281: 125175. https://doi.org/10.1016/j.jclepro.2020.125175.

Lau, H., Khosrawipour, V., Kocbach, P. et al. (2020). The positive impact of lockdown in Wuhan on containing the COVID-19 outbreak in China. *Journal of Travel Medicine*.

Li, M., Lei, P., Zeng, B. et al. (2020). Spectrum of CT findings and temporal progression of the disease. *Academic Radiology* 10: 1–6. https://doi.org/10.1016/j.acra.2020.03.003.

Lipsitch, M., Phil, D., Swerdlow, D.L., and Finelli, L. (2020). Defining the epidemiology of covid-19 — studies needed. *New England Journal of Medicine* 382 (13): 1194–1196.

Liu, X. and Zhang, S. (2020). COVID-19 : Face masks and human-to-human transmission. *Influenza and Other Respiratory Viruses* 14 (4): 472. https://doi.org/10.1111/irv.12740.

Luan, P.T. and Ching, C.T. (2020). A reusable mask for coronavirus disease 2019 (COVID-19). *Archives of Medical Research* 2019: https://doi.org/10.1016/j.arcmed.2020.04.001.

Mas-Comaa, S., Jonesb, M.K., and Martyc, A.M. (2020). COVID-19 and globalization. https://doi.org/10.24327/IJRSR.

Mccloskey, B. and Heymann, D.L. (2020). SARS to novel coronavirus – old lessons and new lessons. *Epidemiology & Infection* 148: 6–9.

Mehran, M.T., Naqvi, S.R., Haider, M.A. et al. (2021). Global plastic waste management strategies (Technical and behavioral) during and after COVID-19 pandemic for cleaner global urban life. *Energy Sources, Part A: Recovery, Utilization, and Environmental Effects* 1–10. https://doi.org/10.1080/15567036.2020.1869869.

Meo, S.A., Al-khlaiwi, T., Usmani, A.M. et al. (2020). Biological and epidemiological trends in the prevalence and mortality due to outbreaks of novel coronavirus COVID-19. *Journal of King Saud University - Science* https://doi.org/10.1016/j.jksus.2020.04.004.

Narayan, R. K., Asghar, A., Parashar, R., & Kumari, C. (2020). A standard operative procedure for safe-handling of remains and wastes of COVID-19 Patients. *Bio-protocol*, e3790–e3790. https://doi.org/10.21769/BioProtoc.3790.

Nghiem, L.D., Morgan, B., Donner, E., and Short, M.D. (2020). The COVID-19 pandemic: considerations for the waste and wastewater services sector. *Case Studies in Chemical and Environmental Engineering* 100006. https://doi.org/10.1016/j.cscee.2020.100006.

Nilashi, P.F.R.M., Asadi, R.A.A.S., and Wang, S.S.S. (2020). Coronavirus pandemic (COVID - 19) and its natural environmental impacts. *International Journal of Environmental Science and Technology* https://doi.org/10.1007/s13762-020-02910-x.

Okoro, O.V., Nkrumah Banson, A.N., and Zhang, H. (2020). Circumventing unintended impacts of waste N95 facemask generated during the COVID-19 pandemic : a conceptual design approach. *ChemEngineering* 4 (3): 54.

Paital, B., Das, K., and Kumar, S. (2020). Inter nation social lockdown versus medical care against COVID-19, a mild environmental insight with special reference to India. *Science of the Total Environment 728*: 138914. https://doi.org/10.1016/j.scitotenv.2020.138914.

Parashar, N. and Hait, S. (2021). Science of the total environment plastics in the time of COVID-19 pandemic : protector or polluter? *Science of the Total Environment* 759: 144274. https://doi.org/10.1016/j.scitotenv.2020.144274.

Patrício, A.L., Prata, J.C., Walker, T.R. et al. (2021). Increased plastic pollution due to COVID-19 pandemic: challenges and recommendations. *Chemical Engineering Journal* 405(August 2020): 126683. https://doi.org/10.1016/j.cej.2020.126683.

Peng, J., Wu, X., Wang, R. et al. (2020). Medical waste management practice during the 2019-2020 novel coronavirus pandemic: experience in a general hospital. *AJIC: American Journal of Infection Control* https://doi.org/10.1016/j.ajic.2020.05.035.

Raja, V.K., Bhakta, S.H., Prakash, R.V. et al. (2021). Challenges and strategies for effective plastic waste management during and post COVID-19 pandemic. *Science of the Total Environment* 750: 141514.

Ramteke, S. and Sahu, B.L. (2020). Novel coronavirus disease 2019 (COVID-19) pandemic: considerations for the biomedical waste sector in India. *Case Studies in Chemical and Environmental Engineering* 2019: 100029. https://doi.org/10.1016/j.cscee.2020.100029.

Ranjan, M.R., Tripathi, A., and Sharma, G. (2020). Medical waste generation during COVID-19 (SARS-CoV-2) pandemic and its management : an indian perspective. *Asian Journal of Environment & Ecology* 13 (1): 10–15. https://doi.org/10.9734/AJEE/2020/v13i130171.

Rothan, H.A. and Byrareddy, S.N. (2020). The epidemiology and pathogenesis of coronavirus disease (COVID-19) outbreak. *Journal of Autoimmunity* 102433. https://doi.org/10.1016/j.jaut.2020.102433.

Rume, T. and Islam, S.M.D. (2020). Heliyon environmental effects of COVID-19 pandemic and potential strategies of sustainability. *Heliyon* 6: e04965. https://doi.org/10.1016/j.heliyon.2020.e04965.

Sangkham, S. (2020). Mask and medical waste disposal during the novel COVID-19 pandemic in Asia. *Case Studies in Chemical and Environmental Engineering* (2): https://doi.org/10.1016/j.cscee.2020.100052.

Sharma, H.B., Vanapalli, K.R., Cheela, V.R.S. et al. (2020). Challenges, opportunities, and innovations for effective solid waste management during and post COVID - 19 pandemic. *Resources, Conservation & Recycling* 105052. https://doi.org/10.1016/j.resconrec.2020.105052.

Shetty, S.S., Wollenberg, B., Merchant, Y., and Shabadi, N. (2020). Discarded Covid 19 gear: a looming threat. *Oral Oncology* 107: 104868.

Singh, N., Tang, Y., Zhang, Z., and Zheng, C. (2020). COVID-19 waste management: effective and successful measures in Wuhan, China. *Resources, Conservation & Recycling* 163: 105071. https://doi.org/10.1016/j.resconrec.2020.105071.

Somani, M., Srivastava, A.N., Gummadivalli, S.K., and Sharma, A. (2020). Bioresource technology reports indirect implications of COVID-19 towards sustainable environment : an investigation in Indian context. *Bioresource Technology Reports* 11: 100491. https://doi.org/10.1016/j.biteb.2020.100491.

Valenzuela, P.L., Santos-Lozano, A., and Simone Lista, J.A.S.-R. (2020). Severe Acute Respiratory Syndrome Coronavirus 2 (SARS-CoV-2)-related deaths in french long-term care facilities: the "confinement disease" is probably more deleterious than the Coronavirus Disease-2019 (COVID-19) itself. *Journal of the American Medical Directors Association* 21 (7): 988–989. https://doi.org/10.1016/j.jamda.2020.03.026.

Van Der Ploeg, J.D. (2020). From biomedical to politico-economic crisis : the food system in times of Covid-19. *The Journal of Peasant Studies* 47 (5): 944–972. https://doi.org/10.1080/03066150.2020.1794843.

Van Fan, Y., Jiang, P., Hemzal, M., and Klemeš, J.J. (2021). An update of COVID-19 in fluence on waste management. *Science of the Total Environment* 754: 142014. https://doi.org/10.1016/j.scitotenv.2020.142014.

Velavan, T.P. and Meyer, C.G. (2020). La epidemia de COVID-19. *Tropical Medicine and International Health* 25 (3): 278–280. https://doi.org/10.1111/tmi.13383.

Villani, F.A., Aiuto, R., Paglia, L., and Re, D. (2020). COVID-19 and dentistry : prevention in dental practice, a literature review. *International Journal of Environmental Research and Public Health* 17 (12): 4609.

Wang, Q. and Su, M. (2020). A preliminary assessment of the impact of COVID-19 on environment – a case study of China. *Science of the Total Environment* 728: 138915. https://doi.org/10.1016/j.scitotenv.2020.138915.

Wang, D., Hu, B., Hu, C. et al. (2020a). Clinical characteristics of 138 hospitalized patients with 2019 novel coronavirus–infected pneumonia in Wuhan, China. *Jama* 323 (11): 1061–1069.

Wang, J., Shen, J., Ye, D. et al. (2020b). Disinfection technology of hospital wastes and wastewater: Suggestions for disinfection strategy during coronavirus Disease 2019 (COVID-19) pandemic in China. *Environmental Pollution* 2019: 114665. https://doi.org/10.1016/j.envpol.2020.114665.

WHO (2005). *Management of Solid Health-Care Waste at Primary Health-Care Centres: a decision-making guide*. WHO.

Wölfel, R., Corman, V.M., Guggemos, W. et al. (2020). Virological assessment of hospitalized patients with COVID-2019. *Nature* 581 (7809): 465–469. https://doi.org/10.1038/s41586-020-2196-x.

World Health Organization, 2020. WHO COVID-19 preparedness and response progress report – 1 February to 30 June 2020.

Xu, Z., Shi, L., Wang, Y. et al. (2020). Case report pathological findings of COVID-19 associated with acute respiratory distress syndrome. *The Lancet Respiratory* 8 (4): 420–422. https://doi.org/10.1016/S2213-2600(20)30076-X.

Yao, Y., Pan, J., Liu, Z. et al. (2020). No association of COVID-19 transmission with temperature or UV radiation in Chinese cities. *The European respiratory journal* https://doi.org/10.1183/13993003.00517-2020.

Zambrano-monserrate, M.A., Alejandra, M., and Sanchez-alcalde, L. (2020). Science of the total environment indirect effects of COVID-19 on the environment. *Science of the Total Environment 728*: 138813. https://doi.org/10.1016/j.scitotenv.2020.138813.

Zhang, W., Zhao, Y., Zhang, F. et al. (2020). The use of anti-inflammatory drugs in the treatment of people with severe coronavirus disease 2019 (COVID-19): the experience of clinical immunologists from China. *Clinical Immunology* 2019: 108393. https://doi.org/10.1016/j.clim.2020.108393.

Zhou, P., Yang, X., Wang, X. et al. (2020). A pneumonia outbreak associated with a new coronavirus of probable bat origin. *Nature* 2019: https://doi.org/10.1038/s41586-020-2012-7.

14

Strategies for Effective Waste Management for COVID-19

Aayush Dey[1], Nitasha Khatri[2], Piyush K. Rao[1], and Deepak Rawtani[3]

[1] School of Doctoral Studies and Research, National Forensic Sciences University (Ministry of Home Affairs, GOI), Gandhinagar, Gujarat, India
[2] Department of Forest and Environment, Gujarat Environment Management Institute (GEMI), Gandhinagar, Gujarat, India
[3] School of Pharmacy, National Forensic Sciences University (Ministry of Home Affairs, GOI), Gandhinagar, Gujarat, India

14.1 Introduction

The advent of the novel coronavirus disease has brought about a radical transformation in the nature of waste generated. Although due to the imposed lockdown on a global scale, the environment has become cleaner (Saadat et al. 2020), the rapid rates of the COVID-19 transmission have brought about an unexpected and grave concern regarding waste generation and management (Vanapalli et al. 2021). The outbreak of the novel coronavirus, when declared a global pandemic, brought a sharp increment in the utilization of protective kits and hand sanitizers that ultimately generates waste. The use of surface disinfectants has also increased, which, like the protective kits and hand sanitizers, generates waste. Solid wastes such as food-packaging materials from households and other residential buildings due to the imposed lockdown are also generated. Wastes from health care facilities, i.e. biomedical wastes along with other types of waste mentioned above have added an extra load to the prevailing waste treatment systems. In household settings, where individuals have been working from home, it is evident that wastes are generated from such sources too. Home-quarantined individuals who are either symptomatic or asymptomatic, generate wastes that require proper handling. Face masks, face shields, body fluids, and tissues can act as the most intricate sources of COVID-19 transmission. When the attention is focused on wastes generated in health care units, prevailing facilities that have been ensuring the safe disposal of wastes, have reported a record-shattering increment in waste production due to the onset of COVID-19. Due to the aforementioned fact, it becomes crystal clear that normal guidelines for waste disposal would not suffice.

As mentioned in the former part of this section, wastes such as solid wastes and biomedical wastes, i.e. wastes generated from health care units and other industrial wastes, are some of the prime sources of waste in the COVID-19 era. A complete depiction of types of COVID-19 wastes is depicted in Figure 14.1. COVID-19 waste disposal and management

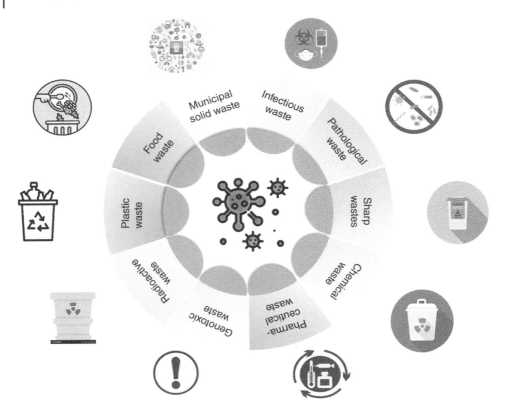

Figure 14.1 Types of COVID-19 wastes.

require proper attention and planning. Further, the use of plastics as the chief material for almost all disposable personal protective equipment (PPE) kits and single-use carry bags for necessary household items have unexpectedly changed the composition of wastes that are being generated (Singh 2020). Although, it must be evident that plastic wastes are not solely responsible for the increase in the level of waste generation. Other types of waste stated in the former part of the introduction also contribute to the overall increment in waste production. The centralizing focus of the general public regarding the recent conditions in increasing waste generation is vital. This chapter aims at exploring the solid and biomedical wastes generated during COVID-19. More importantly, it is suggestive to explain the different potential and novel waste mitigation strategies that would be helpful in curbing the extra waste generation and the overload on prevailing disposal systems.

14.2 Composition of Wastes Corresponding to the COVID-19 Pandemic

The induction of lockdown on a global scale has untethered the organization of waste collection and disposal in different urban and rural environments. Waste sources from households, industries, and other small-scale businesses combined with extra health care or biomedical wastes have not only changed the composition of wastes but also changed the dynamics of waste generation (Naughton 2020). The current statistics and facts regarding the waste generated due to COVID-19 serve as a sole reason to stir up policymakers and even the civilians to take necessary steps that could lead to the mitigation of waste generation due to the COVID-19 pandemic (Sharma et al. 2020). Solid wastes generated due to COVID-19 can primarily be categorized into food wastes, plastic wastes, and municipal solid wastes. The category of biomedical wastes has a broad classification of wastes as described by the Institute of Global Environmental Strategies under the United Nations Environment Programme (IGES 2020).

14.3 Solid Waste

Solid wastes are generally generated in residential and household environments. Materials such as plastics, papers, furniture wood, and glasses contribute to the formation of such wastes. An exemplary shift in the type of solid waste generated has been observed due to the COVID-19 pandemic, for example, the increased usage of plastic packaging material for food and increased usage of disposable items such as PPE kits, face masks, shields, and hand gloves. The local urban and rural authorities and officials in order to maintain health and hygiene must implement and practice solid waste management. Various governmental and private institutions around the globe have stated the concerns related to the overusage of plastic-based masks and other PPE kits that are disposed of in the water bodies without prior planning and treatment. This overuse of plastic-based materials has led to a detonation of plastic pollution in the water bodies. As stated formerly in this particular section, plastics, papers, furniture wood, glasses, etc., are responsible for the generation of solid wastes, but they are not solely affecting the solid waste generation, other types of wastes that contribute to its formation include, food wastes from households, schools, the hospitality sector, etc. Other household wastes that are generated when an individual with a probable possibility of infection is quarantined at a quarantine center or a health care facility also contribute to the formation of solid wastes. It is apparent that if solid wastes are not treated with the utmost care, they can serve as a major entry point for the novel coronavirus into the environment. Due to the aforementioned fact, proper waste disposal strategies are required to curb the spread of COVID-19 in the environment and possibly prevent transmission at the community level.

14.3.1 Food Wastes

The onset of the novel coronavirus disease has provocatively imposed a different trend in the purchasing and consumption habits of the population. The aforementioned fact is justifiable because of the fears of commotion in food supply among people. These fears have stimulated people in purchasing extra supplies of food for their respective households. Stockpiling of extra food supplies can have some drawbacks. Extra consumption of food supplies can affect the environment in terms of groundwater pollution and greenhouse emissions (Pappalardo et al. 2020). The aforementioned sentence can be justified on the basis that when food wastes are dumped off into landfills, they rot, which, in turn, act as a primary source for methane gas, which is a primary contributor to the greenhouse effect

(Scherhaufer et al. 2018). Further, these food wastes undergo chemical changes and various other reactions that form toxic substances, which can leach into the groundwater, hence polluting the water table (Tonini et al. 2018). As the problems related to food waste have been stated, it is important to discuss the relation of the novel coronavirus to food waste generation in detail. According to a report published in the Food and Agriculture Organization (FAO) of the United Nations (Rolle 2020), disruptions in the food supply chain may arise due to the hurdles in the transport routes and other lockdown measures. It is these commotions that result in food loss and waste. Agricultural products such as vegetables and fruits and animal food products such as meat, eggs, etc., and other produces from the dairy such as cottage cheese, milk, and curd etc., are the types of foods that are most likely to perish due to food loss and waste. It is these logistical challenges that primarily contribute to food loss and wastage (Sharma et al. 2020).

In the advent of the digital decade and the COVID-19 pandemic, it has become easy to identify specific regions that exhibit a higher number of individuals with a positive infection. These places have been given the term "hotspot." These hotspots can also be generated in areas with a single case of COVID-19 infection if these areas exhibit a higher potential for a broader spread of the novel coronavirus disease (The Economic Times 2020). Such hotspots also pose as a potential source for the generation of food wastes due to disruption in the food supply chain. Unfitting storage strategies and indecorous means of gaining food resources also constitute probable causes of food wastage (Sharma et al. 2020).

14.3.1.1 Probable Management Strategies

In connection with food wastes generated from households and those generated due to a disrupted food supply chain, it is necessary to innovate a novel solution that could be implemented at the very core of food production (Sharma et al. 2020). If the steps involved in food production are evaluated, it is observed that food supply to consumers begins with obtaining raw materials such as tools for sowing and ploughing, seeds that are to be sown, and other miscellaneous resources. Such resources due to the imposed pandemic measures were not available for the food producers and cultivators to be purchased directly. Hence, these resources can be provided by the local authorities or small scale nongovernmental organizations, in coordination with the government (Parfitt et al. 2010). Storing food after the harvest must be a collaborative initiative amongst cultivators. As the pandemic prevails, storage of the food produce might be done at local storage silos. As a part of the lockdown measures, vehicular movements have been strictly regulated because of which careful transport and supply of food resources must be done. This can be achieved by obtaining proper consent from the concerned authorities. Authorities maintaining the law and order regarding the lockdown must also ensure aspects of transportation of food, which include, food and water supply to the transporters, convenience of PPEs to transporters and support staff working at storage silos (Saini and Kozicka 2014). Such mitigation strategies (Figure 14.2) would definitely help in the reduction of the generation of food wastes and also ensure the availability of food to each and every section of the society in the COVID-19 era. Speaking of hotspots as another major point source of food waste generation, contactless delivery of food via food supply drones can be an appropriate way of ensuring the decline in the generation of food wastes (Porter 2020).

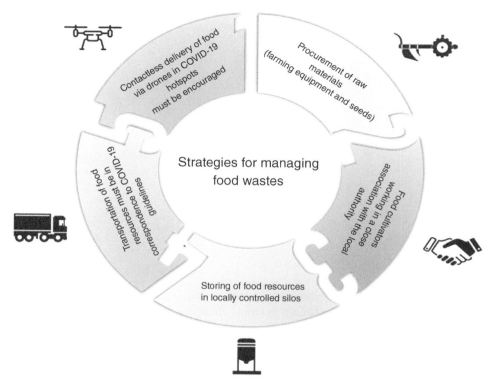

Strategies for managing food wastes

Procurement of raw materials (farming equipment and seeds)

Food cultivators working in a close association with the local authority

Storing of food resources in locally controlled silos

Transportation of food resources must be in correspondence to COVID-19 guidelines

Contactless delivery of food via drones in COVID-19 hotspots must be encouraged

Figure 14.2   Food waste management strategies.

14.3.2   Plastic Wastes

Plastic waste is another category of solid wastem, whose disposal has posed a greater challenge to researchers globally. The hazards posed by the generation of plastic waste have urged authorities and governments to take necessary steps regarding the reduction in plastic waste generation. It is a well-established fact that plastic wastes generated pose a grave threat to the aquatic environment (Schnurr et al. 2018), and the outbreak of the COVID-19 pandemic has just boosted the plastic waste generation. Several ground-breaking complications have emerged in the COVID-19 era regarding plastic wastes and strategies that have been previously formulated for its disposal and management. The onset of the COVID-19 pandemic has made people aware of health and hygiene practices. Also, people who are required to travel to different workplaces are instructed to practice and follow hygienic practices for their personal as well as others' safety (WHO 2020a). A negative influence has been observed on the efforts to curb the generation of plastic wastes due to the onset of COVID-19. The overutilization of disposable gowns, masks, gloves, and face shields as a defence against the transmission of COVID-19 has changed the dynamics of plastic waste generation and their disposal (Sharma et al. 2020). Various other point sources (Figure 14.3) for the plastic waste generation have been identified over time that requires immediate attention by the government, the concerned authorities, and even the general public

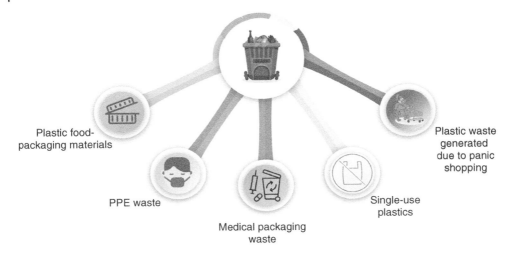

Figure 14.3 Point sources of plastic wastes.

(Vanapalli et al. 2021). E-commerce has gained a huge user base after the COVID-19 outbreak. The packaging material used in online shopping and food delivery incorporates plastic, which also contributes toward the overall plastic waste generation. Additionally, panic shopping, exploitation of single-use plastic bags, and medical supplies using plastic-packaging materials also contribute toward overall plastic waste generation in this ongoing pandemic caused by the novel coronavirus.

14.3.2.1 Plastic Waste Management Strategies

Plastic wastes generated due to the outbreak of COVID-19 require immediate attention. Despite the resources available, a limited number of solutions have been figured out regarding plastic waste disposal and management, due to which there is an urgent need to innovate novel methods and strategies for the disposal of plastic wastes generated in the perspective of COVID-19. The prevailing waste management systems can be integrated with new innovative solutions in order to enhance their capabilities in terms of waste disposal. This would also prepare the existing facilities to prepare themselves for upcoming surges in plastic waste generation (Vanapalli et al. 2021). Feedstock and mechanical recycling (Vollmer et al. 2020) of plastic wastes refer to an innovative method of dealing with surges in plastic wastes. The use of bioplastics such as polylactic acid (PLA) is another innovative method for curbing plastic wastes (Barletta et al. 2020). The treatment of plastic waste is not an easy task, as it involves different steps, such as recognizing the point source of waste generation, classifying the plastic wastes, and collecting them. Further steps include their transportation, treatment, and disposal in accordance with sanitation and safety measures.

14.3.3 Municipal Solid Waste and Management Strategies

Lockdown imposed by governments on a global scale has caused a sporadic collection of wastes by management and treatment facilities. This is the primary reason why an overload upon the prevailing management and treatment facilities is observed in the

COVID-19 era. Commercial and residential wastes in solid or semi-solid form, are generally included in the municipal waste category. Other types of waste such as discards from households and nonhazardous wastes from industries and wastes generated as scrapes in the streets also contribute to this category (Rao et al. 2017). Many international organizations such as the International Solid Waste Association (ISWA) (Scheinberg et al. 2020), Occupational Safety and Health Organization (OSHA) (OSHA 2020a, 2020b), United States Environmental Protection Agency (USEPA) (USEPA 2020), World Health Organization (WHO) (WHO 2020b), and Women in Informal Employment: Globalizing and Organizing (WEIGO) (WEIGO 2020) have put forward a respective set of guidelines to mitigate the generation of municipal solid wastes, which have been summarized in Figure 14.4.

14.4 Biomedical Wastes

Health care wastes according to the WHO have been classified into two primary components, which include hazardous and nonhazardous wastes (WHO 2018). Mostly health care wastes are generated from sources that include hospitals and health care units, laboratories, and research facilities. Biomedical wastes in general can be classified into two broader categories that include hazardous biomedical wastes and nonhazardous biomedical wastes (IGES 2020). A detailed description of the types of biomedical wastes and their suitable mitigation strategies has been given in the preceding sections.

14.4.1 Hazardous Biomedical Wastes

Hazardous biomedical wastes generated due to COVID-19 are classified into the following categories (IGES 2020).

14.4.1.1 Infectious Waste
The infectious waste is one of the categories of hazardous biomedical waste that are suspected to consist of pathogens. In the wake of COVID-19, infectious biomedical or health care wastes can be generated from sources such as fabrics stained with blood and other biological fluids. Diagnostic samples that have to be discarded after analysis also serve as a source of infectious wastes. Cell cultures from laboratory work and other wastes derived after conduction of autopsies and animals infected with pathogens are the primary sources of infectious wastes. Waste derived from patients in health care facilities or infected individuals kept in isolation in houses also serves as a prime source of infectious waste. Swabs or cotton fibres, fabrics, plastics, etc. from such households comprises infectious wastes (IGES 2020).

14.4.1.2 Pathological Waste
While conducting surgery or an autopsy on who might have been potentially infected with the novel coronavirus, generally, remains such as human tissues or organs and other biological fluids are generated, which serve as a primary source of pathological wastes (IGES 2020).

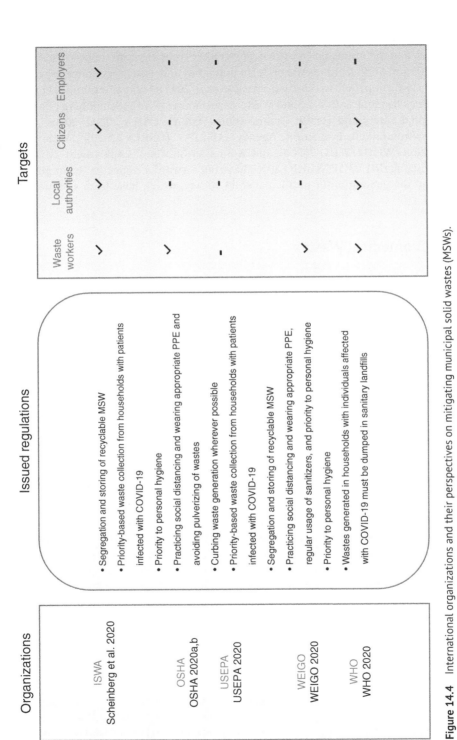

Figure 14.4 International organizations and their perspectives on mitigating municipal solid wastes (MSWs).

14.4.1.3 Sharps Waste

There are certain sharp items that are used to treat patients showing chronic symptoms of COVID-19. Syringes, needles, disposable or metal scalpels, blades, knives, etc., are some of the items that come under the category of sharps waste generated due to COVID-19 (IGES 2020).

14.4.1.4 Chemical Waste

Discards from research facilities and health care units that include chemical solids, liquids, and gases generated from research experiments consist of chemical wastes. Chemical wastes generated due to COVID-19 are recognized as hazardous chemical wastes if they constitute properties such as toxicity, corrosiveness, flammability, and genotoxicity (IGES 2020).

14.4.1.5 Pharmaceutical Waste

These types of wastes are generated when medicines have achieved their particular expiry dates. Unused and other contaminated drugs are also comprised of pharmaceutical wastes. Vials in which unused and expired drugs are stored along with used gloves and masks also account for pharmaceutical waste generated in the wake of COVID-19 (IGES 2020).

14.4.1.6 Genotoxic Waste

Wastes arising from health care facilities and research laboratories that consist of mutagenic, teratogenic, and carcinogenic characteristics are termed genotoxic wastes (IGES 2020).

14.4.2 Probable Mitigation Strategies for Hazardous Biomedical Wastes Generated Due to COVID-19

Prior to opting for a suitable methodology for disposing of biomedical wastes, these wastes must be segregated. After the segregation of different biomedical wastes, appropriate disposal techniques such as incineration, utilization of thermal techniques, and chemical and physical techniques for COVID-19 biomedical waste mitigation have been discussed in detail in the upcoming sections of the chapter. These techniques are useful as they are affirmed to prevent any sort of COVID-19 infection. Such strategies mentioned above would not only curb biomedical wastes but are time-efficient too (Ilyas et al. 2020). If statistics are considered, approximately 85% of the biomedical wastes are nonhazardous and the rest is comprised of hazardous biomedical wastes (Datta et al. 2018). Some of the potent biomedical waste mitigation strategies are discussed in detail next.

14.4.2.1 Incineration

It is one of the most commonly used strategies for pathogen disinfection in biomedical wastes. The combustion temperature of biomedical wastes in this technique lies between the 800 °C and 1200 °C range, which significantly neutralizes any pathogen that might prevail on surfaces. This strategy of waste mitigation has been redesigned keeping in mind the prevalence of the novel coronavirus, where the temperatures for waste disposal have been kept over 1100 °C. This step will ensure that approximately 90% of the organic matter will be burned up during the incineration process (Wang et al. 2020). Although incineration of biomedical wastes as a full-fledged strategy is effective for COVID-19 waste neutralization, it has some disadvantages too. One of the greatest concerns regarding the incineration of biomedical wastes is the generation of CO_2. At temperatures greater than 800 °C, greater amounts of fuel are required to maintain the temperature range and also maintain the stability of the incinerator at such high temperatures, hence its dependency on fossil fuels for combustion (Peng et al. 2020; Purnomo et al. 2021). Generation of polycyclic aromatic hydrocarbons (PAHs) and polychlorinated dibenzofurans (PCDF), polychlorinated dibenzo-p-dioxins (PCDD), chlorophenols and chlorobenzenes have been already reported due to incineration techniques (Font et al. 2010). These chemical compounds have been reported to damage the immune and the endocrine system in humans after getting accumulated to the fatty tissues (Ilyas et al. 2020). These chemicals hence generated act as potent air pollutants. Hence, a proper flue-treatment facility is required for the neutralization of such chemicals. Almost half of the entire budget required to operate an incineration facility is required to keep the flue-treatment facility operational. This makes incineration an expensive procedure, and substituting strategies are required to dispose of biomedical wastes.

14.4.2.2 Thermal Strategies for Biomedical Waste Mitigation

The thermal strategies for COVID-19 biomedical waste treatment have been classified into pyrolysis and microwave techniques. These techniques are suitable for the treatment of biomedical wastes as, unlike incineration, the harmful impact upon the environment in the form of air pollution is minimal.

Pyrolysis: Unlike incineration, pyrolysis, as a strategy for waste management is more feasible. It operates at a lower temperature range when compared to incineration, i.e. 540 °C–830 °C (Kantarelis et al. 2009). Pyrolysis-oxidation, plasma-pyrolysis, induction-based pyrolysis, and laser-based pyrolysis are different pyrolysis processes that have been employed for COVID-19 waste treatment and management. The pyrolysis-oxidation technique is one of the most commonly employed pyrolysis techniques including the burning of wastes in the presence of the excess air/oxygen supply. Solid wastes generated due to COVID-19 are combusted at approximately 600 °C (Datta et al. 2018). In this technique, glass, metallic shards, and ash are the most common residues that are left over after the combustion. The next type of pyrolysis strategy includes plasma-mediated combustion of wastes, which takes place within a temperature range of 982 °C–1093 °C. The plasma-pyrolysis of different wastes generates flammable gaseous residues, which are further neutralized in this step. This plasma-pyrolysis step also neutralizes noxious residues such as dioxins and furans. This neutralization is achieved by dropping temperatures of flammable gases as below as 70 °C. This inhibits the recombination reaction of gaseous molecules to further form poisonous particulates, for example, dioxins and furans as mentioned earlier (Nema and Ganeshprasad 2002). Induction-based pyrolysis technique unlike the pyrolysis oxidation process does not require oxygen for the combustion of waste materials (Nakanoh et al. 2001). Pyrolysis-oxidation and plasma-pyrolysis technique for waste mitigation are more rapid than any other pyrolysis technique and hence these techniques are more commonly used for accelerated waste disposal, corresponding to the transmission speed of SARS-CoV-2 (Ilyas et al. 2020).

Microwave-based techniques: This technique unlike pyrolysis works within a medium temperature range that lies between 177 and 540 °C. Under the influence of an inert atmosphere, the waste materials generated due to COVID-19 interact with high-energy microwave beams. Since such waste materials consist of organic molecules, these molecules break down when they come in contact with the high-energy microwave beams. When the waste materials absorb the microwaves, the internal rubbing of molecules causes the adjacent molecules to vibrate and as a result, the internal energy of the materials increases. This causes the disintegration of the waste materials that require proper management and disposal (Zimmermann 2017; Ilyas et al. 2020). The microwave technique for waste management has numerous advantages that include lower energy and action temperature requirement for disinfection, limited heat loss, and nonformation of toxic residues prior to disposal and management, leaving no burden upon the environment. Microwave-based devices have been reported as an efficient means of SARS-CoV-2 neutralization (Zulauf et al. 2020). Microwave techniques in combination with autoclaves have also been utilized for the mitigation and management of biomedical wastes (Veronesi et al. 2007). The temperatures for this combination generally lie in the range of 93–177 °C.

14.4.2.3   Biomedical Waste Management-Based via Chemical Techniques

All the biomedical wastes generated due to COVID-19 prior to chemical treatment undergo mechanical processing such as physical shredding and crushing. After subsequent mechanical processing of COVID-19 wastes, the biomedical wastes are treated with well-known chemical surface disinfectants such as sodium and calcium hypochlorite and chlorine dioxide (Tsai and Lin 1999). This results in an apt neutralization of infectious pathogens and decomposition of organic components in the waste, if present. Chemical disinfection strategy in the wake of the COVID-19 pandemic has seen a sudden surge. Chemical disinfectants apart from neutralizing COVID-19 causing SARS-CoV-2 exhibit a broad spectrum regarding the inactivation of microorganisms and bacterial spores. Chemical disinfectants such as hypochlorites and chlorine dioxide consist of user-friendly intrinsic characteristics that make them suitable for general usage. These intrinsic characteristics include odorlessness, tastelessness, colorless, safety, and solubility in water. Apart from these characteristics, these chemical disinfectants do not leave behind any residual hazard prior to disinfection (Wang et al. 2020).

14.4.2.4   COVID-19 Biomedical Waste Management via Steam
Sterilization Technique

Another technique for biomedical waste management is high-temperature steam disinfection. This treatment strategy utilizes steam at a high temperature, i.e. >100 °C to kill pathogens. The biomedical wastes generated due to COVID-19 are formerly set in an environment with a definitive temperature of water vapor for a limited time period. The high temperature of water vapor produces the latent heat, which, in turn, causes the denaturation and coagulation of pathogenic/viral proteins, hence resulting in the ceasing of the pathogenic life cycle (Bao et al. 2013).

14.5 A Global Perspective Upon COVID-19 Waste Management

The onset of the global pandemic caused by the novel coronavirus that originated in the Wuhan, Hubei province of China has sent the world to a standstill. Waste collection, transport, disposal, and management have been impacted impromptu. The prevailing waste management systems and guidelines set globally were nullified due to sudden changes in the composition of wastes due to COVID-19. There has been an urgent requirement for an upgrade and validation regarding the prevailing available strategies for waste management. A perspective on the guideline changes outlined by different superpowers around the globe has been outlined as follows.

14.5.1 India's Take on COVID-19 Waste Management

COVID-19 transmission rates in India were very high at the end of the first quarter of 2020. Prompt guidelines regarding COVID-19 waste management were not issued until a sudden surge in the production of solid and biomedical waste generation was observed. Prior to the outbreak of the COVID-19 pandemic, the statistics regarding biomedical waste generation state that approximately 265 tonnes of biomedical waste were generated each day. This numeric figure witnessed a sudden boom up to 463 tonnes of biomedical waste generation per day in India after the COVID-19 outbreak (DNA 2020). The Central Pollution Control Board (CPCB) is the primary constitutional body that is regulated by the Ministry of Environment, Forest and Climate change. This organisation is primarily responsible for environmental protection and controlling all other dynamics that would lead to a better environment. According to the guidelines published by the CPCB regarding waste generation and management due to COVID-19 (CPCB 2020), general solid wastes generated from different households or other urban settings and health care facilities and quarantine centers must be segregated accordingly. Wastes such as food wastes, packaging and plastic wastes, throwaway utensils, etc., can be collected and disposed of by the waste collectors. Apart from these, biomedical wastes from quarantine facilities, hospitals, and research labs must be collected in a separate yellow bag and must be treated accordingly at a common biomedical waste treatment facility (CBWTF). In the wake of COVID-19, a revised version of the duties of local urban bodies, the State Pollution Control Board and the Pollution Control Committee have also been outlined and defined in detail by the CPCB.

14.5.2 COVID-19 Waste Management in Spain

The population of Spain was severely hit by the COVID-19 pandemic. The relationship between the rising number of COVID-19 cases and waste production has been evident. Plastic waste in Spain in particular served as an epicenter of the problem of waste disposal and management. Plastic waste disposal is a serious issue as it is known to adsorb inorganic nutrients, which accomplishes a suitable growth ground for pathogenic viruses such as the SARS virus (Frère et al. 2018). As a protective measure, the concerned authorities of Spain issued several plans to ensure the proper disposal of plastics and domestic wastes generated due to COVID-19. According to the set of rules set by the authorities in Spain, contaminated wastes must be disposed of in sealed and leakproof bags. The preferred strategy for waste disposal and management would be incineration and landfilling (Prata et al. 2020). As for biomedical wastes, high-temperature incineration, landfilling of residual ash, and mechanical processing prior to chemical disinfection are preferred (Windfeld and Brooks 2015).

14.5.3 Practices for COVID-19 Waste Management by the United States

Two of the primary organizations in the United States of America, i.e. Occupational Safety and Health Administration (OSHA) and the Centers for Disease Control and Prevention (CDC) have issued several sets of guidelines for proper waste disposal and management corresponding to COVID-19. OSHA, a statutory body governed by the United States Department of Labor, has issued interim guidelines for proper management of solid and biomedical wastes. In order to properly manage the solid wastes generated in households or any other residential areas, safe work practices must be induced, such as the usage of PPEs. The utilization of puncture-resistant face masks and shields by frontline workers and waste collectors is recommended by OSHA. As far as biomedical wastes are concerned, all hazardous biomedical wastes must be incinerated or disinfected using pyrolysis or microwave exposure strategy. Similar to the handling of solid wastes, the usage of PPEs and face masks and shields is recommended for the handling of biomedical wastes (OSHA 2020a). According to the guidelines set by the CDC, waste generated from testing centers includes infectious wastes such as cotton swabs, biological fluids, and vials that have been utilized to store biological samples such as blood, saliva, etc. Such wastes must be classified as hazardous biomedical wastes (CDC 2020). Risk assessments of wastes must be done according to the protocols provided by the Association of Public Health Laboratories (APHL) (APHL 2016). The assessments must be performed onsite or offsite to mitigate the spread of the COVID-19 disease.

14.5.4 China's COVID-19 Waste Management Strategy

Speaking about the most populated country in the world, China generated about 247 tons of biomedical waste per day at the peak of the COVID-19 pandemic. This statistic of waste generated accounts to be approximately six times more than the amount of waste generated prior to the COVID-19 pandemic (Singh et al. 2020). Post-COVID-19 outbreak, the biomedical waste generation surge was observed and kept on increasing at a rate of 110–150 tons of biomedical waste per day. The concerned authorities involved four companies that specialized in solid and biomedical waste management and claimed to dispose of approximately 30 tons of COVID-19 wastes each day (Wei 2020).

14.6 Conclusion

The rate of waste generation has always exceeded the rate of waste disposal. Be it, any sort of solid and biomedical waste, its management and disposal have always been challenging. The pandemic caused by the novel coronavirus has led the population to rely especially on plastics and other materials that potentially have changed the dynamics of waste generation, and in addition to it, the dynamics of waste management and disposal. Biomedical wastes generated due to COVID-19 in addition to solid wastes also pose a greater challenge to the existing waste management systems. The scenario of waste management due to the viral outbreak has been dismantled to the core due to excessive waste generation. All of these problems need urgent and effective solutions. Novel solutions integrated into the prevailing strategies will not only boost waste disposal but also help in sustaining the environment. The responsibility for the environment sustenance solely does not belong to policymakers, but it is important to change the psychological and behavioural aspects of civilians regarding waste generation. Pertaining to a joint venture between the public–government regarding figuring out novel strategies for sustaining the environment, mitigating COVID-19 transmission and waste management will be resourceful not only for the present generation but also for the upcoming generation.

References

APHL (2016). Risk assessment best practices. https://www.aphl.org/programs/preparedness/Documents/APHL Risk Assessment Best Practices and Examples.pdf (accessed 24 February 2021).

Bao, Z., Jin, D., Teng, H., and Li, Y. (2013). The general process of medical waste high temperature steam sterilization treatment technology. *Adv. Mater. Res.* 807–809: 1160–1163. https://doi.org/10.4028/www.scientific.net/AMR.807-809.1160.

Barletta, M., Aversa, C., and Puopolo, M. (2020). Recycling of PLA-based bioplastics: the role of chain-extenders in twin-screw extrusion compounding and cast extrusion of sheets. *J. Appl. Polym. Sci.* 137: 49292. https://doi.org/10.1002/app.49292.

CDC (2020). Waste management guidance for SARS-CoV-2 point-of-care testing. https://www.cdc.gov/csels/dls/locs/2020/waste_management_guidance_for_sars-cov-2_point-of-care_testing.html (accessed 24 February 2021).

CPCB (2020). Revision 4 Guidelines for Handling, Treatment and Disposal of Waste Generated during Treatment/Diagnosis/ Quarantine of COVID-19 Patients Central Pollution Control Board.

Datta, P., Mohi, G., and Chander, J. (2018). Biomedical waste management in India: critical appraisal. *J. Lab. Physicians* 10: 006–014. https://doi.org/10.4103/jlp.jlp_89_17.

DNA (2020). Half of bio-medical waste not disposed of properly: Study. https://www.dnaindia.com/india/report-half-of-bio-medical-waste-not-disposed-of-properly-study-1370510 (accessed 23 February 2021).

Font, R., Gálvez, A., Moltó, J. et al. (2010). Formation of polychlorinated compounds in the combustion of PVC with iron nanoparticles. *Chemosphere* 78: 152–159. https://doi.org/10.1016/j.chemosphere.2009.09.064.

Frère, L., Maignien, L., Chalopin, M. et al. (2018). Microplastic bacterial communities in the Bay of Brest: influence of polymer type and size. *Environ. Pollut.* 242: 614–625. https://doi.org/10.1016/j.envpol.2018.07.023.

IGES (2020). Waste management during the COVID-19 pandemic.

Ilyas, S., Srivastava, R.R., and Kim, H. (2020). Disinfection technology and strategies for COVID-19 hospital and bio-medical waste management. *Sci. Total Environ.* 749: 141652. https://doi.org/10.1016/j.scitotenv.2020.141652.

Kantarelis, E., Donaj, P., Yang, W., and Zabaniotou, A. (2009). Sustainable valorization of plastic wastes for energy with environmental safety via High-Temperature Pyrolysis (HTP) and High-Temperature Steam Gasification (HTSG). *J. Hazard. Mater.* 167: 675–684. https://doi.org/10.1016/j.jhazmat.2009.01.036.

Nakanoh, K., Hayashi, S., and Kida, K. (2001). Waste treatment using induction-heated pyrolysis. *Fuji Electr. Rev.* 47: 69–73.

Naughton, C.C. (2020). Will the COVID-19 pandemic change waste generation and composition?: the need for more real-time waste management data and systems thinking. *Resour. Conserv. Recycl.* 162: 105050. https://doi.org/10.1016/j.resconrec.2020.105050.

Nema, S.K. and Ganeshprasad, K.S. (2002). Plasma pyrolysis of medical waste. *Curr. Sci.* 83: 271–278.

OSHA (2020a). COVID-19 - Control and prevention - solid waste and wastewater management workers and employers | occupational safety and health administration. https://www.osha.gov/coronavirus/control-prevention/solid-waste-wastewater-mgmt (accessed 12 February 2021).

OSHA (2020b). Worker exposure risk to COVID-19 classifying worker exposure to SARS-CoV-2.

Pappalardo, G., Cerroni, S., Nayga, R.M., and Yang, W. (2020). Impact of Covid-19 on household food waste: the case of Italy. *Front. Nutr.* 7: 1–9.

Parfitt, J., Barthel, M., and Macnaughton, S. (2010). Food waste within food supply chains: quantification and potential for change to 2050. *Philos. Trans. R. Soc. B Biol. Sci.* 365: 3065–3081. https://doi.org/10.1098/rstb.2010.0126.

Peng, J., Wu, X., Wang, R. et al. (2020). Medical waste management practice during the 2019–2020 novel coronavirus pandemic: experience in a general hospital. *Am. J. Infect. Control* 48: 918–921. https://doi.org/10.1016/j.ajic.2020.05.035.

Porter, J., 2020. Alphabet's nascent drone delivery service is booming - The Verge. https://www.theverge.com/2020/4/9/21214709/alphabet-wing-drone-delivery-coronavirus-covid-19-demand-increase-toilet-paper-baby-food (accessed 30 January 2021).

Prata, J.C., Silva, A.L.P., Walker, T.R. et al. (2020). COVID-19 pandemic repercussions on the use and management of plastics. *Environ. Sci. Technol.* 54: 7760–7765. https://doi.org/10.1021/acs.est.0c02178.

Purnomo, C.W., Kurniawan, W., and Aziz, M. (2021). Technological review on thermochemical conversion of COVID-19-related medical wastes. *Resour. Conserv. Recycl.* 167: 105429. https://doi.org/10.1016/j.resconrec.2021.105429.

Rao, M.N., Sultana, R., and Kota, S.H. (2017). Chapter 2 - Municipal Solid Waste. In: *Solid and Hazardous Waste Management* (ed. M.N. Rao, R. Sultana and S.H. Kota), 3–120. Butterworth-Heinemann https://doi.org/10.1016/B978-0-12-809734-2.00002-X.

Rolle, R.S. (2020). Mitigating risks to food systems during COVID-19: Reducing food loss and waste |Policy Support and Governance| Food and Agriculture Organization of the United Nations. http://www.fao.org/policy-support/tools-and-publications/resources-details/en/c/1276396/ (accessed 28 January 2021).

Saadat, S., Rawtani, D., and Hussain, C.M. (2020). Environmental perspective of COVID-19. *Sci. Total Environ.* 728: 138870. https://doi.org/10.1016/j.scitotenv.2020.138870.

Saini, S. and Kozicka, M. (2014). *Evolution and Critique of Buffer Stocking Policy of India*. New Delhi: Indian Council for Research on International Economic Relations (ICRIER).

Scheinberg, A., Woolridge, A., Humez, N. et al. (2020). ISWA's Recommendations.

Scherhaufer, S., Moates, G., Hartikainen, H. et al. (2018). Environmental impacts of food waste in Europe. *Waste Manag.* 77: 98–113. https://doi.org/10.1016/j.wasman.2018.04.038.

Schnurr, R.E.J., Alboiu, V., Chaudhary, M. et al. (2018). Reducing marine pollution from single-use plastics (SUPs): a review. *Mar. Pollut. Bull.* 137: 157–171. https://doi.org/10.1016/j.marpolbul.2018.10.001.

Sharma, H.B., Vanapalli, K.R., Cheela, V.R.S. et al. (2020). Challenges, opportunities, and innovations for effective solid waste management during and post COVID-19 pandemic. *Resour. Conserv. Recycl.* 162: 105052. https://doi.org/10.1016/j.resconrec.2020.105052.

Singh, H. (2020). Lockdown helps bring back plastic bags - The Hindu. https://www.thehindu.com/news/national/telangana/lockdown-helps-bring-back-plastic-bags/article31381638.ece (accessed 27 February 2021).

Singh, N., Tang, Y., and Ogunseitan, O.A. (2020). Environmentally sustainable management of used personal protective equipment. *Environ. Sci. Technol.* 54: 8500–8502. https://doi.org/10.1021/acs.est.0c03022.

The Economic Times (2020). Coronavirus hotspot: The process of identifying a covid "hotspot" is not uniform: Lav Agarwal - The Economic Times. https://economictimes.indiatimes.com/news/politics-and-nation/the-process-of-identifying-a-covid-hotspot-is-not-uniform-lav-agarwal/articleshow/74913130.cms?from=mdr (accessed 30 January 2021).

Tonini, D., Albizzati, P.F., and Astrup, T.F. (2018). Environmental impacts of food waste: Learnings and challenges from a case study on UK. *Waste Manag.* 76: 744–766. https://doi.org/10.1016/j.wasman.2018.03.032.

Tsai, C.T. and Lin, S.T. (1999). Disinfection of hospital waste sludge using hypochlorite and chlorine dioxide. *J. Appl. Microbiol.* 86: 827–833. https://doi.org/10.1046/j.1365-2672.1999.00732.x.

USEPA, 2020. Recycling and sustainable management of food during the coronavirus (COVID-19) public health emergency | coronavirus (COVID-19) | US EPA. https://www.epa.gov/coronavirus/recycling-and-sustainable-management-food-during-coronavirus-covid-19-public-health (accessed 12 February 2021).

Vanapalli, K.R., Sharma, H.B., Ranjan, V.P. et al. (2021). Challenges and strategies for effective plastic waste management during and post COVID-19 pandemic. *Sci. Total Environ.* 750: 141514. https://doi.org/10.1016/j.scitotenv.2020.141514.

Veronesi, P., Leonelli, C., Moscato, U. et al. (2007). Non-incineration microwave assisted sterilization of medical waste. *J. Microw. Power Electromagn. Energy* 40: 211–218. https://doi.org/10.1080/08327823.2005.11688546.

Vollmer, I., Jenks, M.J.F., Roelands, M.C.P. et al. (2020). Beyond mechanical recycling: giving new life to plastic waste. *Angew. Chemie Int. Ed.* 59: 15402–15423. https://doi.org/10.1002/anie.201915651.

Wang, J., Shen, J., Ye, D. et al. (2020). Disinfection technology of hospital wastes and wastewater: Suggestions for disinfection strategy during coronavirus Disease 2019 (COVID-19) pandemic in China. *Environ. Pollut.* 262: 114665. https://doi.org/10.1016/j.envpol.2020.114665.

Wei, G. (2020). Medical waste management experience in COVID-19 outbreak in Wuhan. https://www.waste360.com/medical-waste/medical-waste-management-experience-and-lessons-covid-19-outbreak-wuhan (accessed 26 February 2021).

WEIGO (2020). Recommendations for the prevention of the spread of Coronavirus disease (COVID-19) among solid waste workers.

WHO (2018). Health-care waste. https://www.who.int/news-room/fact-sheets/detail/health-care-waste (accessed 2 January 2021).

WHO (2020a). COVID-19 guidance and information for employers and workers. https://www.who.int/teams/risk-communication/employers-and-workers (accessed 30 January 2021).

WHO (2020b). Water, sanitation, hygiene, and waste management for SARS-CoV-2, the virus that causes COVID-19. https://www.who.int/publications/i/item/WHO-2019-nCoV-IPC-WASH-2020.4 (accessed 12 February 2021).

Windfeld, E.S. and Brooks, M.S.-L. (2015). Medical waste management – a review. *J. Environ. Manage.* 163: 98–108. https://doi.org/10.1016/j.jenvman.2015.08.013.

Zimmermann, K. (2017). Microwave as an emerging technology for the treatment of biohazardous waste: a mini-review. *Waste Manag. Res.* 35: 471–479. https://doi.org/10.1177/0734242X16684385.

Zulauf, K.E., Green, A.B., Nguyen Ba, A.N. et al. (2020). Microwave-generated steam decontamination of N95 respirators utilizing universally accessible materials. *MBio* 11: e00997–e00920. https://doi.org/10.1128/mBio.00997-20.

15

Environmental Policies and Strategies for COVID-19

Vimbai Masiyambiri[1], Piyush K. Rao[2], Nitasha Khatri[3], and Deepak Rawtani[1]

[1] *School of Pharmacy, National Forensic Sciences University, Gandhinagar, Gujarat, India*
[2] *School of Doctoral Studies and Research, National Forensic Sciences University, Gandhinagar, Gujarat, India*
[3] *Department of Forest and Environment, Gujarat Environment Management Institute (GEMI), Gandhinagar, Gujarat, India*

15.1   Introduction

The World Health Organization (WHO) recognized COVID-19 as a pandemic and informed the world on 11 March, 2020 (WHO 2020). There was a rapid spread of the virus to different countries with no cure at hand. There was a spread of the disease with total disregard for race, age and health (Rawtani et al. 2022). Therefore, the WHO had to come up with guidelines fast so as to save people's lives. The urgency exhibited by WHO is the same that should propel the formulation of environmental policy. Human health policymaking and adherence have become the determinant of whether lives are lost or saved. Policymakers are making up policies and strategies as they go, with the public at large looking up to them for guidance in the face of this disaster (Weible et al. 2020). Uniform policy across a nation and the world can save lives. Politics over science has failed in the face of politics guided by science. In the same breath, environmental issues are just as important and should not be marginalized and forgotten. As a policy for human health is being implemented, environmental policy and strategies for COVID-19 should also be integrated.

There has never been a greater opportunity than right now to influence public opinion on environmental issues. A greater sense of human solidarity is emerging. The environmental policy should be used as a tool to link people with nature. Human beings need to cultivate a greater sense of responsibility for the environment vulnerability to COVID-19 has shown the world that despite race, political and economic differences, it is only through uniting that we can manage to build resilience and reduce mortality rate of COVID-19. The opportunity for a great "Do-over" is before the world. Let environmental policy be interwoven with every aspect of human administration. It is an opportunity for scientific research to influence environmental policy because governments draw from different voices when formulating policy (Oliver and Cairney 2019).

15.2   Linking Policy with the Environment

The policy relates to ideas or plans agreed upon to tackle a problem. The environmental policy for land reclamation, reforestation and conservation of biodiversity and ecosystems protects and supports human existence. The aim is to have an umbrella policy that provides for human health as well as ecosystem health (de Wit et al. 2020). The environmental policy refers to measures or guidelines put in place to pave way for environmental legislation. These guidelines are for safeguarding environmental integrity, abatement, and prevention of environmental degradation. It especially targets pollution and emissions control, habitat and species integrity, and decreasing the effects of natural catastrophes. The environmental policy looks at the intersections and incongruent links between society, the economy, and the environment (Benson and Jordan 2015). This makes it exceptional in determining the best fit in policymaking. Therefore, policymakers have a great role in policy formulation because our environment is dynamic. This means that what posed little or no documented threat twenty years ago can have a huge environmental impact present day. An example of this is the emerging threat of chemicals from medication and cosmetics found in treated wastewater that has the ability to disrupt organism endocrine systems and also develop hybrid pathogens that are immune to antibiotics (Deziel 2014; Kumari and Tripathi 2019). Therefore, environmental policy has to be alive, constantly evolving to suit the conditions favorable for environmental sustainability.

There are different types of environmental policies. It can be vertical (for a single entity) or Horizontal (multisectorial) in accordance with shared areas of interest (Torjman 2005), for example, existing of linkages between Transport and Mining, will prompt an umbrella policy (horizontal) instead of writing policy separate for each sector (vertical). The environmental policy can also be proactive or reactive. We cannot predict the future, as seen by the onset and magnitude of COVID-19. The proactive policy is important to counter or reduce risk and vulnerability of ecosystems. It somewhat predicts future impacts using existing data. A reactive policy is formed in reaction to an environmental disaster. This has been the basis for most environmental policies.

The Rio Declaration of 1992 (United Nations 1992) contained 27 principles. Of these, the polluter pays, and precautionary principles have become a prominent actor in the formulation of international and domestic policies. The EU's environmental policy Article 191(2) of the 2007 Treaty on the Functioning of the European Union (TFEU) states that its policy on the environment shall utilize both the polluter pays principle and the precautionary principle so that environmental degradation is prevented and accounted for (UN 2015). The polluter pays principle-based policy uses instruments such as control laws (licensing, bans) and market-based tools, for example, charges, taxes, and tradable permits. The aim of environmental policy is to have equilibrium between the economy, the environment, and society. An example of this is paying for plastics at a supermarket if one wants to carry groceries. Taking the cue from the Rio Declaration, global leaders came together to develop environmental policies, which continue to evolve as and when needed. Figure 15.1 tracks changes that have occurred in the environmental policy.

The evolution of environmental policy described in Figure 15.1 shows the dynamic nature of the environment. Anthropogenic impacts on the environment led to the Montreal Protocol for the protection and rehabilitation of the ozone layer (Ozone Secretariat 2018).

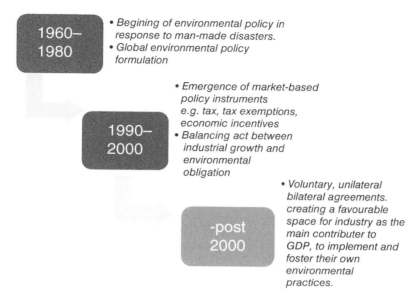

Figure 15.1 Timeline of the development of the global environmental policy.

The success of the Montreal Protocol is mirrored by the reduction of air pollution during the lockdown phase of the COVID-19 pandemic. The timeline and subsequent changes depict the conflict that is between society, economic development, and environmental rehabilitation. To achieve sustainability, a balance must be maintained. Therefore approaching to environmental issues, though stringent, allows for more user-friendly for the industry to incorporate and innovate.

Historically, the environmental policy has been influenced by imminent or onset of disaster, for example, mercury poisoning at Minamata, Japan (Minamata Disease Municipal Museum 2007). This has led to an endemic disease, which has no cure. The global environmental policy for mercury poisoning was put in place in 2017. Another example are the ozone-depleting substances (ODSs) measured in the form of the Montreal Protocol (Ozone Secretariat 2018). The restorative and rehabilitation efforts may cost more than the world is prepared to pay. Therefore, this is the right time to curb environmental degradation that will be caused by COVID-19 and preceding pandemics. The COVID-19 restrictions have helped the environment by clearing the air and aquatic environments as shown in Table 15.1. The issue that arises now is that after the lifting of restrictions on the movement, economic processes spur an increase in production by industry, an increase in combustion emissions as people travel to and from work, and an increase in medical waste from public use of personal protective equipment (PPE). The environmental advantages that have been gained should continue. Streamlining economies to environmental policies that reduce waste, support reforestation and afforestation, eco-friendly tourism, and mitigation of pollution at the point source. Current fiscal policies have not only already started to mitigate economic loss suffered but also catalyzed businesses to go back to pre-COVID-19 conditions. There is disregard toward environmental rehabilitation. The discord stems from policymakers who treat the physical environment as separate from the human

Table 15.1 Response of established environmental policies to COVID-19.

Policy	Response to COVID-19	Citation
• Paris agreement, Montreal protocol	• Initial sharp drop in the emission of air pollutants by industry and transport sector leading to cleaner air	• UNFCC (2016) • Ozone Secretariat (2018) • Saadat et al. (2020)
	• Black carbon and NO_2 reduction	• Tobías et al. (2020)
	• Sharp rise in O_3 due to reduced NO_2	• Dantas et al. (2020) • Shakil et al. (2020)
	• Air pollution reduction by 30% • Long-term GHG emissions are plausible as economic activities and traffic will increase after each lockdown	• Wang and Su (2020)
	• Marked drop in diffuse air pollution in China, the United States, Spain, Italy, and France	• Shakil et al. (2020) • Zangari et al. (2020)
	• PM_{10} and $PM_{2.5}$ reduced to a low level	• Abdullah et al. (2020) • Dantas et al. (2020)
• Healthcare waste management • Basel Convention	• Increased biomedical waste	• WHO (2016)
	• Household waste has now become a source of biomedical waste leading to a sharp increase in pollution	• Bergesen et al. (2019) • Saadat et al. (2020)
	• No segregation of biomedical waste and municipal waste. There is no proper disposal of biomedical waste	• Zambrano-monserrate et al. (2020)
	• Lack of knowledge of biomedical waste disposal by the common man	
	• Increased bulk waste and biomedical waste from households but decreased initiatives toward recycling	
	• Presence of COVID-19 in wastewater recorded in raw sewage and also in post-secondary treatment. Enveloped viruses released from infected human feces can survive for days to months in aqueous environments. For example, SARS-CoV could survive for more than many days in relative temperatures, hospital sewage, municipal sewage, and chlorine-free tap water	• Hu et al. (2021) • Panchal et al. (2021) • Randazzo et al. (2020)
	• It was found that the increase of the SARS-CoV-2 concentration in wastewater was positively correlated with the number of COVID-19 cases	• Kumar et al. (2020)

- Disaster management
- Sendai Framework

- Due to COVID-19 there is an increase in exposure and vulnerability throughout the world
- Environmental impacts are taken into account only in event-specific, hazard-exposure, and vulnerability information
- Threatened habitats and biodiversity because of increased waste generation that is not being properly disposed of
- Disinfection of public places poses a great risk not only to microorganism ecosystems, but there is no evidence suggesting that chemicals used do not damage the environment, birds, aquatic animals, and insects

UN (2015)

environment. Without the physical environment (air, water, soil, flora, and fauna), the human environment will not thrive. It is a documented fact that there is a direct correlation between anthropogenic activity and overall environmental degradation (de Wit et al. 2020). But Montreal's best practices also show that man can also rehabilitate the environment. All it needs is a sound environmental policy.

15.3 Challenges of Creating Environmental Policy for COVID-19 and Subsequent Pandemics

Most environmental policies are guided by the polluter pays and precautionary principle. This means that it either reacts (polluter pays principle) after a disaster or is proactive (precautionary principle). This makes it a difficult process as policy formulation is determined by a number of factors. The main factors are politics and economic and social environment. These factors determine how stringent an environmental policy is and how effective it is. Politics will consider the cost-benefit analysis when looking at environmental issues. If the economy cannot handle stringent environmental legislation, politics will try to delay as it looks for better alternatives (Oates and Portney 2001). This makes it possible for a policy to drag for years without ratification or enactment. With this in mind, following are the challenges in creating COVID-19 environmental policies:

- Reactive policies
- Proactive policy formulation for COVID-19
- Environmental indifference role of media and COVID-19 Environmental Policy

15.3.1 Reactive Policies

Environmental policies are generally reactive. They take into account the immediate and future implications of anthropogenic activities. As discussed earlier, the polluter pays principle is a minefield for policymakers. It is a reactive policy – a response to the stimulus. For example, the immediate effects of air pollution are reduced visibility and poor ambient air to breathe causing a disease. The future effects of air pollution are continued greenhouse gas emissions leading to global warming, which is difficult to quantify. The global near-surface temperature has increased by 0.94–1.03 °C. This has contributed to the melting of the polar icecaps, destruction of polar bear habitats, and a decline in polar bear numbers (loss of biodiversity). The effects are cumulative and policymakers can only hypothesize. Scientific research can only use estimation, but the full implications of environmental degradation can never be realized until it is too late. This is the dilemma environmental policymakers have, trying to formulate a sound COVID-19 environmental policy, which is needed. The policy will consider current anthropogenic activities and monitor them in the event of a subsequent pandemic.

The question then becomes how to harness the polluter pays principle to make the manufacturer of single-use PPE pay for the environmental pollution from discard of PPE. What about the user? And how much do they pay to appease future implications mentioned earlier? After the oil industry, textiles are the biggest polluters despite being recyclable. Textiles are still dumped in landfills (Roy Choudhury 2014; Parikh and Rawtani 2022).

PPEs, for example, gloves, masks, gowns, and hairnets are single-use. What are the implications on energy consumption, carbon footprint, amount of water, and accumulated solid waste if everyone wears these in a single day? The externalities are unknown. What yardstick do policymakers use? It is not enough to predict future consequences.

15.3.2 Proactive Policy Formulation for COVID-19

The COVID-19 health policies have to be aligned with the COVID-19 environmental policy. The decision to save lives during COVID-19 meant introducing restrictions to movement policies, with only essential workers going to work. This was done to break the cycle of infection (Fakir and Bharati 2021). Many countries adopted these policies after seeing the devastation COVID-19 was having on other countries. These nations made pre-emptive moves to protect their populations. Now, the environment should thus be protected, by being proactive during the COVID-19 pandemic. This would be favorable but constraints that have resulted in the economy due to COVID-19 may hinder this. The environmental policymakers work within a political framework. They are endorsed by politics or the government. This means that they have a tight rope to balance. Whilst advocating for a greener environment, environmentalists also take into consideration the impact on the economy any measures they put in place. Conflict results when a balance is sought amongst these three concepts, government, economy, and environment. Caution is thus implemented in such instances.

The precautionary principle encourages that in the absence of scientific data, it is better to wait than to have irreversible environmental damage. Scientific data on COVID-19 is still being collected. There is proof that lockdown, travel bans, and restrictions on movements greatly improved the environmental quality. In a short space of time, nature manages to clean herself. The impetus to resume business as usual now that most restrictions are lifted is as yet unaccounted for. Let proactive policy restrict further the amount of emissions, let it add more animals and plants to the CITES list and encourage innovative ways to deal with waste. The impact of COVID-19 on the environment is as yet unknown. It is predicted to be damaging (Shams et al. 2021). This is the scientific fact that is "absent." This is a technical issue that can delay correct environmental policy formulation for COVID-19.

The environmental policy informs and guides legislation. Adherence to legislation is a huge hurdle to environmental rehabilitation and preservation of environmental integrity. In the face of global warming, directly attributed to anthropogenic activities, some countries have not signed/ratified global agreements, pulled out of the agreements, or are failing to reduce emissions to acceptable levels. A study correlates the ambient weather patterns with increases and intensity of colds/SARS-COV/COVID-19/envelop viruses (Shakil et al. 2020). There is a need to revisit the reasons why countries are failing to agree on global environmental treaties so that the implementation of the COVID-19 environmental policy is adhered to.

15.3.3 Environmental Indifference, Role of Media and COVID-19 Environmental Policy

Environmental indifference refers to the people's lack of concern towards environmental issues. Communities are being affected by adverse weather conditions, leading to the loss of life homes. The depth and frequency of human suffering due to natural disasters have become an everyday occurrence. The media makes it a point to report on this every day. Due to the internet, it has become easy to share news on various platforms reaching a global audience. The advantage is that the vulnerability of a society facing disaster is at the forefront of everyone and aid can be given from different sources throughout the world. The biggest disadvantage is the indifference that occurs with the consistent disaster news people are getting. Climate change and human suffering due to the disaster have become commonplace to the extent that people have become somewhat deadened to others' plight. How then can policymakers harness the media to encourage responsibility for the environment on a world population that has suffered heavy loss of life, economic depression, a sharp rise in unemployment, despondency due to impotency due to the pandemic?

The positive impact attributed to the media during the COVID-19 emergency was shown by promoting emotional health. Social media platforms led the movement to provide videos and like content that was aimed at promoting physical and mental well-being started posting videos regarding physical and mental health. (Anwar et al. 2020; Rao and Rawtani 2022). The media spread the "stay home, stay safe" message. This enabled lockdown and restrictions on movement to be effective, which, in turn, benefitted the environment to rehabilitate itself. This positive reporting in the media can be integrated into environmental policymaking for COVID-19. It is already working for health policies. Let us use it to protect the environment. Healthcare waste management and hazardous waste disposal have always been the domain of medical facilities and like institutions. Due to COVID-19, everyone is in a position to dispose of biomedical and hazardous material because of the use of PPEs. Biomedical waste and municipal waste should not be mixed because biomedical waste carries infectious pathogens. By harnessing the global reach of the media, approaches to educating the citizens can be done in easy language, foster environmental responsibility, and lead to better participation of citizens in environmental issues.

15.4 Environmental Strategies for COVID-19

Plans need to be put in place to tackle environmental issues. There is a huge discrepancy between developed and developing countries. Therefore, tailor-made strategies have to be put in place to maintain environmental integrity (OECD 2020). The burden already experienced is due to poverty, displaced communities, armed conflict, hunger, and poor developmental milestones. The pandemic is an added challenge, which not only threatens lives, but also increases the vulnerability of the physical environment to further mismanagement (de Wit et al. 2020; Dey et al. 2022). Strategies should therefore take in all these factors for better implementation of environmental policies. Proposed strategies include:

- Risk analyses and assessment of COVID-19
- Implementation of early warning systems in the environment
- Post-COVID-19 crisis management of the environment
- Building infrastructure for separation of waste.

15.4.1 Risk Analyses and Assessment of COVID-19

Risk assessment is a requisite for the implementation of satisfactory and successful disaster reduction policies. The environmental protection is an integral part of sustainable development and relief from poverty. Risk assessment is important for anticipating and alleviating the impact of natural disasters. The assessment of the risk to communities and the environment to COVID-19 shows the extent of vulnerability to pandemics. COVID-19 showed that our economies and infrastructures are inadequate to deal with the pandemic. In the face of loss of jobs and income, most people turn to environmental products for resale. Demand for herbal products as treatment and immunity boosters against COVID-19 has risen sharply. Countries in Asia, Africa, and the United States have government endorsement to look for generic drug alternatives, which has led to indiscriminate harvesting of wild herbs (Timoshyna et al. 2020; Omokhua-Uyi and Van Staden 2021).

From the earlier example, strategies to safeguard the environment from indiscriminate harvesting have to be put in place. The environment is everyone's heritage. However, if controlled properly, environmental integrity may be maintained. A clean environment protects human beings from diseases. The more pollution there is in the environment, the higher are the chances of spreading infectious diseases. Environmental rehabilitation is a strategy to minimize the risk of contracting COVID-19. Current research is showing that the spread of COVID-19 is encouraged by the weather obtained in an area. The meteorological factors include humidity, temperature, and rainfall patterns (Bilal et al. 2021). According to UNEP, anthropogenic activities have changed almost every part of the earth, exposing humans to new zoonotic diseases: three-quarters of all developing communicable diseases in humans are being transmitted from animals. We are architects of our own predicament. The systematic destruction of nature due attributable to human activities has led to climate change, ecosystem, and also biodiversity loss. Therefore, risk analysis should be two-fold and simultaneous. There is a two-fold risk analysis of humans from environmental factors and anthropogenic activities that exacerbate environmental degradation (Andersen 2020). A step toward reducing human carbon footprint post-COVID-19 is moving toward virtual platforms to engage all who are part of environmental decision-making, and thus lower environmental footprint. This has already been embraced globally with online business fora, virtual fairs, and even online lessons for school children. This reduces the carbon footprint generated by the use of fossil fuel used just to attend a meeting in person.

15.4.2 Implementation of Early Warning Systems in the Environment

Prediction of adverse environmental disasters is an important strategy to develop against COVID-19. Early warning systems are an essential tool for forecasting the environmental damage due to COVID-19. To predict and track rates of infection and death due to COVID-19, early warning systems are in use. Detecting and monitoring of COVID-19 among patients with early warning systems predicted proximity to infected people, the efficacy of treatment, and patients in need of intensive care among other parameters (Zhou et al. 2020; Rao and Rawtani 2022). The same concept can be developed for the environment. An example is testing and finding the COVID-19 virus in wastewater in India (Panchal et al. 2021). Though this detection shows the failure of wastewater treatment because, after treatment, this wastewater is deposited back into the environment. This can be used as an early warning system for the presence of COVID-19, and also the need for better methods of wastewater treatment. A recent study is also showing that wastewater treatment facilities are failing to thoroughly remove compounds used in making antibiotics and personal care products. These are very soluble in water and pose a risk for aquatic animals (Shraim et al. 2017). Some of the effects include developmental reproductive problems in fish and frogs (Hernando et al. 2006). The number of infected people reached more than 200 million and we are still counting. If all of these people accessed medical assistance and were given antibiotics to fight COVID-19 infection, then the magnitude of pharmaceuticals that have entered wastewater from excretion, if visualized, is enormous. Therefore, technologies to detect the COVID-19 virus and subsequent antibiotics can be used as early warning systems to avert ecological disasters.

Strategies for post-COVID-19 management should target building global resilience to economic recession owing to a pandemic. The sustainable development goals should be closely linked with the recovery of economies post-COVID-19. Sustainable goal number one aims at reducing poverty (Johnston 2016). For this to be achievable post-COVID-19, growth in economies should include all people, be sustained, and address all forms of inequality. An example of the impact of COVID-19 is in Africa as a developing continent. Africa is facing a greater risk. Despite its natural resource wealth, pollution, recession due to COVID-19, extreme weather phenomena, and debt, it will further impoverish the continent. This is the trend that will affect all developing countries (OECD 2020). Strategies should align with making the economy green. It should be central to government plans. Business, industry, and social recovery should target greater environmental outcomes. This is a great opportunity for an economic do-over. The world needs to rectify poverty because the affected communities are the most vulnerable in the case of a pandemic. They cannot adhere to COVID-19 regulations if they are hungry and do not have shelter. This situation opens up the door for unregulated trade in wildlife and herbal plants and pollution (Chomel et al. 2007; Timoshyna et al. 2020; de Wit et al. 2020). Greater commitment is needed for investment in reducing carbon footprint in line with the Paris agreement. This involves looking for and implementing clean energy sources. There is a need to put more advocacy on the use of solar power for energy requirements. This does away with the burning of fossil fuels, which emit GHGs like carbon dioxide and methane. In the same vein, energy consumption must be monitored and be a responsibility of everyone. By investing in green energy, we are financing efforts for a better climate and preservation of environmental integrity. Approaches to green energy are supported by the green recovery of the economy, green technologies, and economic growth that utilizes indigenous investment, labor, and technologies (Andersen 2020).

With a focus to reduce greenhouse gas emissions, innovation and new technologies can be a source of new jobs for people who lost jobs during the pandemic. Research into this shows that more jobs are created when investment into green energy is done in comparison with jobs in nonrenewable energy.

15.4.3 Post-COVID-19 Crisis Management of the Environment

If anything, the emergence of COVID-19 has shown that greater global cooperation is needed to build resilience. With that same concept, more energy should be expended toward fulfilling global commitments such as reducing emission pollution, safeguarding biodiversity, and post-COVID-19 waste supervision. Another reciprocal approach is environment-specific policies, education, and creating awareness among the public of the link between human health and the environment. The public needs to know that climate change is enabling the spread of infectious pathogens. The link between habitat loss, zoonotic disease spread, and humans must also be shown for everyone to understand (Chomel et al. 2007). The more human development intrudes into wildlife habitats, destroying them, the more susceptible humans get to the zoonotic disease. COVID-19 is a disease transmitted by animals to humans. Scientific research attributes the host animal for COVID-19 to be a bat (MacKenzie and Smith 2020). Governments must band together and put restrictions on the wildlife trade. They must create legislation that safeguards biodiversity, which allows it to rehabilitate. There must be policies and strategies that guide scientific study to better comprehend and respond to any threats of zoonotic nature.

15.4.4 Building Infrastructure for Separation of Waste

New infrastructure with the capacity to manage waste should be built. The UNEP is offering support for green technology and eco-friendly infrastructure to governments, which need to create new infrastructure. The increased quantity of biomedical waste means that waste separation, storage, and ultimate disposal are important. The COVID-19 waste generated must be managed correctly to reduce new infections due to improper disposal. Pollution due to plastics is also a threat to environmental health. The use of PPEs has been attributed to an influx of plastic pollution. Plastic does not break down easily. They will break down into micro- and nano-plastics, which will then enter animal systems and cause damage (Shams et al. 2021). The effect of plastic incineration should also be taken into account as it will release greenhouse gases, which contribute to global warming.

15.5 Conclusion

The goal is environmental sustainability. Policy monitoring is important to achieve this goal. The pandemic has come in an environment that is threatened by climate change, pollution, species endangerment, and loss of habitat. It adds another challenge for a man to decipher. There is only one earth for future generations. There is a need to make a futuristic environmental policy. Let it be guided by the best practices. Policy formulation with public participation is important. This creates a sense of ownership and responsibility at the same time fostering effective environmental protection. Environmental policies must address economic externalities with more stringent measures. Transboundary pollution is an example of an unforeseen and uncounted for the circumstance. Waste dumped in oceans or incinerated will cause environmental degradation in different parts of the environment. This becomes difficult for purposes of accountability. The new policy and new approaches to the education on environmental matters need to be adopted.

There is a research gap on the implications of the COVID-19 pandemic on the environment. The current environmental policies seem to be failing to unite governments to focus on one aim – environmental integrity. Given the intensity of the virus, as seen by its short duration and high mortality rate in humans, the existing link between human health and zoonotic disease needs to be investigated. In searching for herbal remedies for COVID-19, the natural plant world is also under threat. The drive to alleviate COVID-19 symptoms and boost immunity has led to a rise in the demand for herbal solutions. Transparent transection in accordance with well-written legislation, certification, and value addition can safeguard wild plants (Timoshyna et al. 2020).

Let policies and strategies for the environment align with economic and health policies. The environment is vital to our survival. It is now time that it is treated as such. Let new technologies mirror the need for environmental sustainability. The new policy and new approaches to education on environmental matters need to be adopted.

References

Abdullah, S., Abu Mansor, A., Mohd Napi, N.N.L., et al. (2020) 'Air quality status during 2020 Malaysia Movement Control Order (MCO) due to 2019 novel coronavirus (2019-nCoV) pandemic', *Science of the Total Environment*, 729, p. 139022. doi:10.1016/j.scitotenv.2020.139022.

Andersen, I. (2020). *Working With the Environment to Protect People*. UNEP.

Anwar, Ayesha Malik M, Raees V, Anwar A. (2020) 'Role of mass media and public health communications in the COVID-19 pandemic', *Cureus*, 12(9) e10453. doi: https://doi.org/10.7759/CUREUS.10453.

Benson, D. and Jordan, A. (2015). *Environmental policy: protection and regulation*. In: *International Encyclopedia of the Social & Behavioral Sciences*, 2e. Elsevier https://doi.org/10.1016/B978-0-08-097086-8.91014-6.

Bergesen, H. O., Parmann, G. and Thommessen, O. B. (2019) 'Convention on the Control of Transboundary Movements of Hazardous Wastes and their Disposal (Basel Convention)', *Yearbook of International Cooperation on Environment and Development* 1998–99, pp. 87–89. doi: 10.4324/9781315066547-15.

Bilal, Bashir, M.F., Shahzad, K. et al. (2021). Environmental quality, climate indicators, and COVID-19 pandemic: insights from top 10 most affected states of the USA. *Environmental Science and Pollution Research International* 28 (25): 32856–32865. https://doi.org/10.1007/s11356-021-12646-x.

Chomel, B. B., Belotto, A. and Meslin, F.-X. (2007) 'Wildlife, exotic pets, and emerging zoonoses1', *Emerging Infectious Disease* 13(1), pp. 6–11. doi: https://doi.org/10.3201/eid1301.060480.

Dantas, G., Siciliano, B., Boscaro França, B. et al. (2020) '*The impact of COVID-19 partial lockdown on the air quality of the city of Rio de Janeiro*, Brazil', (January).

Dey, A., Rao, P.K., and Rawtani, D. (2022). Risk management of COVID-19. In: *COVID-19 in the Environment*, 217–230. https://doi.org/10.1016/B978-0-323-90272-4.00018-X.

Deziel, N. (2014). Pharmaceuticals in wastewater treatment plant effluent waters. *Scholarly Horizons: University of Minnesota, Morris Undergraduate Journal* 1 (2): 12.

Fakir, A.M.S. and Bharati, T. (2021). Pandemic catch-22: the role of mobility restrictions and institutional inequalities in halting the spread of COVID-19. *PLoS One* 16 (6): 1–29. https://doi.org/10.1371/journal.pone.0253348.

Hernando, M. D. Mezcua M, Fernández-Alba AR, Barceló D (2006) 'Environmental risk assessment of pharmaceutical residues in wastewater effluents, surface waters and sediments', *Talanta*, 69(2 SPEC. ISS.), pp. 334–342. doi: https://doi.org/10.1016/j.talanta.2005.09.037.

Hu, L., Deng, Wen-Jing., Ying, Guang-Guo. et al. (2021) 'Environmental perspective of COVID-19: Atmospheric and wastewater environment in relation to pandemic', *Ecotoxicology and Environmental Safety*, 219(January), p. 112297. doi: 10.1016/j.ecoenv.2021.112297.

Johnston, R.B. (2016). Arsenic and the 2030 Agenda for sustainable development. In: *Arsenic Research and Global Sustainability – Proceedings of the 6th International Congress on Arsenic in the Environment, AS 2016*, 12–14. https://doi.org/10.1201/b20466-7.

Kumari, V. and Tripathi, A.K. (2019). Characterization of pharmaceuticals industrial effluent using GC–MS and FT-IR analyses and defining its toxicity. *Applied Water Science* 9 (8): 1–8. https://doi.org/10.1007/s13201-019-1064-z.

Kumar, M., Kumar Patel, A., Shah, A.V. et al. (2020) 'First proof of the capability of wastewater surveillance for COVID-19 in India through detection of genetic material of SARS-CoV-2', (January).

MacKenzie, J.S. and Smith, D.W. (2020). COVID-19: a novel zoonotic disease caused by a coronavirus from China: what we know and what we don't. *Microbiology Australia* 41 (1): 45–50. https://doi.org/10.1071/MA20013.

Minamata Disease Muicipal Museum (2007). *Minamata Disease: Its History and Lessons*, 135–148. *Minimata City Planning Division*.

Oates, W. E. and Portney, P. R. (2001). The Political Economy of Environmental Policy, Resources for the Future, Discussion Paper 01-55, November 2001.

OECD (2020) '*Developing Countries and Development Co-Operation: What is at Stake ?*', (April), OECD Publishing pp. 1–17.

Oliver, K. and Cairney, P. (2019). *The dos and don'ts of influencing policy: a systematic review of advice to academics. Palgrave Communications* Palgrave Macmillan Ltd. https://doi.org/10.1057/s41599-019-0232-y.

Omokhua-Uyi, A.G. and Van Staden, J. (2021). Natural product remedies for COVID-19: a focus on safety. *South African Journal of Botany* 139 (January): 386–398. https://doi.org/10.1016/j.sajb.2021.03.012.

Ozone Secretariat (2018). *Montreal Protocol Handbook*. UNEP.

Panchal, D. Prakash O, Bobde P, Pal S (2021) 'SARS-CoV-2: sewage surveillance as an early warning system and challenges in developing countries', *Environmental Science and Pollution Research*, 28(18), pp. 22221–22240. doi: https://doi.org/10.1007/s11356-021-13170-8.

Parikh, G. and Rawtani, D. (2022). Environmental impact of COVID-19. In: *COVID-19 in the Environment*, 203–216. https://doi.org/10.1016/B978-0-323-90272-4.00001-4.

Rao, P.K. and Rawtani, D. (2022). Modern digital techniques for monitoring and analysis. In: *COVID-19 in the Environment*, 115–130. https://doi.org/10.1016/B978-0-323-90272-4.00015-4.

Rawtani, D., Hussain, C.M., and Khatri, N. (2022). *COVID-19 in the Environment: Impact, Concerns, and Management of Coronavirus*. Elsevier.

Randazzo, W., Truchado, P., Cuevas-Ferrando, E. et al. (2020) 'SARS-CoV-2 RNA in wastewater anticipated COVID-19 occurrence in a low prevalence area', (January).

Roy Choudhury, A. K. (2014) *Environmental impacts of the textile industry and its assessment through life cycle assessment. Roadmap to Sustainable Textiles and Clothing* (pp. 1–39). doi: https://doi.org/10.1007/978-981-287-110-7_1.

Saadat, S., Rawtani, D. and Hussain, C. M. (2020) 'Environmental perspective of COVID-19', *Science of the Total Environment*, 728(January). doi: 10.1016/j.scitotenv.2020.138870.

Shakil, M. H. Munim ZH, Tasnia M, Sarowar S (2020) 'COVID-19 and the environment: a critical review and research agenda', *Science of the Total Environment*, 745, p. 141022. doi: https://doi.org/10.1016/j.scitotenv.2020.141022.

Shams, M., Alam, I., and Mahbub, M.S. (2021). Plastic pollution during COVID-19: plastic waste directives and its long-term impact on the environment. *Environmental Advances* 5: 100119. https://doi.org/10.1016/j.envadv.2021.100119.

Shraim, A., Diab, A., Alsuhaimi, A. et al. (2017). Analysis of some pharmaceuticals in municipal wastewater of Almadinah Almunawarah. *Arabian Journal of Chemistry* 10 (Suppl. 1): S719–S729. https://doi.org/10.1016/j.arabjc.2012.11.014.

Timoshyna, A., Ling, X., and Leaman, D. (2020). The invisible trade in the times of COVID-19 and the essential. https://www.traffic.org/Site/Assets/Files/12955/Covid-Wild-At-Home-Final.Pdf.

Tobías, A., Carnerero, C., Reche, C. et al. (2020) 'Changes in air quality during the lockdown in Barcelona (Spain) one month into the SARS-CoV-2 epidemic', (January).

Torjman, S. (2005) '*What is Policy? by What is Policy?*', (September). The Caledon Institute of Social Policy

UNFCC (2016) - Paris, T. (2016) 'The Paris', 2(4), pp. 78–79.

United Nations (1992). A/CONF.151/26/Vol.I: Rio declaration on environment and development. *Report of the United Nations Conference on Environment and Development* I (August), Rio de Janeiro (3–14 June 1992), pp. 1–5.

UN (2015). *Annex I Sendai Declaration*. www.unisdr.org/we/inform/terminology

Wang, Q. and Su, M. (2020) 'A preliminary assessment of the impact of COVID-19 on environment – A case study of China', *Science of the Total Environment*, 728, p. 138915. doi: 10.1016/j.scitotenv.2020.138915.

Weible, C. M., Nohrstedt, D., Cairney, P. *et al.* (2020) 'COVID-19 and the policy sciences: initial reactions and perspectives', *Policy Sciences*, 53(2), pp. 225–241. doi: https://doi.org/10.1007/s11077-020-09381-4.

WHO (2016) - WHO (2016) 'Management of waste from injection activities at district level Guidelines for District Health Managers', *World Health Organisation*, 54(8), pp. 200–289.

WHO (2020). Coronavirus disease 2019 situation report 51 – 11th March 2020. *WHO Bulletin* 2019 (March): 2633.

de Wit, W., Freschi, A., and Trench, E. (2020). *COVID 19: Urgent Call to Protect*, 3.

Zambrano-monserrate, M. A., Alejandra, M. and Sanchez-alcalde, L. (2020) 'Indirect effects of COVID-19 on the environment', (January).

Zangari, S, D. T., C, A. and Mirowsky, J. E. (2020) 'Science of the Total Environment Air quality changes in New York City during the COVID-19 pandemic', *Science of the Total Environment*, 742(December 2019), p.140496. doi: 10.1016/j.scitotenv.2020.140496.

Zhou, H. Huang H, Xie X, Gao J, Wu J, Zhu Y, He W, Liu J, Li A, Xu Y (2020) 'Development of early warning and rapid response system for patients with novel coronavirus pneumonia (COVID-19): a research protocol', *Medicine*, 99(34), p. e21874. doi: https://doi.org/10.1097/MD.0000000000021874.

16

Environmental Implications of Pandemic on Climate

Sapna Jain[1], Bhawna Yadav Lamba[1], Madhuben Sharma[2], and Sanjeev Kumar[1]

[1] *Department of Applied Sciences and humanities, School of Engineering, University of Petroleum and Energy Studies, Bidholi, Energy Acres, Dehradun, Uttarakhand, India*
[2] *School of Engineering, University of Petroleum and Energy Studies, Bidholi, Energy Acres, Dehradun, Uttarakhand, India*

16.1   Introduction

In December 2019, Wuhan city, China, observed the spread of a pneumonia-like disease that eventually spread across the world. The disease was named COVID-19 and due to its dreadful effect, it was declared a pandemic by the World Health Organization (WHO) in March 2020. All the affected countries reported a huge death toll due to the disease. Till the mid of the month of May 2020, it has caused more than 4.8 million infections and about 3.2 lakh deaths in 216 countries.

In India, at that time, the condition was not as frightening with respect to the population density. The same can be attributed to the initial control measures taken by the government and national agencies. One of the measures taken to control the condition was lockdown. The imposition of the lockdown hampered the normal functioning of many activities, with particularly large impacts on travel, tourism, various retail markets, factories, and power generation. The restricted activities helped in the revival of the environment. The implications of the lockdown created a noticeable effect on the economy at both local and global levels. In India, the fuel growth rate declined dramatically with more than 50% lesser consumption. An increase in the consumption of liquefied petroleum (LPG) gas indicated that the cooking at home increased during the lockdown period. An impact on the environment was also observed in terms of better air quality. The impacts were short term. However, the study can be an indicative measure of strategic planning for the benefit of the environment. The instantaneously measurable factors are emissions of air pollutants, improvement in air quality, water quality, etc.

There are many reports suggesting the improvement in air quality based on various mapping technologies like satellite mapping or direct measurement of the concentration of various air pollutants.

A study conducted on the effect of lockdown on pollution levels in three cities of the central China indicated a significant improvement in air quality in terms of the lower level of a particulate matter, sulfur dioxide, carbon monoxide, and nitrogen dioxide (Xu et al. 2020). Another study reported a prominent decrease in the concentrations of common pollutants in the city of Sao Paulo, Brazil during the lockdown in the months of February, March, and April (Urban and Nakada 2021). They compared the impact with the data of the previous five years.

Similar studies in Barcelona (Tobias et al. 2020) and Rio de Janerio (Dantas et al. 2020) also showed a decline in the pollution level owing to the lockdown in the courtiers.

Scientists in various parts of India also studied a comparable effect on air quality. The later part of the chapter described case studies on two different regions of north India.

16.2 Cast Study 1: Megacities of India (Jain and Sharma 2020)

16.2.1 Methodology

Case study 1 describes the impact of restricted activities amid COVID-19 on the air quality of major cities of India, viz. Delhi, Chennai, Bengaluru, Mumbai, and Kolkata. The real-time air quality data were taken from the Central Pollution Control Board (CPCB)-monitoring stations.

16.2.2 Size Description and Data Collection

The selected major cities of India are the economic centers and thus observe more travel movements both at the national and international levels. Delhi and Mumbai were considered epicenters of COVID-19 in India. Both the cities are analyzed for a link between coronavirus infections and air pollution control. The data on air quality was obtained from the CPCB for all the studied air quality parameters:

i) Particulate matter 2.5
ii) Particulate matter 10
iii) Carbon monoxide
iv) Nitrogen dioxide
v) Ozone

The following three meteorological parameters were also studied:

i) Ambient temperature
ii) Relative humidity
iii) Wind speed

The data from all the monitoring stations of each city was procured, viz. thirty-eight centers in Delhi, ten in Mumbai, ten in Bengaluru, and seven in Kolkata.

The data for two years (2019 and 2020) was considered in each city as 24-hour average data. It was collected for 22 days of the year 2019 [20 March to 10 April] and 32 days for the year 2020 [10 March to 10 April]. The study used a tool to understand the maximum and minimum affected places within the city. The tool helped interpolate pollutant concentrations of the entire city.

16.3   Results and Analysis

Daily and annual variations of results of air quality analysis have been analyzed for the five megacities. An extended study to understand spatiotemporal variation in the concentration of air pollutants has been done for two megacities, Delhi and Mumbai. In order to understand the impact of wind speed, ambient temperature, and relative humidity, a time series analysis of daily variations of air pollutant concentration and meteorological parameters has been studied.

All the air pollutants observed a dip in their concentration and ozone observed a hike in the concentration. The variation in the concentration of air pollutants was observed in all five cities. The trend in the concentration of ozone was on a decline in the year 2019. However, there was an increase in the year 2020. The extent of a decrease in the concentration of other pollutants showed a variable trend in the different cities. The values of concentration of air pollutants were in good agreement with the National Ambient Air Quality Standards (NAAQS). However, only Mumbai, Bengaluru, and Chennai were found to be within permissible limits for $PM_{2.5}$ of the WHO standards. All cities exceeded the value for PM_{10} of the WHO standards. Similarly, all cities were within permissible limits of ozone value of the WHO standards (Table 16.1).

Before the lockdown period, the concentration of all the air pollutants, except for $PM_{2.5}$ for Delhi ($66 \mu g\ m^{-3}$) was within the limit of NAAQS. Similarly, the concentration PM_{10} exceeded the standard values in Delhi ($153 \mu g\ m^{-3}$), Mumbai ($126\ \mu g\ m^{-3}$), and Kolkata ($113 \mu g\ m^{-3}$).

A similar trend was recorded for the lockdown period (March–April 2020) in comparison to the previous year's data except for PM_{10} values of Delhi ($222 \mu g\ m^{-3}$), Kolkata ($102 \mu g\ m^{-3}$), and Bengaluru ($118 \mu g\ m^{-3}$), and $PM_{2.5}$ value for Delhi ($89 \mu g\ m^{-3}$).

As per the WHO, a decrease in the concentration of $PM_{2.5}$ value can reduce the premature deaths by 15%. The impact of a decrease in values of pollutants for such a short duration cannot decide or control the mortality, still it can affect the morbidity and quality of life.

Further, the results in the report showed a percentage change in all criteria pollutants in each of the studied cities, for two years (March–April 2019 and March–April 2020). A high decrease in the concentration of nitrogen dioxide was observed in all the cities, with a maximum reported value of more than 75% in Mumbai. As compared to the previous two

Table 16.1   Values of air pollutants as per the NAAQS standards and the WHO standards.

Air pollutant	NAAQS ($\mu g\ m^{-3}$)	WHO standards
$PM_{2.5}$ (based on 24-hr average)	60	$25 \mu g\ m^{-3}$
PM_{10} (based on 24-hr average)	100	$50 \mu g\ m^{-3}$
Nitrogen dioxide (based on 24-hr average)	80	—
Sulfur dioxide (based on 24-hr average)	80	—
Carbon monoxide (based on 8-hr average)	2	—
Ozone (based on 8-hr average)	100	$100 \mu g\ m^{-3}$

decades, a remarkable decline in the concentration of all the air pollutants was reported in Delhi.

The decrease in values of air pollutants, in Delhi, can be summarized as:

a) PM_{10}: Before lockdown = 153 µg m^{-3}, after lockdown = 73 µg m^{-3}, 52% decline.
b) $PM_{2.5}$: Before lockdown = 66 µg m^{-3}, after lockdown = 39 µg m^{-3}, 41% decline.
c) NO_2: Before lockdown = 39 µg m^{-3}, after lockdown = 19 µg m^{-3}, 50% decline.
d) CO: Before lockdown = 0.9 µg m^{-3}, after lockdown = 0.65 µg m^{-3}, 29% decline.

An increase in the concentration of ozone was observed in Delhi (7%) during the lockdown period as compared to before the lockdown period. A similar decrease in pollutant concentration and an increase in ozone concentration were also reported from other parts of world. Xu et al. stated similar trends in cities of the Hubei province, Wuhan, Jingmen, and Enshi. The report compared the average air pollutant data for three months (January to March) of three years (2017–2019) with three months (January to March) of the year 2020. The report suggested:

i) $PM_{2.5}$ concentration: In Wuhan, the decrease was to 59.6 µg m^{-3} from 88.6 µg m^{-3}; a drop to 38 µg m^{-3} from 67.9, and a drop to 34.5 µg m^{-3} from 53.1 in the three months January, February, and March, respectively.
ii) PM_{10} concentration: In Wuhan, the decline was 30–48%.
iii) Carbon monoxide concentration: In Wuhan, the decline was 7–23%.
iv) Nitrogen dioxide concentration: In Wuhan, the decline was 30–61%.
v) Ozone concentration: In Wuhan, the increase was 9–27%.

Case study 1 reported that in Chennai, the decline in the concentration of $PM_{2.5}$ was by 4 µg m^{-3} (14%), nitrogen dioxide was 3 µg m^{-3} (30%), and carbon monoxide was 0.75 µg m^{-3} to 0.56 µg m^{-3} (25%). A rise in the concentration of ozone was not significant enough in Chennai (only 3%). In Kolkata, the decline in the concentration of $PM_{2.5}$ was from 58 to 46 µg m^{-3}; in Mumbai, $PM_{2.5}$ observed a dip from 37 to 45 µg m^{-3} while in Bengaluru, the decline was from 35 to 27 µg m^{-3}. The other pollutant level also observed a significant decline as high as 75% in the cities. Except for Bengaluru, all selected cities observed an increase in the concentration of ozone during the lockdown period.

a) Kolkata: Increase in the concentration of ozone from 51 to 60 µg m^{-3}
b) Mumbai: Increase in the concentration of ozone from 33 to 36 µg m^{-3}
c) Chennai: Increase in concentration of ozone from 43 to 44 µg m^{-3}

The study also reported spatiotemporal analysis using the GIS technique for Delhi and Mumbai. The two are more populous and polluted cities as compared to the other three.

16.3.1 Meteorology and Air Quality in Megacities

The dispersion of air pollutants is governed by the speed of air, temperature, and relative humidity. High wind speed, high temperature, and lower relative humidity favor dispersion of air pollutants and thus decrease their concentration in the environment. The study showed a time series analysis of all the air pollutants and important meteorological parameters. The analysis shows that the wind speed was less than before the lockdown period (0.5 m s^{-1}) as compared to the wind speed after the lockdown (0.7–1.2 m s^{-1}). Similarly, the relative humidity was 58–78% before the lockdown and 50–64% after the lockdown. The temperature was also high (27–32 °C) after lockdown as compared to the temperature before the lockdown (22–27 °C). The more decline in the pollution level in the northern cities may further be due to wind directions. The wind direction was south and southwest.

16.4 Cast Study 2: Selected Cities of Rajasthan, India

16.4.1 Methodology

Case study 2 describes the impact of restricted activities amid COVID-19 on the air quality of seven cities of Rajasthan, India, viz. Ajmer, Alwar, Bhiwadi, Jaipur, Jodhpur, Kota, and Udaipur. Real-time air quality data were taken from CPCB monitoring stations (CPCB 2020).

16.4.2 Size Description and Data Collection

As per data available, among the top 30 most polluted cities in the world, more than twenty cities are in India alone (WAQR 2019; WAQR 2018; CNN 2020). According to a report, the state of Rajasthan reported a maximum death rate due to air pollution. It was measured per lakh population. The deaths were due to regular exposure to air pollutants for a longer period of time TOI (2018). Rajasthan has the highest death rate per lakh due to air pollution, i.e. because of the exposure to ambient air pollutants over a prolonged period of time (TOI 2018).

The change of economic dependence from agriculture to industries (desired for substantial employment and economy uplifting) has increased the pollution level in the state. The industries were established in selected cities like Bhiwadi, Bhilwara, Jaipur, Kota, and Udaipur. The major industries in Rajasthan are (Maps of India 2011):

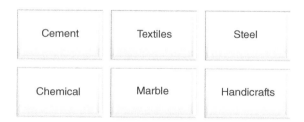

| Cement | Textiles | Steel |
| Chemical | Marble | Handicrafts |

Also, there are a lot of tourist places in the state. These industries and tourism are the main sources of air pollution in the state (Kumar and Sharma 2016; Chauhan 2010).

The data on air quality was obtained from the CPCB for all the studied air quality parameters (CPCB 2020).

  i) Particulate matter 2.5
 ii) Particulate matter 10
iii) Nitrogen dioxide
 iv) Sulfur dioxide
  v) Ozone

16.5   Result and Analysis

Similar to the previous case study, this study also reported a significant decline in the air pollution level during the lockdown period amid the COVID-19 pandemic. All the criteria of air pollutants observed a decrease in concentration except for ozone. The study is divided into different phases of lockdown:

i) Phase 1: 25 March to 14 April, 2020
ii) Phase 2: 15 April to 3 May, 2020
iii) Phase 3: 4 May to 14 May, 2020
iv) Phase 4: 18 May to 31 May, 2020.

The decline in the concentration of pollutants was more significant in the first phase of lockdown. With relaxation in the restrictions, the decline in the air pollutants level becomes less prominent in the later phases of lockdown. The same may be correlated to the extent of restrictions where the later phases of the lockdown observed relaxation. The values of concentration of air pollutants were in good agreement with the NAAQS during the lockdown in the studied cities. (Table 16.1).

The concentrations of all the studied pollutants were within the limit of NAAQS standards, except for the concentration of PM_{10} in four cities – Ajmer ($110.30\,\mu g\ m^{-3}$), Bhiwadi ($178.54\,\mu g\ m^{-3}$), Jaipur ($105.256\,\mu g\ m^{-3}$), and Jodhpur ($154.34\,\mu g\ m^{-3}$).

The results showed the following changes in the percentage of concentration of air pollutants [average of the three phases of lockdown was taken for comparison]:

i) Alwar: A significant decrease of about 47% was observed in $PM_{2.5}$ concentration and about a 42% decline in the concentration of PM_{10}. A decrease in the concentration of nitrogen dioxide by 30% and the concentration of sulfur dioxide by 42%. The ozone concentration was found to increase by 10%.
ii) Ajmer: A significant decrease of about 47% was observed in $PM_{2.5}$ concentration and about a 42% decline in the concentration of PM_{10}. A decrease in the concentration of nitrogen dioxide by 32%. The ozone concentration was found to increase by 1.3% and sulfur dioxide by 2%.
iii) Bhiwadi: A significant decrease of about 58% was observed in $PM_{2.5}$ concentration and about a 44% decline in the concentration of PM_{10}. A decrease in the concentration of nitrogen dioxide by 64% and Sulfur dioxide by 69%. The ozone concentration was found to increase by 45%.
iv) Jaipur: A decrease of about 30% was observed in $PM_{2.5}$ concentration and about a 33% decline in the concentration of PM_{10}. A significant decrease in the concentration of nitrogen dioxide by 56%. The ozone concentration was found to decrease by 25% and sulfur dioxide by 15%.
v) Jodhpur: A decrease of about 30% was observed in $PM_{2.5}$ concentration and about a 33% decline in the concentration of PM_{10}. A decrease in the concentration of nitrogen dioxide by 56% and sulfur dioxide by 38%. The ozone concentration was found to increase by 1%.
vi) Kota: A decrease of about 29% was observed in $PM_{2.5}$ concentration and about a 29% decline in the concentration of PM_{10}. A decrease in the concentration of nitrogen dioxide by 44% and sulfur dioxide by 3%. The ozone concentration was found to increase by 22%.

vii) Udaipur: A decrease of about 29% was observed in $PM_{2.5}$ concentration and about a 29% decline in the concentration of PM_{10}. A decrease in the concentration of nitrogen dioxide by 44% and sulfur dioxide by 3%. The ozone concentration was found to increase by 22%.

As per the results, nitrogen dioxide concentration observed the most significant dip among all the air pollutants. Bhiwadi city observed a maximum dip of 64%. Dutheil and coworkers also reported a similar decline in the concentration of nitrogen dioxide in China (Dutheil et al. 2020).

The concentration of sulfur dioxide also observed a noticeable change in three cities – Bhiwadi, Alwar, and Jodhpur. Similarly, the maximum decline in the concentration of PM_{10} and $PM_{2.5}$ was observed in Bhiwadi.

Similar to case study 1, the ozone concentration witnessed an increase in concentration in all the selected cities except for Jaipur. The maximum increase in concentration was in Kota.

16.5.1 Meteorology and Air Quality: Case Study 2

The study showed a time series analysis of all the air pollutants and available meteorological parameters, wind speed and temperature (Sharma et al. 2020). The average wind speed increased in all except Ajmer.

- Alwar: The wind speed was $1.56\,m\,s^{-1}$ before lockdown and 1.83, 1.69, and $1.67\,m\,s^{-1}$ during the three phases of lockdown, respectively.
- Ajmer: The wind speed was $3.4\,m\,s^{-1}$ before lockdown and 2.5, 2.38, and $3.07\,m\,s^{-1}$ during the three phases of lockdown, respectively.
- Bhiwadi: The wind speed was $0.82\,m\,s^{-1}$ before lockdown and 0.99, 0.82, and $0.82\,m\,s^{-1}$ during the three phases of lockdown, respectively.
- Kota: The wind speed was $1.15\,m\,s^{-1}$ before lockdown and 1.12, 1.46, and $1.4\,m\,s^{-1}$ during the three phases of lockdown, respectively.
- Jaipur: The wind speed was $1.07\,m\,s^{-1}$ before lockdown and 1.27, 1.25, and $1.18\,m\,s^{-1}$ during the three phases of lockdown, respectively.
- Jodhpur: The wind speed was $0.86\,m\,s^{-1}$ before lockdown and 0.77, 0.88, and $0.86\,m\,s^{-1}$ during the three phases of lockdown, respectively.
- Udaipur: The wind speed was $2.34\,m\,s^{-1}$ before lockdown and 2.22, 2.42, and $2.23\,m\,s^{-1}$ during the three phases of lockdown, respectively.

Likewise, all the selected cities observed a hike in the temperature during the lockdown period as compared to before the lockdown period. The high temperature and high wind speed during lockdown favored the dispersion of air pollutants in the selected cities.

16.6 Special Area of Study: Bhiwadi

Bhiwadi is an industrial hub of Rajasthan and is part of the Alwar district. The area has all kinds of industries ranging from small-scale to larger ones. The Rajasthan State Industrial Development and Investment Corporation (RIICO) has facilitated the establishment of various automobile manufacturing enterprises making Bhiwadi an automative hub of

Rajasthan. The air quality of the Bhiwadi region is the poorest owing to high industrialization and urbanization. The most significant effect of lockdown was observed in Bhiwadi. A statistical analysis showed a significant improvement in the quality.

16.7 Conclusion

The contrast in the trend of ozone concentration can be correlated to a decrease in the concentration of nitrogen dioxide, increased solar radiations, and thus modulations in the photochemical reactions involved in the formation and destruction of ozone in the environment. Nitrogen oxides (NOx) and volatile organic compounds (VOCs) are considered ozone precursors. The concentration of ozone depends upon different meteorological parameters like temperature, solar radiations, wind speed, etc., and on the concentration of volatile organic matter and oxides of nitrogen. In the presence of sunlight, the VOC and oxides of nitrogen undergo multiple-step reactions (Srivastava et al. 2005; Lee et al. 2002). The urban area falls under the VOC-limited region and the cities studied in both the case studies are urban and thus can be categorized as the VOC-limited region (Seinfeld and Pandis 1998). The importance of the VOC-limited environment is that the ozone concentration depends upon the emission of nitrogen oxides and ozone, apart from the meteorological parameters. Thus, the increase in the concentration of ozone in these studies could be correlated, safely, with the increase in solar radiations and the decline in the concentration of nitrogen oxides.

The decrease in the concentration of nitrogen oxides in the cities studied in both the case studies is a result of retarded human activities, like transport, industrial processes, and agriculture. These activities are the major sources of nitrogen production in the environment. During the lockdown, all these were put on hold leading to the lowering of the concentration of nitrogen oxides in the VOC-limited environment and thus an increase in ozone concentration. (Sharma and Dikshit 2016; Kim et al. 2018; Sicard et al. 2020; Shrestha et al. 2020).

The reduction in the level of the particulate matter of size 2.5 ($PM_{2.5}$) can also be correlated to a reduction in the concentration of nitrogen dioxide. Nitrogen dioxide plays an important role in the chemistry of the formation of the secondary particulate matter. The other factors that played a role in the reduced level of air pollutants are the closing of industrial areas, the shutdown of constructions, less road dust due to less transport, a decline in the demand for electricity from thermal power plants. The offices, educational institutes, malls, theaters, etc., were shut down during lockdown that resulted in a decrease in the demand for electricity from 20–30% in the various regions of the studied cities.

As per reports, most of the coal power plants were closed in the northern parts of India (Haryana, Uttar Pradesh, and Punjab) except for two at the Dadri power plant in Uttar Pradesh (CREA 2020). The lesser decrease in the concentration of air pollutants in the southern cities like Bengaluru and Chennai can be due to excessive stubble burning owing to the failure of selling agricultural residue. The farmers could not sell the same as the transport facility was stopped during the lockdown period amid the COVID-19 pandemic.

The decline in air pollutant concentrations is also related to the meteorological parameters. Previous reports have suggested that the decrease in relative humidity from 50 to 20%

has increased the concentrations of $PM_{2.5}$ and PM_{10} 1.07 and 1.09 times high, respectively (Putaud et al. 2004). A similar negative correlation between humidity and particulate matters was suggested by Jayamurugan and coworkers (Jayamurugan et al. 2013). Thus, the restricted activity and meteorological parameters both played a role in improving the air quality during the lockdown period.

The chapter gives a clear picture that the imposition of lockdown has affected the environment in a positive manner. However, these are more instantaneously measured factors and highlight the short-term effect on the environment. There is a need to understand and develop sustainable measures to control the pollution and revive the mother earth.

References

Chauhan, S.S. (2010). Mining, development and environment: a case study of Bijolia mining area in Rajasthan, India. *J. Hum. Ecol.* 31 (1): 65–72.

CNN Health (2020). https://edition.cnn.com/2020/02/25/health/most-polluted-cities-india-pakistan-intl-hnk/index.html (accessed 15 April 2020).

CPCB (2020). https://app.cpcbccr.com/ccr/#/caaqm-dashboard-all/caaqm-landing (accessed 5 May 2020).

CREA (2020). Air quality improvements due to COVID 19 lock-down in India. https://energyandcleanair.org/air-quality-improvements-due-to-covid-19-lock-down-in-india/ (accessed 5 May 2020).

Dantas, G., Siciliano, B., França, B.B. et al. (2020). The impact of COVID-19 partial lockdown on the air quality of the city of Rio de Janeiro, Brazil. *Sci. Total Environ.* 729: 139085.

Dutheil, F., Baker, J.S., and Navel, V. (2020). COVID-19 as a factor influencing air pollution? *Environ. Pollut.* (Barking, Essex: 1987) 263: 114466.

Jain, S. and Sharma, T. (2020). Social and travel lockdown impact considering coronavirus disease (COVID-19) on air quality in megacities of India: present benefits, future challenges and way forward. *Aerosol Air Qual. Res.* 20: 1222–1236.

Jayamurugan, R., Kumaravel, B., Palanivelraja, S., and Chockalingam, M.P. (2013). Influence of 484 temperature, relative humidity and seasonal variability on ambient air quality in a 485 coastal urban area. *Int. J. Atmos. Sci* 2013: 1–7.

Kim, S., Jeong, D., Sanchez, D. et al. (2018). The controlling factors of photochemical ozone production in Seoul, South Korea. *Aerosol Air Qual. Res.* 18 (9): 2253–2261.

Kumar, S.S. and Sharma, K. (2016). Ambient air quality status of Jaipur city, Rajasthan, India. *Int. Res. J. Environ. Sci.* 5: 43–48.

Lee, S.C., Chiu, M.Y., Ho, K.F. et al. (2002). Volatileorganic compounds (VOCs) in urban atmosphere of HongKong. *Chemosphere* 48 (3): 375–382.

Maps of India (2011). https://www.mapsofindia.com/maps/rajasthan/quick-facts/area.html (accessed 15 April 2020).

Putaud, J.P., Raes, F., Dingenen, R.V. et al. (2004). A European aerosol phenomenology-2: chemical characteristics of particulate matter at kerbside, urban, rural and background sites in Europe. *Atmos. Environ.* 38: 2579–2595.

Seinfeld, J.H. and Pandis, S.N. (1998). *Atmospheric Chemistry and Physics*. New York: John Wiley & Sons.

Sharma, M. and Dikshit, O. (2016). Comprehensive study on air pollution and green house gases (GHGs) in Delhi. A report submitted to Government of NCT Delhi and DPCC Delhi. 1–334.

Sharma, M., Jain, S., and Lamba, B.Y. (2020). Epigrammatic study on the effect of lockdown amid Covid-19 pandemic on air quality of most polluted cities of Rajasthan (India). *Air Qual. Atmos. Health* 13: 1157–1165.

Shrestha AM, Shrestha U B, Sharma R, Bhattarai S, Tran HNT, Rupakheti M (2020) Lockdown caused by COVID-19 pandemic reduces air pollution in cities worldwide.

Sicard, P., De Marco, A., Agathokleous, E. et al. (2020). Amplified ozone pollution in cities during the COVID-19 lockdown. *Sci. Total Environ.* 735: 139542.

Srivastava, A., Joseph, A.E., More, A., and Patil, S. (2005). Emissions of VOCs at urban petrol retail distribution centres in India (Delhiand Mumbai). *Environ. Monit. Assess.* 109 (1–3): 227–242.

Tobias, A., Carnerero, C., Reche, C. et al. (2020). Canges in air quality during the lockdown in Barcelona (Spain) one month into the SARS-CoV-2 epidemic. *Sci. Total Environ.* 726: 138540.

TOI (Times of India) (2018). https://weather.com/en-IN/india/pollution/news/2018-12-10-rajasthan-highest-death-rate-air-pollution-india (accessed 15 April 2020).

Urban, R.C. and Nakada, L.Y.K. (2021). COVID-19 pandemic: Solid waste and environmental impacts in Brazil. *Sci. Total Environ.* 755 (Pt 1): 142471.

WAQR (2018). World air quality report. https://www.iqair.com/world-most-polluted-countries (accessed 15 April 2020).

WAQR (2019). World air quality report. https://www.iqair.com/world-most-polluted-countries (accessed 20 April 2020).

Xu, K., Cui, K., Young, L.H. et al. (2020). Impact of the COVID-19 event on air quality in central China. *Aerosol Air Qual. Res.* 20 (5): 915–929.

17

COVID-19 Pandemic: A Blessing in Disguise

Pratik Kulkarni[1], Tejas D. Barot[1], Piyush K. Rao[1], and Deepak Rawtani[2]

[1] *School of Doctoral Studies & Research (SDSR), National Forensic Sciences University (Ministry of Home Affairs, GOI), Gandhinagar, Gujarat, India*
[2] *School of Pharmacy, National Forensic Sciences University (Ministry of Home Affairs, GOI), Gandhinagar, Gujarat, India*

17.1   Introduction: A "Make or Break" Perspective

The COVID-19 pandemic or the novel coronavirus infection has created havoc across the globe by disrupting the lives and functioning of human beings. This situation has created a crisis of monumental status. There is a huge amount of loss in terms of human lives. However, its imminent impact on the overall economy and sustainable growth projects is also troublesome. Currently, the world is under a recession period as estimated by the International Monetary Fund and as it is still early to predict the totality of the impact, preliminary estimates suggest it at around 2 trillion USD.

The COVID-19 crisis has exposed many of the fundamental failings in the overall system and has directly shown how the crisis can exacerbate if issues like poverty, lack of health-care facilities, education, and cooperation are prevalent (Power et al. 2020). The notion that our world faces common problems and challenges must be put to rest now as the pandemic has proven it wrong. This crisis has strengthened our interdependence and created a dire need for global action to meet fundamental needs, save our planet, and build a more resilient world than ever before. Therefore, as we all face common challenges, their solutions must also be common, as in a critical situation like this, we are similar in our strengths as our weaknesses and this is what the sustainable development goals (SDGs) are all about which are the foremost pillars to end poverty and ensure the protection and prosperity of our planet.

Unfortunately, at such a crucial time, the pandemic occurred when the SDGs were finally gaining traction, with a significant number of nations making healthy progressions. Thereby, as stringent efforts are underway to curb the spread of the virus and address the negative impacts resulting due to it, the reality is that nations are reprioritizing their goals and are reallocating their sources to deal with the pandemic. However, this is certainly the right thing to do because, as of now, saving human lives must be the highest priority. Thus, as advised by the United Nations, a significant scale-up in the immediate health responses and putting a specific focus on people must be done, such as women, low-wage workers, youth, small, medium enterprises, etc., who are at risk, to end the spread of this deadly virus. Collective efforts to work together can save countless lives, restore livelihoods, and put the declining global economy back on track.

Nevertheless, even in these difficult times, we must not take away necessary resources to move away from crucial SDG actions. Instead, it is certain that achieving SDGs will put us on a firm path to developing a sound plan to address global health hazards and other emerging diseases. For instance, accomplishing SDG-3, i.e. good health will indicate the strengthening capacity of nations to form early warnings, risk reductions, and management of health risks on both national and global levels.

The COVID-19 pandemic has certainly exposed the loss of a structural basis related to global health systems (Kelly et al. 2020). And as it is undermining the prospects to achieve the SDG-3 goal by 2030, some broad effects on all other SDGs can also be expected; e.g. as per the UNESCO estimates, more than 1.25 billion students have been affected, which poses a serious challenge for attaining SDG-4 goal, which stands for quality education. Similarly, as per the early estimates of the International Labour Organization (ILO), more than 25 million jobs are in danger due to the pandemic situation, with those having informal employment at most risk, owing to lack of social protection.

The impact of the pandemic in many parts of the world has been intensified by the crisis in achieving SDG-6 goals, i.e. the provision of clean water and sanitation, SDG-8 goals for fragile economic growth and lack of decent work, SDG-10 goals for omnipresent inequalities and, in particular, SDG-1 and 2 goals, i.e. entrenched poverty and food insecurity. As per the World Bank estimates, up to 11 million could be pushed into poverty. Even under such circumstances, the pandemic is teaching us the importance of unified efforts and the value to become each other's keepers to prioritize the needs of the most vulnerable. Our world has all the necessary knowledge and innovative capacities and if we keep our ambitions well-directed, then the necessary resources can be mustered efficiently to achieve the goals for sustainable living. To achieve that, there is an acute need for a well-enhanced political will and commitment (International Monetary Fund 2020).

The pandemic has made the governments, multilateral organizations, businesses, and civil society raise billions in the shortest span of time to curb the impacts of the pandemic. A similar level of urgency to combat hunger, poverty, and climate change could therefore help us succeed in achieving all the SDGs in this decade of action. As efforts are underway to stop the pandemic and restore global prosperity, a focus on addressing underlying factors must be foremost in achieving SDGs. Our collective efforts must not dampen, even though some SDGs have been attained. Rather, during this span of action, it should help us divert our efforts to improve recovery in order to build a healthier, fairer, safer, and prosperous world in which to live (Risse 2020) (Figure 17.1).

17.2 How Coronavirus Is Shaping Sustainable Development

A major humanitarian crisis is a COVID-19 pandemic, and efforts to contain its spread and support those in dire need must be of paramount importance. Many leaders as a part of their responsibility are looking ahead and assessing the recovery from the pandemic and its

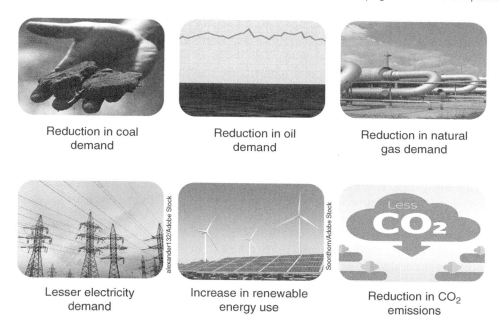

Figure 17.1 A schematic diagram showing reduction in major energy sources leading a shift toward sustainable technologies. *Source:* Risse (2020).

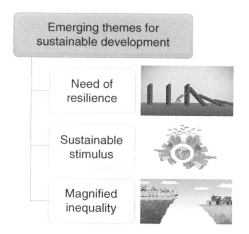

Figure 17.2 A schematic showing the emerging themes for sustainable development.

impact on the future of sustainable development. The view of progress toward the creation of a stable climate, sustainable resource development, and reasonable economies must be practiced firmly (Florizone 2020) (Figure 17.2). From that perspective, currently there are three emerging themes:

Need for resilience: The lack of medical safety equipment for health-care workers, including masks worth less than a dollar, makes it disheartening to see lives at risk.

This highlights a severe lack of planning and preparation to deal with the pandemic crisis and thus shows the need for a resilient plan that allows humans to anticipate, copy, and adapt to the situation (Ross et al. 2015). This resilience is also crucial in how the world responds to climate change, where temperature profiles are now increasing further (Satterthwaite et al. 2020).

A sustainable stimulus: Several economic stimulus and support packages have been implemented by the governments around the world to help individuals, businesses, and economies for their functioning. As this is a necessary step, it must be ensured that these ways ultimately lead to a more sustainable economy in the near future and do not trap us further into a high-carbon world. The COVID-19 pandemic has created a period of high unemployment and low interest rates. So, this may be the right time to invest in low-carbon technologies and infrastructures, which will support a smoother transition toward clean energy (Florizone 2020; Ross et al. 2015).

Magnified inequality: The impact of inequality has been magnified to its limit due to the pandemic leading to an unprecedented global shock, hitting the poor hardest. Frontline workers in the developed countries and poor people in the developing countries are facing the worst of consequences due to the crisis. The frontline workers are exposed to the virus the most and are the least to absorb the resulting financial impact and the poor in developing countries are the ones having no social security net and stimulus packages. Here, the G7 and G20 must step in for an immediate help for financing the flattening the spread of the COVID-19 curve. For a long-term vision, the efforts must be redoubled to foster sustainable economy including fair trade and investments for a better security (Florizone 2020).

17.2.1 Moving Toward a Sustainable Future

Recently, a policy note released by the UN Economic Commission for Asia and the Pacific (ESCAP) highlighted the key impacts of COVID-19 in the Asia-Pacific region by offering them ways to build strength across the development of robust and systemic healthcare and measures of social security for everyone. More than two-thirds of the world's population live in this region, and it is home to much of the world's energy and manufacturing activity. In these countries, therefore, the initial steps to stop the spread of the pandemic have affected all the service sectors such as aviation, hospitality, retail, tourism, and, more significantly, the foreign market for fossil fuels such as (Satterthwaite et al. 2020).

Hence, immediate and fiscal measures that ensure the economic and financial stability of people must be undertaken. For example, in countries like Hong Kong and Singapore, funds for proper subsidization of sectors like food, retail transport, and tourism have been successfully done. The policy also suggests countries employ cross-border movements to facilitate the delivery of necessary drugs, machinery and equipment, and other things. Removing tariffs and measures of nontariffs could also be practised (Satterthwaite et al. 2020; ExoShock.com 2020).

On the environmental front, the note states that pandemic containment measures have led to a drastic reduction in global levels of CO_2 emissions and decreased demand for fossil fuels such as coal, oil, etc. For instance, China reported a 15–40% reduction in the industrial outputs where a 3% reduction in coal and NO_2 levels was observed (Wahlén 2020). This highlights the importance of how the reduction in industrial and transport activities impacts the emissions in a drastic way. The note recommends that governments develop stimulus packages to address climate change and sustainable development that can accelerate decarbonization, such as sustainable mobility, and make the economy greener. Stimulus packages that contribute to environmental degradation should be highly discouraged. The note also recommends a region-wise ban on the illegal wildlife trade, habitat loss, and the adoption of international standards for sanitation and hygiene (Satterthwaite et al. 2020; Wto.org 2020).

Due to health inequalities in the Asia-Pacific region, lack of clean water access can be a major problem (Jones 2020). Also, older people, migrant workers, and disabled are more vulnerable to the virus (Khatib-Othman and As 2020; Asia 2020; Ilo.org 2020). Hence, the note suggests placing this group of people in the center of social policy reform measures by establishing universal health-care systems and social protection. In the viewpoint of long term, the countries should strengthen emergency preparedness to enhance the resilience of the economy and minimize the risks of future health-related emergencies. Investments in digital communication should also be increased as it has proven its might in enabling social distancing. In the end, the note also stresses the establishment of emergency funds and debt relief measures. UN and ESCAP could act here to organize monetary resources at a regional level and provide dedicated backing to the most affected countries (Satterthwaite et al. 2020).

17.2.2 Building Back Better After COVID-19

Green building programs can simultaneously achieve environmental and social goals by stimulating economic activities and creating jobs. For instance, small additional investments in green buildings will lead to massive long-term costs and greenhouse gas (GHG) emissions. Sustainable buildings are estimated to save a staggering 1.1 trillion USD by 2050 as per the International Energy Agency (IEA) report. The coronavirus pandemic has presented a great chance to change the building sector's path toward green construction. If "business-as-usual" is what we are striving for, the same errors will inevitably be repeated. Therefore, to move toward green building construction or even zero-carbon buildings, we need to change the course of the building sector. Some promising examples of the past during the financial crisis in 2008 can be given (Hageneder 2020).

For example, the Republic of Korea implemented strict policies with additional financial support to develop green buildings. The government also provided financial incentives for those with retrofitting of their houses. Also, a "Building Energy Certificate Programme" was extended for all the forms of construction (Republic of Korea 2020). Programs for energy-efficient building and refurbishment have been developed in Germany. Refurbishment loans for newer residential buildings set higher expectations for energy quality. In 2016, for example, more than 400 000 private residential units were funded, leading to 286 000 jobs. Reports suggest that in 2017, 1730 GWh unit worth of final energy was saved from the subsidized buildings and 619 000 tons of GHG emissions (Hageneder 2020).

Knowledge transfer and the growth of local green building and construction skills can promote policies and standards for green building construction. There are some fundamental requirements that can be applied to support sustainable development at the national level, such as (i) rewarding higher energy and low carbon goals with financial incentives; (ii) providing incentives for project certification and labeling by systemic inclusion of energy efficiency techniques; (iii) giving high priority to green construction projects, for instance, fast-track processing of the permits, and (iv) accelerating national climate policies for better sustainable development of the country (Hageneder 2020).

17.2.3 Global Shift to Renewable Energy. Is COVID-19 Slowing It?

As noted earlier, the renewable energy industry was expected to increase in recent demand owing to a significant roadblock, which is due to three main reasons: the COVID-19 pandemic, the resultant global financial crisis, and a dramatic drop in oil and gas prices (Fox-Penner 2020a). As they are interrelated, such events can, therefore, be termed mutually reinforcing. Moreover, it is too early to assess its impact on the socioeconomies and the environmental sectors of the world. However, a significant catch-up period of recovery after this meltdown is projected but in a prospective way.

A reduction in the demand for renewables in the world is likely due to the crippling economy and will supposedly hurt new renewable installations. For example, businesses are certainly tightening their budgets and stopping the construction of new plants. Moreover, companies producing solar cells, wind turbines, and other green technologies may take strict measures to delay their development (Fox-Penner 2020b). Cleantech analysts at the Morgan Stanley project declines of 17–48% in the US solar photovoltaic setups in the upcoming quarters of 2020 (Capital Budgeting Techniques 2020; Fox-Penner 2020c).

17.2.4 Clean Energy Momentum

In the movement for a move toward renewable energy, there have been some countervailing factors that will partly counterpoise this momentary decline, at least in rich industrialized nations. As part of a clean energy target in state regulations, many renewable plants have already been constructed for reasons other than demand growth (Oil & Gas 360 2015). Public pressure and different government policies are also forcing a shift toward renewable energy utilization and stop coal-run power plants. It is projected that in the United States, by 2025, more than one-third of the coal-generating capacity will be reduced and is likely to get replaced with solar, wind, and hydropower technologies (Capital Budgeting Techniques 2020).

Despite the current pandemic, there is continuing pressure to adapt to cleaner energies and carbon-free energy. Several utilities in the world have already committed to a specific carbon reduction goal and have pledged to become carbon-free soon (Mokurai 2020). There has been an almost 50% rise in voluntary green purchases by many companies in the leading nations. Moreover, residential customers are opting to buy renewables via options of community solar programs, which seems to be a good sign (Capital Budgeting Techniques 2020; Pichler et al. 2017).

17.3 Reverting to Dirty Fuels

Widely used to generate electricity, affordable natural gas would fuel demand, resulting in economic growth. However, during this period, a decline in oil and gas prices will impact the use of renewables in quite an unconventional and sophisticated way. But this may substantially vary in different markets and regions of the world (Capital Budgeting Techniques 2020). In comparison, if there is no effective requirement for the use of renewable energy, it would be cheaper to look at continuing or new forms of oil and gas production (Romano 2020).

For example, it would not look good now, as it did years ago, to replace dirty diesel with solar power in conjunction with some other form of energy storage. Furthermore, this is very crucial and alarming for emerging nations, where a constant need to expand the electricity supply and that too in cheaper ways is imperative (Capital Budgeting Techniques 2020). As these economies are still low on resources and sensitive to energy prices, it would eventually be bad for air quality and climate policy to opt for more affordable fossil fuels instead of green technologies (Yamineva and Liu 2019).

Renewables usually require high capital costs, and thus, to make their installation cheaper, central banks have started promoting meager and negative interest rates to tackle the economic meltdown and crisis (World-nuclear.org 2020). There needs to be a complete discouragement for a wholesale shift to produce newer fossil fuels to make renewable technologies prosper (Morgan Stanley 2020).

17.3.1 Part Shortages

The supply chain part of the renewable industry has been most affected by the pandemic (Pichler et al. 2017). Executives antedating delivery and slowdowns in construction have stalled the progress even further due to the nationwide lockdown of industries to curb the viral spread among the workers. As most renewable energy projects come from China, a substantial decrease in the production of various products has resulted, such as solar panel materials in countries like India and Australia. In addition to renewable components, this disruption is projected to contribute to a one- or two-year dip (Capital Budgeting Techniques 2020). Emerging markets that generate a decade of carbon dioxide emissions from a new fossil fuel plant can have a much more significant impact and are therefore very worrying (Lim 2020). These effects are not uniformly adverse and harmful, however, and the COVID-19 pandemic will not alter carbon-free energy long-term objectives and make the earth more sustainable (Capital Budgeting Techniques 2020; Scales 2020). As the global economy recovers, this pandemic episode is expected to persuade world leaders to make climate policy efforts more quickly to avoid the next climate-induced disease-causing vector or a weather event that shocks the global economy again (Capital Budgeting Techniques 2020; Canadell 2020; Mylenk 2020).

17.4 Consequences of the Pandemic on Fragile States

17.4.1 Food Systems and the Biodiversity Connection

Effects of the COVID-19 pandemic could have severe implications on the environment in fragile states due to challenges faced by their populations and governments. The socioeconomic status of the fragile states due to the pandemic is of immediate nature and potentially devastating. Both domestic and international food systems in fragile countries have been disrupted and could subsequently increase food insecurity for poor and most vulnerable humans. Agriculture is the most dominant source of livelihood in most fragile states. Cutting off farmers from their markets and their fields owing to lockdowns could threaten the local food supplies, and, hence, lead to a price hike despite contracting incomes. The shutdown of fisheries could also increase the risks to food security. Repetition of the food price crisis during 2008 and social instability is a glooming concern. Correspondingly, this could cause a rapid increase in the land to agriculture conversion; local subsistence hunting; and illegal, unregulated, and unreported fishing. Such issues must be sustainably managed and controlled in order to prevent harmful implications on local biodiversity, ecosystem and community health (Crawford 2020).

17.4.2 Mining, Conflict, and Land Rights

Besides food, many fragile states rely on the mining sector as a key pillar for sustaining their economies. The pandemic has caused a shutdown of several mining operations through governmental orders and corporate policies. This could increase the number of workers in the artisanal and small-scale mining (ASM) sector, which is already crowded at large-scale mines. Governments are unable to enforce regulations for these remote operations some examples of which are water pollution, deforestation, and increased use of cheap mercury leading to health and safety risks to large numbers of untrained miners, and use of child labor due to school closures and reduced incomes. Women will also bear many ill effects of these actions. ASM operations springing up in close proximity to large-scale mines may increase tensions and conflicts between miners and companies (Crawford 2020).

17.4.3 Prevention of Pandemic and Its Cost Measures

Research suggests that an increased level of deforestation and human activity in tropical forests is responsible for increased transmission of the virus from animals to humans. Also, wildlife hunting and selling their meat in livestock markets propel their transmission further. Due to the coronavirus pandemic, there has been a failure in protecting tropical rainforests amounting to a cost of trillions of dollars. The pandemic has resulted in historic levels of unemployment and economic havoc in major parts of the world (Schwab 2020).

Scientists and environmentalists have been trying to warn about the ill effects of tropical forest deforestation for decades (Figure 17.3). The emergence of new diseases is an example of those harms due to transmission between wild animals and humans. SARS-CoV-2 is also postulated to be transmitted from the livestock market in China from bats to humans and has affected more than 70 million people in the world till now. Researchers highlight the indifference that has occurred at the edges of these forests. An interesting study with the aim to understand the overall economic costs to reduce the transmission of such novel viruses was done recently with some stark outcomes (Schwab 2020). It was discovered that it would cost approximately between $22.2 and $30.7 billion every year globally, in order to reduce the transmission of such new diseases significantly. In contrast, it has been estimated that controlling the COVID-19 pandemic would end up costing between $8 trillion and $16 trillion worldwide, which represents almost 500 times that of investing in avoiding the same. The financial cost of COVID-19 was estimated on the basis that many thousand

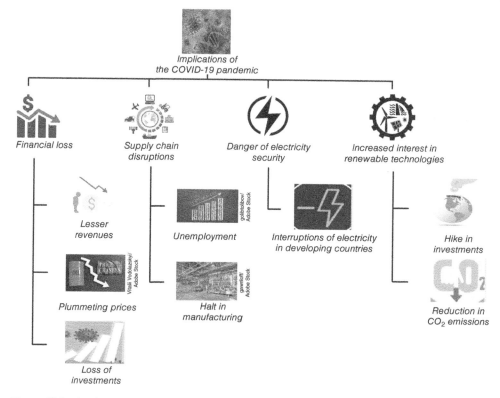

Figure 17.3 A schematic diagram showing the implications of COVID-19 on the environment.

deaths occurred worldwide, including the lost gross domestic product, labor force, and economic costs (Schwab 2020).

Researchers have suggested that disease transmission increases from wild animals to humans because of increased human invasions at the edges of tropical forests. Excessive logging, cattle ranching, exotic animal trade, and other livestock enterprises are examples of such incursions. The cutdown of the woods in patterns resembling patchwork or checkerboard is due to this increased danger of transmission. This reduction exposes the amount of land at the edges and thus increases the rate of transmission of diseases between organisms usually living in different habitats (Schwab 2020).

17.4.4 Prevention of New Pandemics

In order to reduce disease transmission, many researchers have collaborated to promote the monitoring of wildlife trade, investments in efforts to ban the wild meat trade in China and other places around the world, policies to reduce deforestation by at least 40%, and preventing the transmission of diseases from the wild animals to livestock and subsequently to humans. China alone accounts for $20 billion in wildlife farming, which is a government-monitored effort for sustainable hunting practices to avoid overhunting. This billion-dollar industry employs nearly 15 million people. Many communities in China consider the purchase of wildlife and their meat a symbol of status (Schwab 2020).

In order to develop an open-source library containing the specific genetic signatures of all recognized viruses, researchers have proposed that the source of emerging diseases be determined and prevented more effectively until they spread. According to researchers, every two years, two new viruses are transmitted from animals to humans. The viruses that have been included are SARS-CoV1, MERS, HIV, H1N1, and the recent SARS-CoV-2 virus that causes COVID-19. The team behind this study hopes that their research will help policymakers around the world finance these preventive measures, including the US government. Recently, a ray of hope was issued by the Standing Committee of the National People's Congress when it declared a ban on the consumption of wildlife in China for food or any related trade. The COVID-19 pandemic has given an incentive to act on addressing concerns that are and may become immediate threats to individuals (Schwab 2020).

17.4.5 Climate Change and Wildlife

Some positive implications of COVID-19 are an increase in wildlife sightings, improved air quality, and reduced carbon emissions. Despite these positive outcomes, the eclipsing tragic cost for humans due to the coronavirus cannot be sidelined. Many experts are wondering what the pandemic will mean for global wildlife. In recent years, it has been well understood that bumblebees and many other species have been steadily declining. It has become very important to find the reason behind these declines, especially for the pollinator groups, which are responsible for performing irreplaceable ecosystem and agriculture services (Soroye 2020).

Recent evidences have shown that climate change has been instrumental in the huge decline of bumblebees' population across Europe and North America. The study has also revealed the mechanism that leads to these pollinator declines and its link with climate change termed climate chaos. Usually, the wildlife tolerates some degree of warming, either by moving away from risky weather or adapting to evolutionary changes. However, tolerating chaotic and increasing extremes of weather like prolonged drought, heatwaves, or tropical storms makes it much more difficult for the species to adapt and survive (Soroye 2020).

This study was focused on bees, regarding the effects of increasing extremes and resulting climate change. In principle, such extremes should affect other species as well in a similar way. If that becomes true, then the extremes of either temperature, precipitation, or both above (or below) their limits of what the species could tolerate will cause an abrupt reshaping in the ecosystems around the globe by 2030 (Soroye 2020).

17.4.6 Necessary Responses Needed

Despite facing the detrimental consequences of climate change over decades, though we still have some fair prospects for minimizing its worst impacts, it is critically important to resolve the triggers. The provision of well-maintained protected microhabitats to provide cover or shade and the diversification of habitats in some landscapes will minimize species' exposure to climate extremes. Due to the pandemic, as human activity has reduced, it is estimated that more species will traverse landscapes in less disturbed regions. For instance,

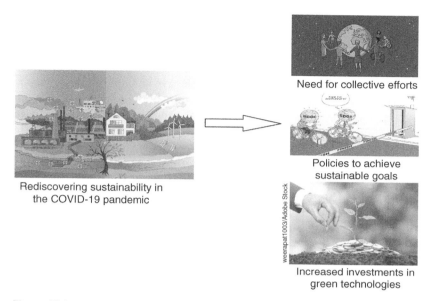

Rediscovering sustainability in
the COVID-19 pandemic

Need for collective efforts

Policies to achieve
sustainable goals

Increased investments in
green technologies

Figure 17.4 A schematic diagram depicting the need for sustainable efforts for combatting future pandemics.

unmaintained roadside verges have caused the profusion of wildflowers, which could lead to excessive nesting and foraging activity for pollinators, if left idle for the remaining year. Similarly, the increasing number of gardens due to less human activity will provide an equal benefit (Soroye 2020).

If the current reduction in emission levels is practiced for long even after lockdown, then it is poised to be beneficial for pollinators and other wildlife and will act as a deciding factor for their survival. The environment and species are bouncing back in many areas, but not everywhere because poachers are destroying protected wildlife because of the economic burden. The incalculable human toll, or its economic costs, will never account for these glimmers of hope. Nevertheless, optimism is the only instrument that can inspire us to take the requisite steps to combat climate change. There is no need for climate change to get locked down and practice social distancing. A decline in species without which human coexistence will be difficult and an accelerating rate of erosion of the planet's life support systems call for concerted global action to improve harmful situations (Soroye 2020) (Figure 17.4).

17.5 Energy Security

Energy security in terms of oil and gas markets has been tested as simultaneous supply and demand concerns have created turmoil in the oil markets (IEA 2020a). As both a share of foreign trade and a government revenue stream for primary producers, oil is part of global macrofinance. There has been an unprecedented reduction in its demands due to lockdown measures. The speed and magnitude of this decline have exceeded the normal market flexibility in terms of supply (Truter 2020). Hence, it is projected that even a coordinated management plan is likely to shut down production in several places. Subsequent macro-economic and financial disruptions can also undermine the ability of the industry to increase production as demands recover (IEA 2020b).

For many industries, the supply of natural gas is critical, including residential and heating services and electrical supplies. There have been a massive amount of investments in recent years, and a sudden slump in the demand for gas during the pandemic situation has increased the supply of the global gas markets immensely. Their storage levels have been occupied to the maximum limit (Ozili and Arun 2020; IEA 2020a). Likewise, an increase in financial strain has hurt several industries badly, including companies that run critical infrastructure facilities. Therefore, there is a need to prioritize the maintenance of operational and safety expenditures by policymakers and regulatory personnel (Bureau 2020).

The COVID-19 crisis has underscored electricity security (Ortiz-Ospina and Beltekian 2020). A robust, uninterrupted supply of electricity is a prerequisite for the operational health care system, social welfare maintenance, and online economic activity. The crisis has been eased by robust power systems, including a vast expansion of tele-networking activities, mainly in advanced economies, to allow for adaptation to this situation. However, in certain regions across the globe (IEA 2020a), a stable supply cannot be taken for granted. Several hospitals and health care facilities in Africa have limited or no access to electricity; therefore, such problems restrict social distancing (UniversalClass.com 2020).

Still, electricity security has remained sufficient as the use of renewable energy has increased due to the pandemic situation. Ahead of the COVID-19 pandemic, the shares of renewables like solar and wind have jumped to an exceptional level, including the shares of curbing CO_2 emissions and air pollution. This can pose a problem for electricity security, but in progressive economies, blackouts' primal cause is due to improper maintenance of sudden power flows and network issues (IEA 2020b). As a result, combined with the steady growth of renewable technologies, the lower demand for electricity has increased its share, creating greater flexibility to keep the lights on. But at the same time, due to the shutdown of industries, this flexibility has been limited, which helps provide a response to demand. Similarly, dispatchable power plants have been idle due to dropping prices (Paterson et al. 2014). Therefore, as financial challenges for the energy industry grow, restarting the dispatchable power plants can become a security concern for industries as the economy and electricity demands recover. Major world economies have maintained their reliability for the energy systems; however, constant vigilant efforts will be needed from the personnel, regulators, and the governments (IEA 2020a).

The COVID-19 crisis, on the positive side, is leading to a pathway for clean energy transitions, as evidenced by the reduction of global CO_2 emissions, which is the lowest year-to-year record so far (Irena.org 2020; Dietz and Venmans 2019). This transition, however, requires a planned government strategy, as it calls for ongoing efforts and commitment, and this sudden drop in emissions can only be temporary without well-planned structural reforms (Tyilo 2020). This is to avoid the sudden rise in CO_2 levels again once the pandemic subsides, as demonstrated by the highest year-to-year increase back in 2010 (Climatecentral. org 2020). In a way, the pandemic provides a way for policymakers to design an economic stimulus plan that ties economic recovery efforts with renewable energy transformations, paving the way for a more prosperous future (Climatecentral.org 2020; IEA 2020b). To do this, in order to take advantage of its possibilities, a concerted strategy needs to be built, leading to a new, safer, and more resilient energy market for all (Reubold 2020).

17.6   Conclusion

As the COVID-19 situation unfolds further, achieving goals of sustainable development should not be overlooked despite the primary measures to save human lives remaining the utmost priority. The pandemic has proved itself as a blessing and a strict lesson for us all to rectify our past mistakes and work in unison globally for developing sustainable earth where solutions could be devised way before any other crisis of this magnitude takes place. This chapter gives a detailed insight into the measures needed to be taken from the perspective of future sustainable development and how our collective efforts can actually benefit in the long term. It also discusses the positive and negative impacts of the pandemic on various other sectors like wildlife, energy, climate change, and prospective ways to overcome the pitfalls once we recover from this situation.

References

Asia, W. (2020). Water pollution in Asia. Recap.asia. www.recap.asia/climate-asia/Water-Pollution-in-Asia.html (accessed 13 December 2020).

Bureau, F. (2020). 60,000 govt canteens should be set up to feed 3 crore urban migrants: National Institute of Public Finance and Policy. The Financial Express. www.financialexpress.com/india-news/60000-govt-canteens-should-be-set-up-to-feed-3-crore-urban-migrants-national-institute-of-public-finance-and-policy/1988743/ (accessed 13 December 2020).

Canadell, P. (2020). Fossil fuel emissions hit record high after unexpected growth—Global Carbon Budget 2017. Phys.org. www.phys.org/news/2017-11-fossil-fuel-emissions-high-unexpected.html (accessed 13 December 2020).

Capital Budgeting Techniques (2020). Independent and mutually exclusive projects. www.capitalbudgetingtechniques.com/independent-and-mutually-exclusive-projects/ (accessed 13 December 2020).

Climatecentral.org. (2020). The 10 Hottest Global Years on Record. www.climatecentral.org/gallery/graphics/the-10-hottest-global-years-on-record (accessed 13 December 2020).

Crawford, A. (2020). The Environmental Consequences of COVID-19 in Fragile States. www.iisd.org/articles/impact-covid-fragile-states (accessed 13 December 2020).

Dietz, S. and Venmans, F. (2019). Cumulative carbon emissions and economic policy: in search of general principles. *Journal of Environmental Economics and Management* 96: 108–129.

Exoshock.com (2020). Aiding the transition from fossil fuels to renewable energy. www.exoshock.com/2018/06/aiding-the-transition-from-fossil-fuels-to-renewable-energy/ (accessed 13 December 2020).

Florizone, R. (2020). Three ways the coronavirus is shaping sustainable development. IISD. www.iisd.org/library/coronavirus-shaping-sustainable-development (accessed 13 December 2020).

Fox-Penner, P. (2020a). Coronavirus will slow—not stop—the total dominance of renewable energy. The National Interest. www.nationalinterest.org/blog/buzz/coronavirus-will-slow%E2%80%94not-stop%E2%80%94-total-dominance-renewable-energy-139602 (accessed 13 December 2020).

Fox-Penner, P. (2020b). Will the COVID-19 pandemic slow the global shift to renewable energy? Boston University. www.bu.edu/articles/2020/will-the-covid-19-pandemic-slow-the-global-shift-to-renewable-energy/ (accessed 13 December 2020).

Fox-Penner, P. (2020c). COVID-19 will slow the global shift to renewable energy, but can't stop it. The Conversation. www.theconversation.com/covid-19-will-slow-the-global-shift-to-renewable-energy-but-cant-stop-it-133499 (accessed 13 December 2020).

Hageneder, C. (2020). Guest article: COVID-19 stimulus spending for green construction means building back better | SDG Knowledge Hub | IISD. Sdg.iisd.org. www.sdg.iisd.org/commentary/guest-articles/covid-19-stimulus-spending-for-green-construction-means-building-back-better/ (accessed 13 December 2020).

IEA (2020a). Energy efficiency – topics - IEA. www.iea.org/topics/energy-efficiency (accessed 13 December 2020).

IEA (2020b). Global energy review 2020 – analysis - IEA. www.iea.org/reports/global-energy-review-2020 (accessed 13 December 2020).

Ilo.org (2020). The ILO's policy framework to respond to the COVID-19 crisis. www.ilo.org/global/topics/coronavirus/impacts-and-responses/WCMS_739047/lang--en/index.htm (accessed 13 December 2020).

IMF (2020). Policy responses to COVID-19. www.imf.org/en/Topics/imf-and-covid19/Policy-Responses-to-COVID-19 (accessed 13 December 2020).

Irena.org (2020). Global renewable generation capacity (GW). www.irena.org/-/media/Files/IRENA/Agency/Publication/2019/Dec/IRENA_Demand-side_flexibility_2019.pdf (accessed 13 December 2020).

Jones, D. (2020). Global coal generation fell by a record amount in 2019, while COVID-19 may cause bigger fall in 2020 - Institute for Energy Economics & Financial Analysis. Institute for Energy Economics & Financial Analysis. www.ieefa.org/global-coal-generation-fell-by-a-record-amount-in-2019-while-covid-19-may-cause-an-even-bigger-fall-in-2020/ (accessed 13 December 2020).

Kelly, N., Majka, D., and Samaris, D. (2020). Monitoring the financial implications of COVID-19 on hospitals & health systems. Kaufmanhall.com. www.kaufmanhall.com/ideas-resources/article/monitoring-financial-implications-covid-19-hospitals-health-systems (accessed 13 December 2020).

Khatib-Othman, H. and As, S.E. (2020). Guest article: Achieving public health Equity – Start with Sanitation and Hygiene for all | SDG Knowledge Hub | IISD. Sdg.iisd.org. www.sdg.iisd.org/commentary/guest-articles/achieving-public-health-equity-start-with-sanitation-and-hygiene-for-all/ (accessed 13 December 2020).

Lim, J. (2020). The Big Read: Global supply chain shock has farmers dumping food as consumers fret over shortages, price hikes. TODAY online. www.todayonline.com/big-read/big-read-global-supply-chain-shock-has-farmers-dumping-food-while-consumers-fret-over (accessed 13 December 2020).

Mokurai (2020). Renewable friday: Covid-19 vs. renewable energy again. Daily Kos. www.dailykos.com/stories/2020/4/10/1934480/-Renewable-Friday-Covid-19-vs-Renewable-Energy-Again (accessed 13 December 2020).

Morgan Stanley (2020). Is the climate changing for fossil fuel investments? | Morgan Stanley. www.morganstanley.com/articles/fossil-fuels (accessed 13 December 2020).

Mylenk, T. (2020). Impact of Covid-19 on the global energy sector. www.pv-magazine.com/2020/04/24/impact-of-covid-19-on-the-global-energy-sector/ (accessed 13 December 2020).

Oil & Gas 360 (2015). Oil and gas bankruptcy climbs to more than $16 billion in 2015 - Oil & Gas 360. www.oilandgas360.com/oil-and-gas-bankruptcies-climb-to-more-than-16-billion-in-2015/ (accessed 13 December 2020).

Ortiz-Ospina, E. and Beltekian, D. (2020). Trade and globalization. Our World in Data. www.ourworldindata.org/trade-and-globalization (accessed 13 December 2020).

Ozili, P.K. and Arun, T. (2020). Spillover of COVID-19: impact on the global economy. Available at SSRN 3562570.

Paterson, J., Berry, P., Ebi, K., and Varangu, L. (2014). Health care facilities resilient to climate change impacts. *International journal of environmental research and public health* 11 (12): 13097–13116.

Pichler, P.P., Zwickel, T., Chavez, A. et al. (2017). Reducing urban greenhouse gas footprints. *Scientific reports* 7 (1): 1–11.

Power, M., Doherty, B., Pybus, K., and Pickett, K. (2020). How COVID-19 has exposed inequalities in the UK food system: the case of UK food and poverty [version 2; peer review: 5 approved]. *Emerald Open Research* 2: 11.

Reubold, T. (2020). OPINION: What does a sustainable future actually look like? Ensia. www.ensia.com/voices/what-does-a-sustainable-future-actually-look-like/ (accessed 13 December 2020).

Risse, N. (2020). Policy brief: Getting up to speed to implement the SDGs: Facing the challenges | SDG Knowledge Hub | IISD. Sdg.iisd.org. www.sdg.iisd.org/commentary/policy-briefs/getting-up-to-speed-to-implement-the-sdgs-facing-the-challenges/ (accessed 13 December 2020).

Romano, A. (2020). The role of renewable energy certificates in community solar. Guidehouseinsights.com. www.guidehouseinsights.com/news-and-views/the-role-of-renewable-energy-certificates-in-community-solar (accessed 13 December 2020).

Ross, A.G., Crowe, S.M. and Tyndall, M.W. (2015). Planning for the next global pandemic. *International Journal of Infectious diseases* 38: 89–94.

Satterthwaite, D., Archer, D., Colenbrander, S. et al. (2020). Building resilience to climate change in informal settlements. *One Earth* 2 (2): 143–156.

Scales, M. (2020). Making the Earth more sustainable: One customer (manufacturer) at a time - sight machine blog. Sight Machine. www.sightmachine.com/blog/making-the-earth-more-sustainable/ (accessed 13 December 2020).

Schwab, J. (2020). Fighting COVID-19 could cost 500 times as much as pandemic prevention measures. www.weforum.org/agenda/2020/08/pandemic-fight-costs-500x-more-than-preventing-one-futurity/ (accessed 13 December 2020).

Soroye, P. (2020). COVID-19 has helped the environment, but it can't save us from climate change. www.weforum.org/agenda/2020/06/covid19-coronavirus-lockdown-nature-environment (accessed 13 December 2020).

Sustainabledevelopment.un.org (2020). Republic of Korea: Sustainable development knowledge platform. www.sustainabledevelopment.un.org/memberstates/republicofkorea (accessed 13 December 2020).

Truter, C. (2020). COVID-19: impact on businesses and investments in South Africa - Bowmans. Bowmans. www.bowmanslaw.com/insights/mergers-and-acquisitions/covid-19-impact-on-businesses-and-investments-in-south-africa/ (accessed 13 December 2020).

Tyilo, M. (2020). Climate cMalibongwe Tyilohange: could the 2020 drop in CO_2 emissions be a game changer? MSN. www.msn.com/en-za/news/world/climate-change-could-the-2020-drop-in-co2-emissions-be-a-game-changer/ar-BB13JsZc?li=BBqfP3n (accessed 13 December 2020).

UniversalClass.com (2020). Identifying and prioritizing needs and risks in strategic planning. www.universalclass.com/articles/business/identifying-and-prioritizing-needs-and-risks-in-strategic-planning.htm (accessed 13 December 2020).

Wahlén, C. (2020). ESCAP reviews COVID-19 impacts, recommends regional actions I News I SDG Knowledge Hub I IISD. Sdg.iisd.org. www.sdg.iisd.org/news/escap-reviews-covid-19-impacts-recommends-regional-actions/ (accessed 13 December 2020).

World-nuclear.org (2020). Renewable energy and electricity I sustainable energy I renewable energy. World Nuclear Association. www.world-nuclear.org/information-library/energy-and-the-environment/renewable-energy-and-electricity.aspx (accessed 13 December 2020).

Wto.org (2020). WTO I goods measures - COVID-19: Trade and trade-related measures. https://www.wto.org/english/tratop_e/covid19_e/trade_related_goods_measure_e.htm (accessed 13 December 2020).

Yamineva, Y. and Liu, Z. (2019). Cleaning the air, protecting the climate: policy, legal and institutional nexus to reduce black carbon emissions in China. *Environmental Science & Policy* 95: 1–10.

Index

Note: Page numbers in *italics* refer to figures; page numbers in **bold** refer to tables.

The Environmental Impact of COVID-19, First Edition. Edited by Deepak Rawtani and Chaudhery Mustansar Hussain.
© 2024 John Wiley & Sons Ltd. Published 2024 by John Wiley & Sons Ltd.